ENHANCING MOBILITY IN LATER LIFE

Assistive Technology Research Series

Volume 17

Previously published in this series

Vol. 16. A. Pruski and H. Knops (Eds.), Assistive Technology: From Virtuality to Reality – AAATE 2005
Vol. 15. S. Giroux and H. Pigot (Eds.), From Smart Homes to Smart Care – ICOST'2005
Vol. 14. D. Zhang and M. Mokhtari (Eds.), Toward a Human-Friendly Assistive Environment
Vol. 13. H. Mollenkopf, F. Marcellini, I. Ruoppila and M. Tacken (Eds.), Ageing and Outdoor Mobility – A European Study
Vol. 12. M. Mokhtari (Ed.), Independent Living for Persons with Disabilities and Elderly People – ICOST'2003
Vol. 11. G.M. Craddock, L.P. McCormack, R.B. Reilly and H.T.P. Knops (Eds.), Assistive Technology – Shaping the Future
Vol. 10. C. Marincek, C. Bühler, H. Knops and R. Andrich (Eds.), Assistive Technology – Added Value to the Quality of Life
Vol. 9.   M. Mokhtari (Ed.), Integration of Assistive Technology in the Information Age
Vol. 8.   H.-W. Wahl and H.-E. Schulze (Eds.), On the Special Needs of Blind and Low Vision Seniors
Vol. 7.   N. Katevas (Ed.), Mobile Robotics in Healthcare
Vol. 6.   C. Bühler and H. Knops (Eds.), Assistive Technology on the Threshold of the New Millennium
Vol. 5.   L.H.V. van der Woude, M.T.E. Hopman and C.H. van Kemenade (Eds.), Biomedical Aspects of Manual Wheelchair Propulsion
Vol. 4.   I. Placencia Porrero and E. Ballabio (Eds.), Improving the Quality of Life for the European Citizen
Vol. 3.   G. Anogianakis, C. Bühler and M. Soede (Eds.), Advancement of Assistive Technology
Vol. 2.   K. Cullen and S. Robinson, Telecommunications for Older People and Disabled People in Europe
Vol. 1.   I. Placencia Porrero and R. Puig de la Bellacasa (Eds.), The European Context for Assistive Technology

ISSN 1383-813X

Enhancing Mobility in Later Life

Personal Coping, Environmental Resources and Technical
Support. The Out-of-Home Mobility of Older Adults in
Urban and Rural Regions of Five European Countries

Edited by

Heidrun Mollenkopf

*German Centre for Research on Ageing at the University of Heidelberg
(DZFA), Heidelberg, Germany*

Fiorella Marcellini

*INRCA, Istituto Nazionale Riposo e Cura Anziani, Dipartimento Ricerche
Gerontologiche, Ancona, Italy*

Isto Ruoppila

Department of Psychology, University of Jyväskylä, Jyväskylä, Finland

Zsuzsa Széman

*Institute of Sociology, Hungarian Academy of Sciences HAS, Welfare Mix
Team, Budapest, Hungary*

and

Mart Tacken

*Faculty of Architecture, Delft University of Technology, Delft,
The Netherlands*

IOS
Press

Amsterdam • Berlin • Oxford • Tokyo • Washington, DC

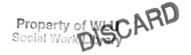

ISBN 1-58603-564-9
Library of Congress Control Number: 2005933296

Publisher
IOS Press
Nieuwe Hemweg 6B
1013 BG Amsterdam
The Netherlands
fax: +31 20 687 0019
e-mail: order@iospress.nl

Distributor in the UK and Ireland
IOS Press/Lavis Marketing
73 Lime Walk
Headington
Oxford OX3 7AD
England
fax: +44 1865 750079

Distributor in the USA and Canada
IOS Press, Inc.
4502 Rachael Manor Drive
Fairfax, VA 22032
USA
fax: +1 703 323 3668
e-mail: iosbooks@iospress.com

Contents

Preface   xi

Chapter 1.   The Significance of Out-of-Home Mobility in Modern Society   1
             Heidrun Mollenkopf

1.1   Mobility as a component of life quality in older adults   1
1.2   Background and goals of the MOBILATE Project   2
1.3   Towards a comprehensive understanding of mobility   5

Chapter 2.   Background Conditions for Outdoor Mobility in Finland, Germany, Hungary,
             Italy, and the Netherlands   11
             Cristina Gagliardi, Nina Hirsiaho, Csaba Kucsera, Fiorella Marcellini,
             Heidrun Mollenkopf, Isto Ruoppila, Zsuzsa Széman and Mart Tacken   11

2.1   Welfare regimes and mobility   11
2.1.1   Changes in the welfare regimes   12
2.1.2   Connection between the welfare regimes and mobility of elderly people   14
2.2   Demographic trends in the MOBILATE countries   17
2.2.1   Demographic changes   18
2.2.2   Social ageing   19
2.3   Traffic and transportation systems   20
2.3.1   Mobility and transportation systems   22
2.4   Traffic characteristics of the participating countries   23
2.4.1   Finland   23
2.4.1.1 Driver licences regulation   24
2.4.1.2 Traffic accidents   24
2.4.2   Germany   26
2.4.2.1 Driver licences regulation   26
2.4.2.2 Elderly persons and the traffic system   26
2.4.2.3 Traffic accidents   27
2.4.3   Hungary   28
2.4.3.1 Driver licences regulation   29
2.4.3.2 Traffic accidents   29
2.4.4   Italy   31
2.4.4.1 Driver licences regulation   32
2.4.4.2 Traffic accidents   32
2.4.4.3 Improvements in public transport   33
2.4.5   The Netherlands   34
2.4.5.1 Driver licences regulation   34
2.4.5.2 Elderly persons and the traffic system   34
2.4.5.3 Problems and impairments   35
2.5   Conclusions   36

Chapter 3.   Methodology   43
             Stephan Baas, Fiorella Marcellini, Heidrun Mollenkopf, Frank Oswald,
             Isto Ruoppila, Zsuzsa Széman, Mart Tacken and Hans-Werner Wahl

3.1   Methods and research instruments   43
3.1.1   The MOBILATE Survey Questionnaire   43
3.1.2   The MOBILATE Diary of out-of-home mobility   45
3.2   The research areas   45
3.2.1   Finland   46
3.2.1.1   Urban area: Jyväskylä   46
3.2.1.2   Rural area: Karstula, Kivijärvi and Nilsiä   47
3.2.2   Germany   48
3.2.2.1   Urban areas: Chemnitz (eastern Germany) and Mannheim (western Germany) 48
3.2.2.2   Rural areas: District of Jerichow and District of Vogelsberg   50
3.2.3   Hungary   51
3.2.3.1   Urban area: Pécs   51
3.2.3.2   Rural area: Jászladány   52
3.2.4   Italy   52
3.2.4.1   Urban area: Ancona   52
3.2.4.2   Rural areas: Municipalities of Mondavio, Montefelcino and Orciano 53
3.2.5   The Netherlands   54
3.2.5.1   Urban area: Maastricht   54
3.2.5.2   Rural (non-urban) area: Margraten   55
3.3   Fieldwork and sample   55
3.3.1   Fieldwork   56
3.3.2   Drop-out   59
3.3.3   Weighting the data   60
3.4   Basic description of the samples   62
3.4.1   Mean age   62
3.4.2   Marital status   64
3.4.3   Education   64
3.4.4   Occupation and status of employment   66
3.4.5   Financial situation   70
3.4.6   Health status   72
3.5   Summary   73

Chapter 4.   Physical Health and Mobility   77
             Nina Hirsiaho and Isto Ruoppila

4.1   Introduction   77
4.2   Health and mobility in the MOBILATE study   82
4.2.1   Research question and hypotheses   82
4.2.2   Methods   82
4.2.3   Statistical analyses   85
4.3   The relation between health and outdoor mobility   86
4.3.1   The relation between health and single outdoor mobility variables 86
4.3.2   The relations between health and outdoor mobility indicators 90
4.4   Regression analyses of health variables explaining outdoor mobility
          indicators   94
4.4.1   Regression analyses of transport modes used   94

4.4.2	Regression analyses of outdoor activities subjects take part in	95
4.4.3	Regression analyses of means of trips from the trip-diary	96
4.5	Discussion	97
4.6	Conclusions	98

Chapter 5. Transport Behaviour and Realised Journeys and Trips 105
Mart Tacken and Ellemieke van Lamoen

5.1	Mobility and behaviour	105
5.1.1	Introduction	105
5.1.2	Satisfaction with mobility	106
5.1.3	Availability and use of a car as driver and passenger	107
5.1.4	Not driving a car	111
5.1.5	The use of a bicycle	112
5.1.6	Elderly people as pedestrians	113
5.1.7	The role of public transport	114
5.1.8	Relative importance of transport modes	115
5.1.9	Accidents	116
5.1.9.1	Experience with traffic today	117
5.2	Journeys in the MOBILATE diary	118
5.2.1	General information on journeys	118
5.2.1.1	Chaining of trips in journeys	119
5.2.1.2	Motives	119
5.2.1.3	Choice of mode	120
5.2.2	Temporal aspects of the mobility behaviour of older people	121
5.2.3	Distribution of mobility over a day	122
5.2.4	Comfort of journeys	127
5.3	Trips made by elderly people	128
5.3.1	Trips in the diary	128
5.3.2	Means of transport for trips	129
5.3.3	Motives for the trip	130
5.4	Spatial aspects of out-of-home behaviour	132
5.5	Possible solutions for experienced mobility problems	133
5.5.1	Improvements in the transport system in general	133
5.5.2	Flexible demand responsive (public) transport	134
5.5.3	The use of new technology	135
5.6	Conclusions	136

Chapter 6. Health and Leisure Activities 141
Isto Ruoppila, Mart Tacken and Nina Hirsiaho

6.1	Introduction	141
6.2	Health and leisure activities in the MOBILATE study	147
6.2.1	Research questions and hypotheses	147
6.2.2	Methods	148
6.3	Leisure activities: description and explanation	150
6.3.1	Satisfaction with leisure and sport activities	150
6.3.2	Participation in leisure activities	151
6.3.3	Variety in indoor and outdoor activities	153

6.3.4	Comparison of the variety in outdoor activities in survey and in diary	157
6.3.5	Changing leisure behaviour	158
6.3.6	Travel and satisfaction with this activity	159
6.4	The relationship between health and leisure time activities	161
6.4.1	Health and satisfaction with possibility to participate in leisure activities	161
6.4.2	Health and indoor leisure activities	162
6.4.3	Health and outdoor leisure activities	163
6.4.4	Health and holiday trips lasting at least one week during the last year	165
6.5	Discussion	166
6.6	Conclusions	167

Chapter 7.   Psychological Aspects of Outdoor Mobility in Later Life   173
Frank Oswald, Hans-Werner Wahl and Roman Kaspar

7.1	Introduction	173
7.2	In-depth description of psychological measures, psychometric analyses, and basic intercorrelations	177
7.2.1	Description of measures and their psychometric properties	177
7.2.2	Intercorrelations of psychological constructs, age, and gender	180
7.3	Psychological constructs and outdoor mobility: bivariate relations across geographical locations	181
7.3.1	Psychological constructs as predictors of outdoor mobility	182
7.3.1.1	Psychological constructs as mediators of outdoor mobility	184
7.3.1.2	Psychological constructs as outcomes of mobility	189
7.4	Psychological constructs and outdoor mobility: multivariate relations across countries	190
7.5	Summary and conclusions	191

Chapter 8.   Social Relations and Mobility   195
Stephan Baas, Csaba Kucsera, Heidrun Mollenkopf and Zsuzsa Széman

8.1	Introduction	195
8.2	Characteristics of the household	197
8.2.1	Average household size	197
8.2.2	Composition of household	197
8.3	Number of children	200
8.4	Social relations outside the household	201
8.4.1	Overview about the important persons outside the household	202
8.5	Further aspects about older persons' social networks outside the household	205
8.6	Living distance to the most important persons	208
8.7	Intensity of contact and used means of transportation	210
8.7.1	Used means of transportation	212
8.7.2	What does the frequency of personal contact depend on?	212
8.8	Difficulties in meeting important persons	214
8.9	Summary and conclusions	216

Chapter 9. Mobility and the Built-Up Environment   221
            Fiorella Marcellini, Heidrun Mollenkopf, Zsuzsa Széman,
            Sabina Ciarrocchi, Csaba Kucsera, Andrea Principi and Liana Spazzafumo

9.1   Introduction   221
9.2   Housing conditions in urban and rural areas   222
9.2.1   Duration of residence   222
9.2.2   Type of home and ownership   223
9.3   Neighbourhood conditions in urban and rural areas   225
9.3.1   The use of services   226
9.3.2   Feelings of security   237
9.3.3   Environmental features   238
9.4   Summary and conclusions   239

Chapter 10. Main Issues of Older People's Out-of-Home Mobility   243
            Mart Tacken and Heidrun Mollenkopf

10.1   Introduction   243
10.2   Older people's actual mobility   243
10.3   The mobility needs of older people   246
10.3.1   Barriers and hindrances in the mobility of people of old age   247
10.3.1.1 Hindrances in the spatial environment   248
10.3.1.2 Hindrances in the social context   249
10.3.1.3 Hindrances in the transport system   250
10.3.2   Coping behaviour of elderly people   251
10.4   Improvement of the mobility conditions   254

Chapter 11. A New Concept of Out-of-Home Mobility   257
            Heidrun Mollenkopf, Stephan Baas, Fiorella Marcellini, Frank Oswald,
            Isto Ruoppila, Zsuzsa Széman, Mart Tacken and Hans-Werner Wahl

11.1   Introduction   257
11.2   Mobility indicators   258
11.2.1 The options of transport modes   258
11.2.2 Options of outdoor activities   259
11.2.3 Extent of realised mobility   261
11.3   Explaining out-of-home mobility   262
11.3.1 Transport options   263
11.3.2 Options of outdoor activities   268
11.3.3 Number of trips/realised mobility   273
11.4   Summary and conclusions   277

Chapter 12. Mobility and the Quality of Life   279
            Heidrun Mollenkopf, Stephan Baas, Fiorella Marcellini, Frank Oswald,
            Isto Ruoppila, Zsuzsa Széman, Mart Tacken and Hans-Werner Wahl

12.1   Introduction   279
12.2   The conceptual MOBILATE-model: extension to quality of life   280

12.2.1	Results of structural equation modelling	283
12.2.1.1	Overall model fit evaluation	283
12.2.1.2	In-depth consideration of measurement models	285
12.2.1.3	In-depth evaluation of the structural model	286
12.3	Summary and Conclusions	287

Chapter 13. The Mobility Rich and Mobility Poor   289
Heidrun Mollenkopf, Roman Kaspar and Hans-Werner Wahl

13.1	Introduction	289
13.2	Identifying the 'Mobility rich' and 'Mobility poor'	289

Chapter 14. Summary and Conclusions   295
Heidrun Mollenkopf, Fiorella Marcellini, Isto Ruoppila, Zsuzsa Széman and Mart Tacken

14.1	Overview on the main MOBILATE findings	295
14.1.1	The basic goals and background of the MOBILATE project	295
14.1.2	The mobility patterns of older men and women in urban and rural areas	298
14.1.3	The prerequisites and problems of older men's and women's out-of-home mobility	302
14.2	Methodological challenges of a cross-cultural project	305
14.3	Conclusions and Outlook	309

Annex	317
The MOBILATE Consortium	319
Europe (Map)	320
The MOBILATE Diary	321
Addresses	324
Author Index	325

Preface

Outdoor mobility in old age, the focus of this book, is a complex phenomenon. On the one hand, it is a basic human need and means the physical ability to move. On the other, it means the realisation of all types of trips outside the home, either by foot or by any means of transportation. In addition, societal and individual necessities, modern values and economic interests mutually reinforcing each other have resulted in mobility as an ever more important precondition of ensuring the ability to lead an autonomous life and participate actively in society according to their individual needs. Mobility also promotes healthy ageing, delays the onset of disabilities, and postpones frailty, thereby contributing to subjective well-being and life satisfaction. With advancing age, however, maintaining mobility may become jeopardized because of the increasing risk of physical and sensory impairments.

Hence, the research theme of the comparative European project "MOBILATE - Enhancing outdoor mobility in later life: Personal coping, environmental resources, and technical support", that is, the detailed analysis of outdoor mobility in old age as well as its potentials and hindrances, is highly relevant for a 'good life' (Lawton, 1983) for today's and tomorrow's ageing adults. This interdisciplinary project was funded by the European Commission in the context of the Fifth Framework Programme (Key Action "The ageing population and their disabilities", programme area no 6.3, Project QLRT-1999-02236) and aimed to better understand the complex interplay between personal competencies and aspects of the physical and social environment, all of which significantly impinge upon the mobility of older people. It combined different data-sources (person, environment, including urban versus non-urban regions) as well as different data-collection strategies in order to contribute to the societal challenge of how mobility, an important aspect of life-quality in old age, can be maintained or enhanced.

This book compiles the main results of this research. It includes information on the transportation tools used, the prevalence of typical problems associated with out-of-home mobility, the impact of health, social networks, the home and neighbourhood environments, and psychological aspects on the mobility and activities of older people, differences between urban and non-urban areas, and age and gender differences. In addition, a new model of mobility is suggested and the relation between mobility and quality of life is analysed. Each participating research team focused on one or several specific topics and was responsible for the respective chapters, as well as the analyses and interpretations provided therein.

The following institutes and universities have contributed to the project from the beginning:

The *German Centre for Research on Ageing at the University of Heidelberg (DZFA), Department of Social and Environmental Gerontology*, was the main contractor and co-ordinator of the project that began in January 2000 and lasted until December 2002.

Dr. Heidrun Mollenkopf was the co-ordinator and scientific leader of the project in conjunction with Prof. Dr. Hans-Werner Wahl and Dr. Frank Oswald, assisted by Dipl. Soz. Stephan Baas as the principal researcher and Dipl. Soz. Dinah Kohan and Roman Kaspar as research assistants. The fieldwork was carried out by sub-contractor USUMA GmbH, Berlin, in the cities of Mannheim and Chemnitz and the rural areas of Vogelsbergkreis and Jerichower Land.

In Finland, the research project was conducted under the scientific direction of Professor Isto Ruoppila at the *Department of Psychology, University of Jyväskylä*, and managed by the principal researcher, M.S. Nina Hirsiaho. The fieldwork was performed by 17 research assistants hired to carry out the data collection (most of them psychology students) in the city of Jyväskylä and the rural areas of Karstula, Kivijärvi and Nilsiä.

In Italy the research project was carried out under the direction of Dr. Fiorella Marcellini, chief of the Social Gerontology Unit (Department of Research) at the *Italian National Research Institute on Aging* (*Istituto Nazionale Riposo e Cura Anziani - INRCA - Ancona*). Assistance was provided by senior researcher Dr. Cristina Gagliardi, and Dr. Andrea Principi regarding the social aspects, as well as by senior researcher Dr. Liana Spazzafumo and Dr. Sabina Ciarrocchi for the statistical analysis. Subcontractor CSRSS (Centro Studi Ricerche Scienze Sociali) had the task of carrying out the interviews in the city of Ancona and in the rural villages of Mondavio, Orciano and Montefelcino.

The *Urban and Regional Planning Group, Faculty of Architecture, Delft University of Technology*, the Netherlands. The project was coordinated by Dr. Mart Tacken. Ellemieke van Lamoen assisted in the development of the common database and the analysis of these data. Remon Rooij performed the geographical analysis of the data and conducted work on the demand-responsive transport system in Maastricht. Fieldwork was carried out by the subcontractor "Research and Marketing" (R & M). The municipality of Maastricht (except for the villages Borgharen and Itteren) was chosen as the urban area, and the municipality of Margraten as the non-urban (rural) area.

In Hungary, the research project was carried out under the direction of Dr. Zsuzsa Széman, head of the Welfare Mix Team at the *Institute of Sociology of the Hungarian Academy of Sciences, Budapest,* and assisted by senior research fellow Dr. László Harsányi and research assistant Csaba Kucsera. Subcontractor Szonda-Ipsos investigated the planned sample between October and December of 2000 in the rural area of Jászladány and the city of Pécs.

We would like to thank Dr. David Burmedi, Dr. Michael Freeman and Dr. Monica Glebocki for substantially improving our English language style. We are also grateful to Ursula Koenig for preparing the manuscript in camera-ready form.

The project group received valuable support from the municipality administrations of the cities and rural areas included in the research: they provided us with important information on the respective settlement and transport infrastructure and enabled us to select sample populations representative for men and women aged 55 to 74 years and 75 years or older.

A further important prerequisite for a valid and reliable database is a high participation rate. For this, we thank the older women and men who gave both their time and knowledge to be used not only for national purposes but also for providing valuable information on the outdoor mobility of elderly people from a European perspective. With this book we hope to contribute to the final goal of the MOBILATE project, that is, to improve the possibilities for out-of-home mobility of older adults. Comparison of diverse European countries with diverging geographic, climatic, economic and cultural conditions may allow for a better understanding of varying patterns of mobility in different regional actualities.

Reference

Lawton, M. P. (1983). Environment and other determinants of well-being in older people. *The Gerontologist, 23*, 349-257.

Heidrun Mollenkopf
Fiorella Marcellini
Isto Ruoppila
Zsuzsa Széman
Mart Tacken

Enhancing Mobility in Later Life
H. Mollenkopf et al. (Eds.)
IOS Press, 2005

1

Chapter 1
The Significance of Out-of-Home Mobility in Modern Society

Heidrun Mollenkopf

1.1   Mobility as a component of life quality in older adults

Mobility as movement in time and space is necessary in order to overcome   distances, improve accessibility to essential commodities, and pursue activities outside the home. It can be manifested in many different ways, can be motivated by diverse, often inseparably intertwined motives, and have distinct features. Over the course of the 19th century, industrial development opened up new opportunities for individual mobility and traffic. Technological advances have made high speed and flexible transportation systems possible, enabling long distance trade and travel. At the same time, the provision of extended road infrastructure accelerated the functional and spatial separation between the occupational, commercial, and private spheres of life and of extensive suburban development. The outward relocation of private households, in turn, increased the necessity to commute and dependency upon access to cars. The shift to individual modes of transport often coincided with cutbacks in public transportation, and the once dense network of retail shops gave way to suburban supermarkets and downtown shopping centres oriented to car users as customers. Therefore, for every member of society, mobility is not only a basic human need for physical movement. Out-of-home mobility and the use of the transport system, whether by foot or with private or public means of transportation, have become major prerequisites for maintaining autonomy, independence, and quality of life for as long as the mental and physical capacities permit a person to participate actively in society. Empirical research has stressed the importance of outdoor mobility for the maintenance of independent living in old age (e.g., Berlin & Golditz, 1990; Heikkinen, 1997; Mollenkopf, Marcellini, & Ruoppila, 1998, 2004; Ruuskanen & Ruoppila, 1995; Spirduso & Asplund, 1995; Tacken, 1998). Mobility is crucial to ensure that people can obtain their daily necessities, make use of neighbourhood facilities and access health care. It is essential for keeping up social relations and taking part in everyday activities as well as in community life according to their individual needs (Schaie, 2003). Mobility also promotes healthy ageing, delays the onset of disabilities, and postpones frailty, thereby contributing to subjective well-being and life satisfaction. Hence, it is of great importance to know the needs and problems that older people meet in moving about outside their homes.

1.2   Background and goals of the MOBILATE Project

With regard to out-of-home mobility in old age, a great deal of descriptive information on the trip behaviour of older people has been gathered. Data available in national travel surveys have been used to describe their outdoor mobility and to analyse their trip making (Centre d'études sur les réseaux, les transports, l'urbanisme et les constructions publiques (CERTU), 2001; Chu, 1994; European Conference of Ministers of Transport (ECMT), 2000; Tacken, 1998). The Transportation Research Board (TRB) studies 'Transportation in an ageing society' (1988, 2004) are good examples of comprehensive studies of older people's mobility. However, social, psychological as well as environmental aspects have been largely neglected in earlier research approaches. In this regard, the authors of this book were the first to describe the mobility-relevant personal, social and environmental conditions of older people as well as their mobility needs and the hindrances they experience while taking trips (Mollenkopf & Marcellini, 1997; Mollenkopf, Marcellini, & Ruoppila 1998; Mollenkopf, Marcellini, Ruoppila & Tacken, 2004; Tacken et al., 1999). Our previous findings illustrate both important similarities and differences in mobility between different European countries (only European cities were involved) and how elders cope with outdoor mobility-related obstacles. However, important differentiations on the personal level (such as a broad mobility-related psychological assessment), on the environmental level (such as the consideration of urban versus non-urban regions), and analysis of the long-term course of outdoor mobility capability as well as a detailed analysis of the opportunities and challenges of transport technologies for the older persons were not possible in this earlier research.

The key to maintaining out-of-home mobility lies within the interaction between each individual and his or her immediate surroundings, significant others, and family. The consideration of living and neighbourhood environments, social and spatial environments, as well as technological environments (including transport facilities) is thus crucial for a comprehensive understanding of outdoor mobility. Therefore, the goal of the interdisciplinary project entitled "MOBILATE. Enhancing Outdoor Mobility in Later Life—Personal Coping, Environmental Resources, and Technical Support", funded within the European Commission's 5th Framework Programme, was to better understand the complex interplay between personal competencies and aspects of the physical and social environments of older adults. Its main objective was to provide a comprehensive and detailed description and explanation of their actual outdoor mobility by means of mobility-related personal as well as environmental factors and to identify specific ways to facilitate mobility in later life in order to help them participate in society. This included a fine-tuned documentation of outdoor mobility patterns, the frequency of use of the whole range of transportation devices and technology resources, and typical problems with out-of-home mobility. Emphasis was placed upon environment-related competencies (physical capacity, vision, etc.) and psychological coping strategies to deal with functional limitations. Regarding the environment, variables cover - from the macro- to the meso- and micro-level - urban versus non-urban regions, the level of motorisation in the country in question, the social network, and the physical, spatial, and technical infrastructure.

In industrialised countries, mobility is aided largely by technical means of transportation. Therefore, the availability and accessibility of these technologies for older persons - which is a function of personal coping efforts as well as potential constraints inherent to the physical and social environment - was a major focus of the investigation. New technologies in the transportation domains make new solutions possible, but we must ensure that they really fulfil the demands of older users and provide them with acceptable, accessible solutions. More tailor-made, public, and shared transport alternatives can provide solutions to the diminishing functioning of older (and particularly old-old) persons. To prevent older people from becoming victims of restrictive measures, technology must develop new, efficient and sustainable alternatives which successfully meet the needs of older persons (OECD, 2001; OECD Working Group on Human Factors, 2003). Therefore, an analysis of the mobility behaviour of older users and non-users of a demand responsive transport system at one project site (Maastricht, the Netherlands) was also included in the project (Tacken & van Lamoen, 2002).

A central tenet of the project was that resources for mobility on the personal, environmental and technological level are distributed very differently among European countries in general and among urban and non-urban regions within these countries in particular. Therefore, countries from northern, southern, and different parts of central Europe as well as an eastern European country were included in the investigation. These countries represent five socially, geographically and economically different areas in Europe. Thus, the data from the research project reflect diverse European realities in which today's and tomorrow's ageing takes place.

In addition to national differences, various kinds of residential, traffic, and resource structures, including public services, social relationships, and support potentials differ greatly between urban and non-urban areas (Beaulieu, Rowles, & Myers, 1996; Golant, 2004; Mollenkopf, Marcellini, & Ruoppila, 1998). These conditions made it necessary to obtain samples in clearly defined urban and non-urban (rural) areas. Furthermore, subtly differentiated local data on the diverging social and spatial environment conditions of mobility and of the spatial patterns of the actual trip-making behaviour were needed in order to better understand how older people stay active and mobile. This enabled us to assess the effects of the diverging traffic infrastructures, neighbourhood resources, and other services on mobility; it also uncovered divergent needs between older inhabitants of urban, non-urban and rural areas and between differing European regions. The findings are thus a valid indication of the experiences, behaviours, and needs of men and women who are examples of the ageing population in urban and non-urban areas of northern, central, and southern Europe.

The final goal of the MOBILATE project was to id*entify how subjective well-being, a key indicator of life-quality in old age, depends on outdoor mobility as well as on mobility-related personal and environmental factors.* In particular, the impact of different coping strategies - including personal-, environment- and technology-based compensations - on subjective life-satisfaction was examined. Again, the role of urban versus non-urban regions on these relationships was given particular attention.

Further objectives of the MOBILATE project were to *describe and explain individual change and constancy* in mobility patterns in old age as a function of chronological age. In this regard, a 5-year follow-up data collection of persons first investigated in 1995 (Mollenkopf, Marcellini, Ruoppila, & Tacken, 2004) allowed us to describe change and constancy as well as inter-individual variability in these patterns. In addition, the question of *whether new cohorts of older people reveal different mobility patterns, as well as different needs and expectations* as end-users of transport technology compared to older cohorts with differing technological experiences and resources was addressed. The findings of these analyses are compiled in special reports (Mollenkopf, Marcellini, Ruoppila et al., 2003; Ruoppila, Marcellini, Mollenkopf et al., 2003).

Figure 1.1 gives an overview on the project structure. It shows the main assessed aspects in the MOBILATE 2000 study (personal, socio-economic, and structural / regional resources assumed to have an effect on mobility and quality of life), as well as the Follow-up part (data collected of persons first investigated in the Outdoor Mobility Survey 1995). With regard to the latter we assumed that changes during the period 1995 - 2000 might also affect quality of life in 2000.

Figure 1.1:   The MOBILATE Project Structure

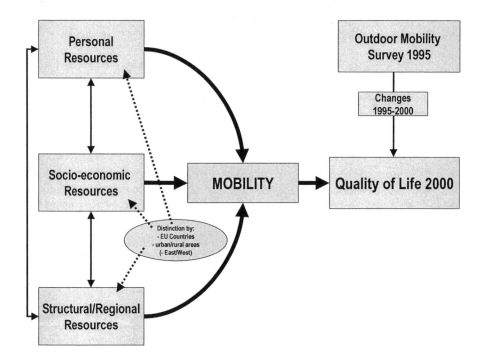

This book marks the conclusion of work on this project. After this first introductory chapter we present the conditioning societal, demographic, and mobility related background conditions relevant for better understanding the outdoor mobility options and constraints of older persons in the countries that were part of the investigation (Chapter 2). We then explain the methodological structure and design of the study and describe the urban and rural regions in which the survey was conducted, as well as the basic characteristics of the national samples (Chapter 3). The individual physical, technical, psychological, social and environmental determinants of mobility among older adults and the key results of the research are then presented by topic (Chapters 4 through 9). Each of these topics was written by one or two research teams, taking the specific disciplinary viewpoints of the researchers and the appropriate theoretical and methodological approaches into consideration. Therefore, the structure, type and level of analyses, and way of reporting may vary by chapter and topic.

The focus and aim of Chapters 10 – 14 is to integrate the several aspects of outdoor mobility. Chapter 10 compiles the main issues of older adults' out-of-home mobility. We continue in chapter 11 with explaining and developing our holistic concept of mobility further and examine its validity by using its components as predictors of subjective quality of life (Chapter 12). Chapter 13 continues with the key results of a cluster analysis, conducted in order to identify specific groups of persons showing different patterns of outdoor mobility. The book concludes with some reflections on the challenges of comparative research, with an overview of the key results of the project, and the implications resulting for social policy, traffic coordination, urban and regional planning, and industrial pursuits for better meeting ageing adults' mobility needs (Chapter 14).

First of all, however, we present and explain our understanding of mobility.

1.3   Towards a comprehensive understanding of mobility

Mobility is a complex phenomenon. On the one hand, it just means the physical ability to move. On the other, it means the realisation of all types of trips outside the home, either by foot or by any means of transportation. In addition, societal and individual necessities, modern values and economic interests mutually reinforcing each other (Burkhardt, 2000; Lash & Urry, 1994; Rammler, 1999) have resulted in mobility as an ever more important precondition of ensuring the ability to lead one's everyday life. This includes such fundamental activities as keeping up social relations, taking part in every kind of activity outside one's home, and seeking out places subjectively significant or objectively central to meeting daily material needs and guaranteeing access to health care. The automobile, in particular, has become a key to mobility. Despite a growing awareness of the problem posed by motorized traffic, it has lost little of its allure and symbolises more than ever the modern values of freedom, competence, and flexibility.

In traffic and transport research, mobility usually has been defined as locomotion, as a movement in time and space. It is measured in terms of trips (= from a place of departure to a destination, ending with an activity), or journeys (= leaving a place of departure, usually the home, until coming back), and reported in standardised diary forms. Information is generally collected and provided on distances, travel modes used, periods of time, and objectives or motives of the trips or journeys (the activity pursued at the destination reached) (ECMT, 2000; CERTU, 2001; Litman, 2003; OECD, 2001). The limitation of this type of methodology is that small trips and non-motorised means of locomotion are under-estimated (round trips are counted as only one trip; trips which are combined of several modes are judged only by the 'main' mode); the categories of activities usually are very rough - 'leisure activities', for instance, don't tell anything about the characteristics of the activity.

This approach is certainly suited if one is interested in travel behaviour, travel flow, etc. as it is the case for traffic and transport planning. It is not sufficient, however, if the focus of research is characterised by social science oriented interests. For instance, if one is interested in the main objectives of mobility, namely all kinds of activities, then probably activities that might be subjectively very important but pursued only once or twice a year risk being neglected in one- or two-day diaries. People's experiences made when venturing out are not assessed at all.

Some of the shortcomings of the traffic oriented type of mobility research could be compensated for in the MOBILATE project by elaborating a diary form guaranteeing the provision of basic information on the respondents' travel behaviour, on the one hand, and the assessment of individual objectives and experiences, on the other. This was achieved by differentiating between more types of activities than usual, and asking for the positive or negative circumstances of the journeys.

Moreover, in a broader sense - including sociological and psychological meanings - mobility comprises much more than just the functional aspect of travelling from a place A to a destination B under certain conditions. In modern society, mobility is associated with highly appreciated values like freedom, autonomy, flexibility, and the variability of behaving and thinking. The same holds true for the so-called information or knowledge society, the main affordances of which are high levels of flexibility, of permanent adaptation to the rapid pace of technological and organisational change, of life-long learning, and mobility. One might argue that these competencies are not relevant for older persons who no longer participate in the labour market of globally acting companies. Even though, they are members of current societies and therefore are affected by these societies' "Zeitgeist", values, and expectations. This can be derived from the high importance older people attribute to leisure time activities. Satisfaction with leisure time possibilities revealed to be a significant predictor of satisfaction with life in general for older adults living in a western German city and rural area (Mollenkopf, 2002). Similarly, Farquhar (1995) found in a study focusing on elderly people's definitions of quality of life that in addition to health status, family relationships and social contacts, activities are important components of a good quality of life.

The assessment of older men's and women's out-of-home mobility should, therefore, include the ability of physical movement, but also, as much as possible, modern characteristics of mobility such as self-determination, flexibility, and variability.

The MOBILATE project team aimed at elaborating such a comprehensive concept. Our understanding of out-of-home mobility, going beyond the common notion of trip-making behaviour, simultaneously considers three basic integral parts: the variety of transport modes used, the diversity of outdoor activities performed, and the extent of realized mobility (actual trip-making).

The amount of *transport modes used* shows the variety of options a person has at hand. The number of used options per person will differ depending on personal conditions (health, competencies, attitudes, economic resources, and private means of transportation available), and depending on environmental and structural conditions (the public transport system available in the area and country of living). In the German cities under investigation, e.g., the public transport systems include buses as well as trams. On the other hand, ships play a certain role for the inhabitants of Jyväskylä, the urban Finnish research region. In some research areas, both modes are not available. The use of more or less options does not necessarily mean that a person is more or less mobile in a quantitative sense. Instead, using a large number of transport modes indicates that the person has a large variety of mobility options at his or her disposal and thus is more or less mobile (flexible) in a qualitative sense.

The amount of options of *outdoor activities performed* shows the variety with respect to the motivational aspect of a person's mobility. Again, the number of used options per person will differ on personal aspects as well as on environmental aspects (availability and accessibility of the necessary facilities, services, and supply provided). The pursue of more or less activities does not necessarily mean that a person is more or less active or mobile in a quantitative sense, but that he or she can pursue a certain variety of activities and thus is more or less mobile (flexible) in a qualitative sense.

The number of actual trips made per day and per person is an expression of a person's extent of *realised mobility*, based on her or his concrete travel behaviour as reported in the mobility diaries.

In other words, flexibility regarding different transport modes and a wide range of leisure time interests as motives for mobility are taken into consideration. All three aspect of mobility were included in the analyses of the Survey data (see in particular Chapters 11, 12 and 13). The goal of this endeavour is a comprehensive Model of Mobility, including the most important components, oriented at modernisation theories.

References

Beaulieu, J. E., Rowles, G. D., & Myers, W. W. (1996). Long-term care for the rural elderly: toward the twenty-first century. In G. D. Rowles, J. E. Beaulieu & W. W. Myers (Eds.), *Long-term care for the rural eldery* (pp. 170-192). New York: Springer.

Berlin, J. A., & Golditz, G. A. (1990). A meta-analysis of physical activity in the prevention of coronary heart disease. *American Journal of Epidemiology, 132,* 612-621.

Burkhardt, J. E. (2000). Limitations of mass transportation and individual vehicle systems for older persons. In K. W. Schaie & M. Pietrucha (Eds.), *Mobility and transportation in the elderly* (pp. 97-123). New York, NY: Springer Publishing Company.

Centre d'études sur les réseaux, les transports, l'urbanisme et les constructions publiques (CERTU) (2001). *La mobilité des personnes âgées - Analyse des enquêtes ménages déplacements* [The mobility of older people. Analyses of household travel research]. Rapport d'étude. Lyon: CERTU.

Chu, X. (1994). *The effects of age on the driving habits of the elderly. Evidence from the 1990 National Personal Transportation Study.* (DOT-T-95-12).Washington, D.C.

ECMT (European Conference of Ministers of Transport) (2000). *Transport and aging of the population.* Report of the 112th round table on transport economics. Paris Cedex, France: OECD Publications.

Farquhar, M. (1995). Elderly people's definitions of quality of life. *Social Science and Medicine*, 41(10), 1439-1446.

Golant, S. M. (2004). The urban-rural distinction in gerontology: An update of research. In H.-W. Wahl, R. J. Scheidt & P. G. Windley (Eds.), *Aging in context: Socio-physical environments (Annual Review of Gerontology and Geriatrics, 2003)* (pp. 280-312). New York: Springer Publishing.

Heikkinen, E. (1997). Background, design and methods of the project. In E. Heikkinen, R.-L. Heikkinen, & I. Ruoppila (Eds.), Functional capacity and health of elderly people - The Evergreen project. *Scandinavian Journal of Social Medicine, Suppl 53,* 1-18.

Lash, S., & Urry, J. (1994). *Economies of signs and space.* London: SAGE.

Lawton, M. P. (1983). Environment and other determinants of well-being in older people. *The Gerontologist, 23,* 349-357.

Litman, T. (2003). Measuring Transportation. Traffic, Mobility and Accessibility. *The ITE Journal*, 73(10), 28-32.

Mollenkopf, H. (2002). Mobilität und Lebensqualität im Alter - objektive Voraussetzungen und subjektive Bedeutung in der mobilen Gesellschaft [Mobility and quality of life in old age – objective conditions and subjective meanings in mobile society]. In W. Glatzer, R. Habich, & K. U. Mayer (Eds.), *Sozialer Wandel und gesellschaftliche Dauerbeobachtung* (pp. 255-271). Opladen: Leske + Budrich.

Mollenkopf, H., & Marcellini, F. (Eds.). (1997). *The outdoor mobility of older people - technological support and future possibilities.* European Commission, COST A5. Luxembourg: Office for official publications of the EC.

Mollenkopf, H., Marcellini, F., Ruoppila, I., & Tacken, M. (Eds.)(2004). *Ageing and Outdoor Mobility. A European Study.* Amsterdam: IOS Press.

Mollenkopf, H., Marcellini, F., & Ruoppila, I. (1998). The outdoor mobility of elderly people - a comparative study in three European countries. In J. Graafmans, V. Taipale & N. Charness (Eds.): *Gerontechnology. A sustainable investment in the future* (pp. 204-211). Amsterdam: IOS Press.

Mollenkopf, H., Marcellini, F., Ruoppila, I., Baas, S., Ciarrocchi, S., Hirsiaho, N., Kohan, D. & Principi, A. (2003). The MOBILATE Follow-up Study 1995-2000. Enhancing Outdoor Mobility in Later Life: Personal Coping, Environmental Resources, and Technical Support. *DZFA Research Report No. 14.* Heidelberg: German Centre for Research on Ageing (DZFA).

OECD (Organisation for Economic Co-operation and Development) (2001). *Ageing and Transport. Mobility needs and safety issues.* Available at http://oecdpublications.gfi-nb.com/cgi-bin/OECDBookShop.storefront/655091789/.

OECD Working Group on Human Factors (2003). New Transportation Technology for Older People. An OECD-MIT International Symposium. Summary Report. Cambridge, Massachusetts: MIT AgeLab.

Rammler, S. (1999). Die Wahlverwandtschaft von Moderne und Mobilität - Vorüberlegungen zu einem soziologischen Erklärungsansatz der Verkehrsentstehung [Affinity between modernity and mobility – considering a sociological explanation of the emergence of traffic]. In R. Buhr, W. Canzler, A. Knie & S. Rammler (Eds.), *Bewegende Moderne. Fahrzeugverkehr als soziale Praxis* (pp. 39-71). Berlin: edition sigma.

Ruoppila, I., Marcellini, F., Mollenkopf, H., Hirsiaho, N., Baas, S., Principi, A., Ciarrocchi, S., & Wetzel, D. (2003). The MOBILATE Cohort Study 1995 – 2000: Enhancing Outdoor Mobility in Later Life. The differences between persons aged 55-59 years and 75-79 years in 1995 and 2000. *DZFA Research Report No. 17.* Heidelberg: German Centre for Research on Ageing (DZFA).

Ruuskanen, J. M. & Ruoppila, I. (1995). Physical activity and psychological well-being among people aged 65 to 84 years. *Age and Ageing, 24,* 292-296.

Schaie, K. W. (2003). Mobility for what? In K. W. Schaie, H.-W. Wahl, H. Mollenkopf, & F. Oswald (eds.), *Aging independently: Living arrangements and mobility* (pp. 18-27). New York: Springer Publishing.

Spirduso, W. W., & Asplund, L. A. (1995). Physical activity and cognitive function in the elderly. *Quest, 47,* 395-410.

Tacken, M. (1998). Mobility of the elderly in time and space in the Netherlands: an analysis of the Dutch National Travel Survey. *Transportation, 25,* 379-393.

Tacken, M., & van Lamoen, E. (2002). *Transport and mobility, differences between European countries in transport behaviour and in realised journeys and trips.* Delft: University of Technology. Info: http://www.bk.tudelft.nl/users/tacken/internet/

Tacken, M., Marcellini, F., Mollenkopf, H., & Ruoppila, I. (Eds.) (1999). *Keeping the Elderly Mobile. Outdoor Mobility of the Elderly: Problems and Solutions.* The Netherlands TRAIL Research School Conference Proceedings Series P99/1. Delft: Delft University Press.

Transportation Research Board (TRB)(2004). *Transportation in an Aging Society. A Decade of Experience.* Washington D.C.: TRB.

Transportation Research Board. National Research Council (TRB)(1988). *Transportation in an aging society. Improving mobility and safety for older persons.* TRB Special report 218. Washington D.C.: TRB.

Chapter 2

Background Conditions for Outdoor Mobility in Finland, Germany, Hungary, Italy, and the Netherlands

Cristina Gagliardi, Nina Hirsiaho, Csaba Kucsera, Fiorella Marcellini,
Heidrun Mollenkopf, Isto Ruoppila, Zsuzsa Széman and Mart Tacken

The preconditions for outdoor mobility of older people vary considerably between European regions. Apart from common tendencies in demographic trends and the generally increasing number of men and women who are able and willing to drive an automobile, this is true for geographic conditions, welfare regimes and the traffic and legislative actualities. In this chapter the general societal, demographic, and mobility related background of each country will be presented together with some specific information about the situation of older adults: General demographic information, characteristics of the welfare regimes, and mobility and transportation systems. The way these external preconditions can affect the traffic participation of older men and women have to be kept in mind when we talk about their mobility in the following chapters.

2.1 Welfare regimes and mobility

There has been much discussion among experts about different types of welfare states. Based on the *classical* definitions elaborated by Esping-Andersen (1990, 1999), which have been used as a basic model by many other authors (e.g. Ferge, 1990; Deacon & Szalai, 1990; Ferge & Lévai, 1991; Széman & Harsányi, 2000, etc.), the following welfare models could be distinguished.

The *residual model* provides social welfare when the market and the family are not capable of meeting social needs (e.g., in Britain, Canada, Australia, and the USA). In this model an attempt is made to solve the problems with means-tested aid, a modest level of universal transfers, and social insurance systems also on a modest level. According to the *industrial performance-result* type social institutions are functions of the economy and social needs adjudged on the basis of merits, work performance, and productivity. The welfare systems of the former Federal Republic of Germany (FRG), Austria and Italy operate according to such a model. These countries have built up welfare states on the basis of the *corporatist-etatist* legacy. It is traditionally characteristic of these countries that the *church* plays a *significant role* in the provision of welfare services (Bartal, 1998). The principle of subsidiarity determines the *philosophy* and practice of social policy; the state intervenes only in cases where the *possibilities of the family or the immediate community* have been entirely exhausted in helping its members. However, none of the models exists in such a clear form.

The present health insurance or pension insurance scheme in Germany, for example, does not contain every element of this model. The transfers of the health and the pension insurance are paid independently from the family income. Hence, it is a good example showing that models do not exist in a 'theoretically pure' form.

In the *institutionalist redistribution model,* the social institutions are integral parts of society and provide universal services outside the market on the basis of needs. This group includes the (social democratic) Scandinavian countries, where universalism and social rights have been extended to the middle classes. In contrast with the subsidiarity principle of the corporatist model, the aim here is to socialise the family's costs in advance (Esping-Andersen, 1999).

Other definitions divide welfare models in a different way, putting southern European countries into a different group: a) the modern universalistic system, in the Nordic countries; b) the liberal free market-based system, in the United Kingdom and Ireland; c) continental labour market participation in Germany, France, Austria, the Netherlands and Belgium; d) the Latin-rim or rudimentary system in Italy, Spain and Portugal (and perhaps in Greece) (Olsson Hort, 1993; Pestoff, 1995). Even newly presented definitions classify European societies into only three types: the Nordic countries, the Southern European countries and the continental countries in between, emphasising that the United Kingdom constitutes a special case (Vogel, 1998).

However, whatever definitions were presented above, none of them mentioned another type, the socialist welfare model - found in both Hungary and the former German Democratic Republic (GDR) before 1990 - which proclaimed equality in its ideology and certain universal services (free health care, free education, a secure livelihood in old age through the pay-as-you-go pension system, etc.). Just recently a new article on welfare regimes treats the two types of German welfare models, the conservative-corporatist type (GFR) and the former GDR model, as inherently distinct (Scheepers, Grotenhuis, & Gelissen, 2002). At the same time, the 'command economy' led to shortages in the infrastructure and services, causing serious problems in the housing sector. There were long waiting lists for cars, a very important factor for mobility. Obtaining a telephone was a similar problem. The latter was related to the lack of democracy which did not allow a free flow of information and communication: the fewer telephones there were in the country, the less problem there was controlling those with a phone.

2.1.1   Changes in the welfare regimes

By the 90s there was a significant change in this situation. With the crisis of the welfare state in the Western societies, the non-profit sector also appeared in the definitions of welfare regimes (Salamon & Anheimer, 1995, 1996). Depending on the nature of the division between the central state and non-profit organisations, the following welfare regimes were distinguished: a) the *social democratic model* which continued to provide services with universal rights (Finland, Sweden, etc.). Despite erosion in the amount and kind of benefits in recent years, state social services provide extensive aid and even include, for example, taxi service (Vaarama, Törmä, Laaksonen, & Voutilainen, 1999), b) the *corporatist non-profit model*, where state funds play a decisive role in the sources of the non-profit sector. In the *corporatist-etatist* model, a quite large non-profit sector can be found together with high welfare expenditures. Government sources are the major factor in the revenue sources of the non-profit sector (especially in Germany). Because of the characteristic processes that have occurred in the development of society (workers' movements and the working class), the state has been forced to co-operate with non-profit organisations (Germany, Italy). In the 19th century, the state came into confrontation with radical demands from below and formed an alliance with the main churches. As a result, non-profit organisations, as service providers, financed by the state and for the most part religiously committed, continue to play an important role in welfare provision (Seibel, 1992), c) the *liberal non-profit model* with low state/governmental spending and a relatively large non-profit sector (USA); d) *state authority* where limited governmental social and welfare protection occur together with a limited non-profit sector (Japan); e) although many countries could be classified into the different models pure models are a rarity. In some places there is a *mixture of the liberal and social democratic models* (e.g., Great Britain). The Netherlands cannot be regarded as a pure model either.

Each of the particular models described above is also marked by *contradictions* since they were produced from empirical investigations and are thus based on the concrete findings of surveys in a given period. Moreover, these model-definitions do not take into consideration that another important type, the *former socialist welfare model,* collapsed and has been replaced by a new, radically different model that only partly adheres to Western notions and demonstrates its own peculiarities.

In Hungary as well as in eastern Germany (the former GDR), there has been a complete chage of system, involving extremely rapid change in legislation (Grabher, 1995; Gyulavári, 2000), the economy, society, social structures and finally, the welfare model. The so-called socialist welfare state including many universal elements was transformed into a welfare-non-profit model best compared to the *corporatist* type (German), with the remark that both similarities and differences can be found between the two. The most striking similarity is that the size of the non-profit sector within the welfare model is also very large in Hungary and the proportion of welfare expenditures - together with a decline in universal benefits - is relatively high. In Hungary both the non-profit organisations and the churches - much like in the southern part of Italy - played an important role in the historical development (and after the change of regime they flourished again) and began to provide social services (Széman & Harsányi, 2000).

Why is it important to have at least a general knowledge of European welfare models and the differing cultural developments? We are convinced that our analyses of the out-of-home mobility of elderly people can only be evaluated if we place them in a broader economic, social, ideological, political and social policy context. Moreover, we must also take into account the cultural and religious customs found in any given country which are important even if they appear in society not at the religious level but transformed into tradition. In addition to all these factors the economic situation of the country has a great influence on the quality of life, including mobility of older people. According to the European Quality of Life Survey (Whelan, Fahey, & Maître, 2004), 28 European countries can be classified into four big categories. Among the old EU member countries, 12 were among the richest, including Finland, Germany, Italy and the Netherlands. The so-called EU Six are lagging behind (six of the ten new member states: Hungary, the three Baltic countries, Slovakia and Poland) (Whelan, Fahey, & Maître, 2004).

2.1.2   Connection between the welfare regimes and mobility of elderly people

In the following, we attempt to trace processes, pointing out the cultural and economic differences, which directly or indirectly explain the different results found between the countries in our investigations or which help to understand the identical or different features emerging from the project. The models outlined above and the differences in the economic status of the countries have been and still are in constant change, and there are also 'soft' elements within the different models which were present invisibly but which exert an influence that can still be felt. We need to acknowledge these elements in order to understand the differences observed in many important indicators in the MOBILATE project.

One such indicator is the *health status* where there is an especially marked deviation between the Western societies and Hungary. Since this is an important point of analysis, we need to deal in somewhat greater depth with its explanation. Behind this lies the fact that in Hungary in the second half of the 80s, the state socialist welfare model began to fall apart under the influence of economic liberalisation. At that time, the economy began to modernise and open up. Most of the state firms purchased advanced Western technology and installations. Nevertheless, the modernisation was carried out in half measures. For example, firms purchased the latest technology but without health protection devices, causing great harm to the workers' health, especially among men (who often did heavier work or worked long overtime hours). As a result of the change, the employees ended up in worse working conditions which is reflected in the state of their health. While life expectancy at birth was 66.3 years for men in 1970, it was 65.5 years in 1980 and by 1994, it had fallen to 64.8 years. A slight increase followed this low point, but the 66.1 years life expectancy at birth in 1998 was still lower than life expectancy in 1970. Although the elder age groups had a somewhat better chance of a longer life, here too it was only in the second half of the 90s that the indicators improved. (The privatisation of the state enterprises, which was followed by full modernisation, almost certainly played a role in this; Tardos, 1993; Széman, 1999). As a consequence, life expectancy for those in their sixties remained low in Hungary. According to comparative forecasts, the indicators will remain low in 2000-2005 for both men and women compared to the figures for Western, Southern and Northern Europe, although Hungary will probably rank around the middle of the field in Central and Eastern Europe. According to the United Nations publication (2002), between 2000-2005, life expectancy at age 60 for men will be 19 years in Germany, the Netherlands and Finland and 20 years in Italy. In contrast, it will only be 16 years in Hungary. Women at 60 can expect another 24 years in each of the four countries just mentioned and only 20 years in Hungary.

Parallel to half-hearted modernisation, other factors also contributed to the deterioration of the health status of Hungarians. In the 80s, the Hungarian economy was marked by double-digit inflation, but wages lagged behind. At the same time, the earlier state subsidies on many products (such as children's clothing and food) were terminated or reduced. Because wages did not ensure a normal living standard, many people, especially men, began to work part-time in the second economy (not the state sector) on a mass scale. Even in the state sector, overtime work became widespread. Agricultural work done in household plots of land and overtime in factories were all activities that extended beyond normal working hours. In other words, people exploited themselves during their off hours in order to earn extra income. Political change brought a further deterioration in that the promotion and restoration of health (medicines, therapeutic aids) became more costly and serious financial problems arose within the health care system. All this was accompanied by the traditional, unhealthy nutrition habits of the Hungarian population (a diet rich in animal fat leading to a high incidence of cardiovascular disease), a lack of exercise, recreation and rest, and a high level of alcoholism. Especially in the early 90s, when unemployment exceeded 10%, many men sought escape in heavy drinking. In the year 1994 the number of alcoholics was estimated at 1,048,000, or one out of every ten persons (Hungarian Central Statistical Office (KSH)[Központi Statisztikai Hivatal], 1996).

Since the 90s, European countries have been making increasing efforts to meet the expectations of the European Union (European Foundation on Social Quality, 2001) and, perhaps even more important, to respond to the challenges they perceive in society. These challenges can be very complex: they touch upon many different social services, and at the same time they can also be directed at eliminating inequalities in social provision between different regions within the country, where disadvantages arose from earlier cultural or welfare systems.

For example, after reunification, Germany transferred € 3.3 billion for care purposes to the former GDR to improve the standard of services (Gennrich, 1994). These funds were not only intended to make up for deficits in the existing system, but to cover costs for a new pillar to the German social insurance structure. After introduction of care insurance (Pflegeversicherung), the notion of care expanded to include a variety of new services, such as "Wohnungsanpassung" (home modification) introduced in 1995. This was a form of support for the conversion of the architecture and installations of the home in order to facilitate independent living for persons in need of care (elderly persons, disabled people). Where necessary, advice is also provided.

Why is this important for our study, and how is it related to the corporatist German non-profit model? The goal of home modification is to allow older people to continue living in their own homes in conditions which promote mobility. Furthermore, data on relocation show that in the eighties and nineties, relocation within cities was stronger in the eastern than in the western cities because the housing stock of the eastern inner city areas was in need of renovation (Mollenkopf & Flaschenträger, 2001). The MOBILATE survey conducted in 2000 found that 25% of eastern Germans compared to only 7% of western Germans moved into their present apartment after 1995 (see the Chapter on Housing). The national data for the Netherlands show more mobility for dwelling and to some extent reflect the effect of the policy that people had to adapt their housing situation to their actual needs (77% of the sample lived in the same dwelling since 1990; van Lamoen & Tacken, 2001).

Once again, how is this related to the welfare system? Many members of the West German non-profit system worked persistently for years to expand the services for elderly persons, including this particular service, moving to a new apartment or giving advice on converting the apartment. After lengthy debates, the uniform federal act mentioned above was adopted in 1995. In this way, within the German corporatist model an initiative from below influenced the behaviour of the state at the macro level. As a consequence the state launched powerful changes in the law and services which have had an appreciable influence on the life of older people.

The Italian service structure also struggled to cope with problems similar to the East-West problem perceived in Germany, except that here the problems arose from economic, social, welfare and political differences between the North and South. There has been a crucial North-South division in social care services as well. The Constitution entrusted the various regions of Italy with legislative power in the field of social services. But from the 1970s onwards, southern regions largely continued to rely on services linked to religious orders and charity services, especially in institutional care, while northern and central regions committed their course of action to innovation. Finally, in November of 2000, Parliament approved law No. 328 which provided a comprehensive framework for regional legislation in the overall field of social care services. For the first time, the new rules established a responsibility on the part of municipal governments for guaranteeing a well-defined set of social care services and benefits within their jurisdiction. Particularly, the list includes home help, sheltered housing and professional counselling by social workers, which are still unknown in the vast majority of southern municipalities.

The law increased the National Social Fund by an extra 930 Million € for 2000-2002 to be distributed primarily but not exclusively to regional governments. Special priority was given to the funding of local projects aimed at building services for the frail elderly. The goal was to establish a mix of public, private and non-profit services, placing the greatest emphasis on the latter but at the same time clearly stating a public responsibility in the field and opting for services rather than cash benefits (Fargion, 2001). This is an indication that the process which took place in the German care structure in the mid-90s began somewhat later in Italy. Because of this delay, are elderly people in Italy at a disadvantage in terms of mobility? We can only interpret the 'objective welfare/service' indicators correctly if we also take into account other indicators, such as social relations. In Italy, the family is very important and within it, there is great solidarity between generations (Mengani & Gagliardi, 1993). Due to this strong tie, most of the respondents have children living nearby (Marcellini, Gagliardi, Spazzafumo, & Leonardi, 1997). These strong family ties also explain things which are otherwise difficult to understand. Family ties are very important in Hungary, too. In rural areas family ties extend not only to direct kin but also to in-laws and close friends. In addition, as in the case of Italy, the Catholic religion is also strong here as well. There is a whole series of related traditions, including the role of godparents and godchildren, even in families that are not otherwise religious.[1]

Through such ties, elderly people receive help that directly or indirectly promotes their mobility outside the home. It was because of this extensive helping background that the Hungarians ranked third in answers of the 'no need for help' type (home help/meals). In connection with the Netherlands, it is important to stress that the 'no need for help' reply was the lowest here (0). It should be added that in the Netherlands, the services with automatic entitlement are very strong in other areas too: Each citizen of the country is entitled to a place to live as a basic right of citizenship, complete with a daily newspaper, a phone, transportation to and from the home, and so on (Harrington, Heys, Koster, & Westra, 2000).

There are also differences between the various countries arising from cultural factors and the outside environment, including neighbours. Neighbours are very important in Hungary, especially in rural areas. In the Hungarian countryside, for example, houses almost always have benches in front, in the street. Elderly people feel that they are mobile even if they simply sit out on the bench because the whole village passes in front of them. They are not segregated, and even feel that they play an important part by spreading news.

Our intention in this introduction has been to point out that, in addition to the statistical data, it is always worth taking into account the shifts in welfare policy, and the culture and traditions of the given country.

---

[1] This means that in Hungary and Italy, the notion of family and its role in a very broad sense is important when considering those whom the elderly regard as important persons. See the Chapter on Social Relations.

2.2   Demographic trends in the MOBILATE countries

Historical events, turning points and transitions influence people's life course. Therefore it is important to know that the oldest subjects of the MOBILATE study experienced both World War I and World War II. In fact, many men (and many women, too) born before 1930 were affected by World War II; many were forced to relocate, pursued a different line of work, and suffered from lack of food. After World War II, new regimes were set up with new ideologies, economies and politics. For example, many new socialist regimes (such as the ones in Hungary and the German Democratic Republic) were born at a time when people, both men and women, experienced different roles on the labour market, in the family and society; moreover, these new (and different) societies also had a strong influence on demographic trends. The world wars, especially World War II, can therefore be considered as major factors influencing demographic trends in Europe and starting transitions. It goes without saying that the youngest subjects (the post-war generation) underwent a completely different life course than the oldest subjects.

However, we should emphasise that the group of phenomena known to demographers as the "second demographic transition"[2] started in the countries of Western Europe in the eighties, while in the Eastern and central parts of Europe, political and economic transitions began in the nineties and can be explained in part by differing causes (material and numerous others in addition to the cultural causes).

Table 2.1:   Population change in 2000 (first estimates), per 1000 population

	Live births	Deaths	Natural increase	Net migration	Total increase
Finland	10.8	9.5	1.3	0.6	1.9
Germany	9.2	10.5	-1.2	2.4	1.2
Hungary	9.6	13.3	-3.8	0.0	-3.8
Italy	9.7	9.8	-0.1	3.5	3.4
The Netherlands	13.0	8.8	4.1	3.3	7.4
EU-15	10.8	9.8	0.9	2.2	3.1

Note. EUROSTAT (2000a, p.2)

Among the countries participating, the greatest increase in population was in the Netherlands (Table 2.1). Based on the rates per 1000, the number of live births was the highest here, the number of deaths the lowest and migration (mainly from the former colonies) among the highest (in 2000). Each of these phenomena contributed to the high growth rate. The 7.4 rate of total increase is also more than double the average for the EU countries. The slight growth of the population of Germany in 2000 was partly caused by migration from southern Europe. Without this, the population would have declined to the same extent that it grew (1.2). Hungary was not able to recover in 2000 from the steady population decline that has characterized its demography for decades (since 1980).

---

[2] The demographic transition has four components (Hablicsek, 2000): very low number of children, very high and further increasing duration of life (ageing), stagnation and decline of the population, and intensive immigration.

2.2.1   Demographic changes

The demographic ageing of society is a general trend in the countries examined. The main cause is the declining trend in both fertility and mortality rates. This trend impacts on the pension system, the service systems and raises health care expenditures.

Among all EU countries, Italy had the second lowest total fertility rate (i.e., the number of children per woman) in 1998 (1.19). The EU average was 1.45, and the highest rate (1.95) was observed in Ireland (EUROSTAT, 2000c). Based on current projections, demographers expect substantial further ageing of society in the coming decades.

Hungary has long stood out among the former socialist countries due to its deteriorating demographic indicators. Around the time of the disintegration of the socialist block (in 1990), the proportion of elderly persons in the general population was the highest in Hungary compared to other post-socialist countries: persons 65 years and over represented 13.4%, and those 85 years and over 2.6% of the population (U.S. Department of Commerce, 1993), while the median age was 36 years. Demographic ageing continued in the second half of the nineties, despite the very high mortality rate, particularly among middle-aged men (related to many factors which have already been discussed in the section on Welfare Regimes). Table 2.2 gives comparative data for the year 2000.

Table 2.2:   Distribution of the population by main age group and dependency ratios, percentages, in 2000

	0-14	15-44	45-64	65+	Row Total	ADR	OADR
Finland	18	40	27	15	100	49	22
Germany	16	43	26	16	100	47	23
Hungary	17	43	26	15	100	46	21
Italy	14	43	25	18	100	48	27
The Netherlands	19	44	24	14	100	47	20

Note. KSH (Központi Statisztikai Hivatal [Hungarian Central Statistical Office]), 2001, p. 444
Date: 01.01.2000 (except Germany: 01.01.1999)
ADR = Age Dependency Ratio (population aged 0-14 and 65+ in relation to the population 15-64; authors' own calculations)
OADR = Old Age Dependency Ratio (population aged 65+ in relation to the population 15-64; authors' own calculations)

In 2000, Italy had the highest proportion of older persons in the general population (18%) (Table 2.2). The lowest proportion was in the Netherlands, while Hungary and Finland had slightly higher figures. The relatively lower proportion of elderly persons (65+) within Hungarian society is due principally to the higher mortality rates already mentioned. Nevertheless it is interesting that the indicators for persons over 65 years differ only slightly between the two countries - this, despite the fact that Hungary and Finland had two entirely different general welfare models. Beginning in the 80s, however, under the influence of the Nordic welfare models, Hungarian services for the elderly gradually became more open: they were modernised, technical standards were improved, new links were added, and many Scandinavian, German and Anglo-Saxon elements were adapted to Hungarian conditions and incorporated into the Act on Social Welfare. By the second half of the nineties, all these factors together made it possible to improve living conditions and increase life expectancy among elders. As we have already shown (Table 2.1), the Dutch situation can be attributed principally to natural growth. Germans will keenly experience the ageing of society in the coming decade(s).

In ten years (which is a very short period of time in the social and demographic sense) present forecasts show that the shift in the present proportion of the elderly in the general population (OADR - Old Age Dependency Ratio) will be the greatest in Germany (23% / 29%)(Tables 2.2 and 2.3). Italy can be expected to retain its leading position: the proportion of those 65 years and over compared to the 15-64 years age group in Italian society will be 31%. The Dutch will continue to be the youngest, substantially below the expected EU average).

Table 2.3:   Dependency ratios in 2010, "baseline" demographic scenarios, percentages

	ADR 2010	OADR 2010
Finland	50	25
Germany	51	29
Hungary	n.a.	n.a.
Italy	54	31
The Netherlands	49	23
EU-15	52	27

Note. EUROSTAT, 2000b, p. 102

2.2.2   Social ageing

The proportion of pensioners within the total population is also a source of serious tension regarding social ageing. In all countries, forms of early retirement (as an alternative to unemployment) represented an escape route from the labour market for many of those faced with redundancy. In the countries in transition, the two main types of 'soft dismissal' were retirement on disability pension and retirement before the normal age limit. In 1990 (at the beginning of the transition) disability/early retirees made up 4.2% of the 15-54/59 years age group,[3] and by 1994 this figure was already 6.0% (World Bank, 1995).[4]

Table 2.4:   Inactivity rate, 55-64 years

Country***	1970	1975	1980	1985	1990	1995*	2000
Finland	25.1	34.4	43.1	48.3	52.9	55.4	54.6
Germany	19.8	30.2	32.7	38.4	39.5		
The Netherlands		27.8	36.8	53	54.3	57.7	
Hungary							23.5**

Note. Source for western countries: Guillemard, A-M., 2001, presentation at Cost A13 (Cooperation between Science and Technology) Conference Aalborg.
* Data are available only for other cohorts.
** Data from 1999, KSH, 2000, p. 32
*** We have not found coherent data for Italy.

---

[3] The retirement age was 55 years for women and 60 years for men.
[4] The number of persons on early retirement does not simply accumulate, because when such persons reach the normal retirement age they are classified as old-age pensioners in the statistics. This means that the growth was higher than 1.8% by 1994 (this 1.8% being the difference between the two figures).

In Finland, inactivity among those aged 55-64 years was already quite high by the second half of the seventies; it strengthened in the eighties and remained unchanged for the ten years after 1990. In the Netherlands, the trend toward early retirement was already very strong in the second half of the eighties. In eastern Germany, early withdrawal was an important part of labour policy in order to conceal true unemployment figures. In Hungary, there was no unemployment under socialism. The process outlined above began with the systemic change. Especially in the early nineties, there was mass unemployment which encouraged active members of the labour market to choose early withdrawal. But as already noted, other countries such as Germany, Italy and Finland also made use of this humane form of economic downsizing, and traces can also be found in the MOBILATE Survey made in 2000 (see Chapter 3).

Table 2.5:   Inactivity rate, 45-54 years

Country***	1970	1975	1980	1985	1990	1995*	2000
Finland	9.4	12.8	12.9	11.4	11	12.6	12.1
Germany	4	5.3	5.7	3.7	3.3		
The Netherlands		9	11.4	14.2	11.7	10.3	
Hungary*						13.9**	

Note. Source for western countries: Guillemard, 2001, presentation at Cost A13 Conference, Aalborg
* Data available for the age group of 40-45 years.
** Together with the unemployed; without the unemployed 10.4%, KSH, 1996, p.48.
*** We have not found coherent data for Italy.

2.3   Traffic and transportation systems

According to the Universal Declaration of Human Rights approved by the United Nations in 1948, mobility is a human right. More recently, in 1990, the ADA (American with Disabilities Act) guaranteed all disabled citizens complete and equal protection and full access to public institutions, both in the abstract and physical sense. The European Conference of the Ministers of Transport defined mobility as a fundamental part of all activities performed away from home. Thus, mobility is considered a prerequisite for successful ageing; the freedom to move as one likes is a necessary prerequisite for health and well being, both physical and psychological.

In order to keep older people mobile and allow them to be independent, it is important to know their mobility patterns, attitudes regarding transport, and different needs: those elements are related to different ages, social and economic characteristics and lifestyle, which can vary a lot among the various groups of elderly. Developing effective transport policies responsive to an ageing society requires recognition of the needs of different groups within the older European population. At a demographic level, two sub-divisions have to be stressed: between men and women and between the old and the very old. Within the ageing phenomenon, the varying male and female life expectancies have considerable consequences for older people, creating a feminization of the older generation (Table 2.6). Ageing rates (percentage ratio between the elderly population of 65 year olds and over and the young generation of under 15 year olds) by gender give an overall dimension of the phenomenon: in 1998 it was equal to 72.7% for men and to 114.2% for women according to Eurostat (1997).

Table 2.6:　General statistics of the MOBILATE regions under investigation

	Finland	Germany	Hungary [3]	Italy	The Netherlands
Population (1000) at 2000 [1]	5 171	82 164	10 086	57 680	15 864
Population aged 65+ (%) [2]	14.1	15.4	14.6	16.4	13.2
Mean life expectancy at birth [1] at 1998					
Males	73.5	74.5	67.1	75.5	75.2
Females	80.8	80.6	75.6	81.8	80.6
Mean life expectancy at 65 years at 1998 [1]					
Males	14.9	15.3	15.3-9.9*	16.0	15.1
Females	19.1	19.0	20.0-12.6*	19.8	19.2
Mean size of households at 1998 [1]	2.1	2.2	2.6**	2.7	2.3

Note. [1] EUROSTAT yearbook: the statistical guide to Europe, edition 2001b;
　　　[2] EUROSTAT, Demographic statistics 1997;
　　　[3] Statistical Yearbook of Hungary 2000, Hungarian Central Statistical Office (KSH), 2001b
　　　* There are no figures available for life expectancy at 65 years, the table contains life expectancy at 60 and 70 years.
　　　** Data referred to 1996

Another substantial difference within the older population is linked to the different stages of age; with a general distinction between those who are still healthy and have a good level of autonomy and those who need treatment and care. Even if the majority of elderly people are healthy and can perform their activities of daily living without help, and can therefore be considered to be active citizens and new consumers in the future, one must consider the needs of the growing population of very old. Related to this aspect, many studies in the geriatric field have shown that an ageing population means there will be an increase in older persons with disabilities, whether as an absolute number or as a percentage over the total population (Ferrucci et al., 1996).

Figure 2.1:　Age structure of the population groups reporting severe, moderate and no disability, EU - 14 1996

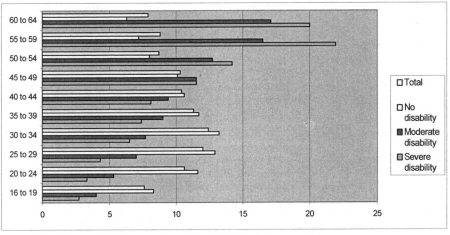

Note. Eurostat, Disability and social participation in Europe, 2001a

Eurostat estimates that almost 60% of the population reporting no disability is under 40 years old, while it is only 24% for those reporting a severe disability. More than 40% of those reporting severe disability and 14% of those reporting no disability are 55 years or older (Figure 2.1). People with reduced physical and mental capacities that hamper their lifestyle probably have also the desire to engage in outdoor activities (Mollenkopf, Marcellini, Ruoppila et al., 1997). However, their transportation possibilities are dramatically reduced, and they thus require viable alternatives. Solutions to the problem involve not only novel forms of public transport but, as often occurs for the disabled, the employment of special cars.

In conclusion, a number of factors have made the elderly population a heterogeneous lot. One can assume that in the future, these factors will tend to accentuate the differences, as new generations of elderly will have lifestyles greatly different from the present ones. For example, many elderly women today have low incomes, they often don't have a car or a driving licence, and their needs and schedules are mostly based on their role as caregivers. Such persons need a public transport service that is flexible, accessible, and cheap. On the other hand, elders who drive (including new generations of women, well acquainted with the labour market) require a series of technological innovations that can adapt the vehicle to their safety needs, especially regarding their reduced physical abilities. For the very old, public transportation becomes important. Moreover, the outdoor environment must be assessed and redesigned with a series of improvements so that they feel safer when walking or driving in areas with busy traffic.

2.3.1   Mobility and transportation systems

The car has become essential to modern daily life due to the flexibility and independence it offers. In Europe today, about 80% of goods and passengers-km are by road (EUROSTAT, 2001b). European citizens travel more than they used to (Table 2.7), especially by car, which is the transport mode used most frequently: the number of passenger cars has risen to more than 270 million.

Table 2.7:   Transport modes of passengers (EU 15). Million passenger kilometers 1994-1998

Modes	1994	1995	1996	1997	1998	1994-1998
Car	3 533 656	3 607 691	3 673 155	3 731 209	3 775 806	242 150
Bus	390262	401053	404000	409700	415385	25 123
Rail	268931	270521	279600	282158	289781	20 850

Note. EUROSTAT yearbook: the statistical guide to Europe, edition 2001b

In recent decades, the number of private cars has notably increased in all the EU countries. Moreover, because most young and middle-aged men and women possess a driving licence, and because the standard of living has continually improved, most of tomorrow's elders will possess a car. This development is not without drawbacks. The increasing use of private cars results in an increasing risk of accidents. The number of people killed is over 40,000 each year. The EU figure for road deaths per 10,000 inhabitants is 1.35, ranging from 0.65 in the United Kingdom to 2.51 in Portugal (EUROSTAT, 1996).

The percentage of older drivers involved in traffic accidents is relatively low in the European Union countries. This is not only due to the fact that the elderly drive less; older individuals are statistically less at risk of being involved in an accident in a car. However, when they are involved in accidents, older car drivers and passengers do have a higher risk of death than younger car drivers and passengers (ISTAT, 1997, 1999, 2000c).

Table 2.8:   Transport statistics

	Finland	Germany	Hungary	Italy	The Netherlands
Number of motor vehicles per 1000 inhabitants	460	617	268	657	485
Number of passenger cars and station wagons [1]	2021	42324	2218	31371	6343
Killed per 100 000 population aged 65+	12.6	10.6	15.9	13.8	11.4
Death rate [2]	9.4	12.2	-	-	9.3
Injury accidents [3]	0.15	0.62	-	-	0.36

Note. IRTAD International Road Traffic and Accident Database (OECD), March 2001
[1] in 1000
[2] killed per 1 billion veh/km
[3] per 1 million veh/km

It is interesting to note that Hungary has the highest number of people killed in accidents per 100,000 of the 65 and over population, despite the fact that the number of motor vehicles here is the lowest of the five countries (Table 2.8). Italy has the highest number of motor vehicles and Germany the second highest. Directly related to this phenomenon, Germany and Italy have the highest number of car passengers.

2.4   Traffic characteristics of the participating countries

2.4.1   Finland

What differentiates Finland from most Central European countries is low population density; Finland has only 15 inhabitants per km². The population centres with higher population density are located in the southern part of Finland, leaving the majority of the country thinly populated. This entails great differences in the availability of public transportation between population centres and the more sparsely populated areas. In areas with less public transportation, owning a car is almost a fundamental necessity. In the population centres, however, the car has also maintained its position as the dominant means of transportation. To entail and make private motorization safer, numerous steps have been taken to develop the traffic environment. Crossroads are more often built as round abouts which effectively prevent high speeds. Speed limits are also adjusted to the season. Speed limits on main roads and motorways are often set 20 km/h lower during the winter (e.g., from 100 km/h to 80 km/h). In town centres and narrow suburban roads, speed limits are generally set to 30-40 km/h throughout the year. In suburban areas with low speed limits, also speed ramps have been and are being built to prevent speeding. Blocking is used in suburban areas to hinder passing (to increase traffic safety). Public transportation services have been improved in several towns, including Jyväskylä, by making special service routes for smaller (12 meter) buses and for door-to-door services. Also an ever increasing number of normal-sized low-floor buses are used on regular routes.

2.4.1.1   Driver licences regulation

Finland became a member of the European Union in 1995, and driving licence regulations were changed in the beginning of 1998 in line with a EU directive. Currently, the right to drive a motor vehicle of a given type is valid until the age of 70 years. However, from the age of 45 onwards, this right is conditional. At the age of 45, the licence holder must pass a vision check-up every five years administered by an optician or a physician. At the age of 60 and thereafter every five years the licence holder must pass a medical examination covering general health status and vision. Previously, this medical examination was given already at age 45 and continued every five years until the age of 70. After the age of 70, the licence expires and drivers who wish to continue driving must pass a medical review and apply for an extension of their licence. In addition two people must confirm that the person has kept up his/her driving abilities. For persons aged 70 years or more, the driver's licence is issued for periods of five years or less, depending on the evaluation of the physician. In the year 2000, the so-called M-class licence was invented as a kind of moped-licence. In 2001, the Cabinet also confirmed the decision to enforce the safety of the road traffic by including the acceptance of the new traffic safety strategy.

2.4.1.2   Traffic accidents

In the whole of Finland in 1995, 16% of all people killed in road traffic were pedestrians, 17% were cyclists, 35% were car drivers, 17% were car passengers, 4% were moped riders and 3% were motorbike riders. During the year 2000, pedestrians made up 16% of all those killed in road traffic accidents, cyclists 13%, car drivers 40%, car passengers 16% and both moped riders as well as motorbike riders 2%. Personal injuries in road traffic in that same year were distributed among traffic users as follows: pedestrians 10%, cyclists 13%, car drivers 34%, car passengers 24%, motorbike riders as well as moped drivers 5% (and bus passengers 1%). In 1995, these figures were very similar: 10%, 15%, 34%, 25%, and 4%, respectively (grouping both motorbike and moped riders together).

Table 2.9:   Volume of domestic passenger traffic. Years 1985, 1995 and 2000
Passengers transport. Billion passenger-km (%)

| Years | By road | | | | By rail* | Other** | Total |
	Private car traffic and mopeds	Bus	Motorcycles	Total			
1985	43.7 (76.1)	8.6 (15.0)	0.8 (1.4)	53.1 (92.5)	3.5 (6.0)	0.8 (1.4)	57.4
1995	50.1 (78.8)	8.0 (12.6)	0.9 (1.4)	59.0 (92.8)	3.6 (5.7)	1.0 (1.6)	63.5
2000	55.7 (79.9)	7.7 (11.0)	0.9 (1.3)	64.3 (92.2)	3.9 (5.6)	1.5 (2.2)	69.7

Note   Statistical Yearbook of Finland 2001. Helsinki: Statistics Finland
* includes railway, tramway and underground traffic
** includes shipping and air traffic

In 1995, 32% of all deaths and 55% of all injuries in road traffic accidents took place in built-up areas. Of all accidents with personal injury or death, 86% involving pedestrians took place in built-up areas. For cyclists this ratio was 88% and for passenger cars 59%. Out of all the road traffic accidents, 26% resulting in death and 52% resulting in injury occurred in the urban areas in 2000. Of all fatal road accidents involving cyclists, 58% occurred in urban areas, and 88% of all personal injuries experienced by cyclists also occurred in built-up areas.

Table 2.10: Persons killed and injured in road traffic accidents per mean population, number of automobiles and automobile kilometres

Years	Killed			
	Number	inhabitants /100 000	automobiles /100 000	automobile-km /100 million
1980	551	11.5	42	2.1
1995	441	8.6	20	1.0
2000	396	7.7	16	0.8
Years	Injured			
	Number	inhabitants /100 000	automobiles /100 000	automobile-km /100 million
1980	8442	177	606	32
1995	10 191	199	467	24
2000	8508	165	n.a.*	18

Note. Road Accidents in Finland 1993, Transport and Tourism 1994: 13. Helsinki: Statistics Finland;
Road Accidents in Finland 1995, Transport and Tourism 1996:15. Helsinki: Statistics Finland;
Road Accidents in Finland 2000, Transport and Tourism 2001:13. Helsinki: Statistics Finland;
Statistical Yearbook of Finland 2001. Helsinki: Statistics Finland
* n.a. refers to the info being not available.

For passenger cars these percentages were 18% and 57%, respectively. Accidents involving cyclists in the built-up areas comprised 23% out of all the road casualties in built-up areas in 2000; for car passengers, the figure was 43%. Regarding personal injury accidents in the built-up areas, 16% involved cyclists and 63% car passengers (Statistical Yearbook of Finland, 2001).

Table 2.11: Elderly (65+) killed or injured in 1993, 1995 and 2000 by road user category, absolute values and percentages on the total of dead and injured people

	Total (all ages)of		As car drivers*		As passengers*		As pedestrians		As cyclists	
	Dead	Injured	Dead	Injured	Dead	Injured	Dead	Injured	Dead	Injured
1993	484	7806	27	189	16	186	36	210	32	210
%			5.6	2.4	3.3	2.4	7.4	2.7	6.6	2.7
1995	441	10191	36	307	14	238	26	223	32	237
%			8.2	3.0	3.2	2.3	5.9	2.2	7.3	2.3
2000	396	8508	28	267	13	225	32	225	28	185
%			7.1	3.1	3.3	2.6	8.1	2.6	7.1	2.2

Note. Road Accidents in Finland 1993, Transport and Tourism 1994:13. Helsinki: Statistics Finland;
Road Accidents in Finland 1995, Transport and Tourism 1996:15. Helsinki: Statistics Finland;
Road Traffic Accidents 2000. Transport and Tourism 2001:13. Helsinki: Statistics Finland.
* includes passenger cars, buses, lorries and vans
Age-grouped information available only since year 1993

In 1995 out of all the road traffic deaths, 11% involved people aged 55-64 years, 14% those aged 65-74 years old, and 13% those over 75 years old. In 2000, these figures were rather similar: 12%, 13% and 13% respectively. Of all injuries in road traffic accidents in 1995, 8% involved people aged 55-64 years, 6% those aged 65-74 and 4% for the over 75 year olds. In 2000 the figures were fairly similar, namely 8%, 7% and 4%, respectively. People aged 65 and over made up 22% of pedestrians injured and 36% of pedestrians killed in road accidents in 1995 (Road Accidents in Finland, 1995). Among all the pedestrians killed in road traffic in 2000, 52% were aged 65 and over, whereas regarding pedestrians' injuries, 26% of them involved people aged 65 and over. Among cyclists these figures were, respectively, 53% and 17%, among car drivers they were 17% and 8% and among car passengers 20% and 10% (Road Traffic Accidents, 2000).

2.4.2   Germany

The dominant means of transportation in Germany is the automobile. As in most industrialized nations, transport policy and planning have been shaped since the 1950s primarily by growing motorization. This orientation has led to massive projects for building new roads, upgrading old ones and reducing the Federal General railroad network. With one passenger car (including station wagons) for about every two inhabitants, the old German Länder today have the highest density of motorization in Europe.

Since the regime shift in Germany, traffic volume has expanded enormously in the new Länder as well. Of the 52.5 million officially licenced motor vehicles in Germany in early 2001, 44 million were passenger cars (including station wagons) - which comprises 83% of all vehicles (Statistisches Bundesamt [Federal Statistical Office of Germany], 2001).

Despite a growing awareness of the problem posed by motorized traffic and even the looming collapse of the entire transport system, the car has lost little of its allure, and the total density and volume of traffic has continued to grow in recent years. Whereas total passenger transport amounted to 854 billion person-kilometres in 1991, this figure had risen to 895 billion six years later. Local public transportation accounted for only 15.7% of the total, with tram, buses and subways contributing 76.3 billion person-kilometres (8.5%) and the railroads 64 billion (7.2%). The percentage of total traffic volume accounted for by local public transport in Germany in 1997 was thus 0.8% lower than it had been in 1991 (Statistisches Bundesamt, 2000).

2.4.2.1   Driver licences regulation

Driving licences do not expire in Germany unless the driver severely contravenes traffic regulations or is declared to be unfit to drive by an expert (medical doctor or traffic psychologist). There are no routine evaluations of driving skills after a person obtains a driving licence.

2.4.2.2   Elderly persons and the traffic system

The number of passenger cars in Germany will continue to rise in the coming years (Statistisches Bundesamt, 2001). The impact that the abrupt increase in private means of transportation has on elderly people varies. On the one hand, the greater variability of private cars increases the mobility of elderly people. On the other hand, the growing volume of traffic also increases potential hazards of such travel. Traffic congestion, particularly in urban centres, has reached an extent that may unsettle elderly people and eventually prevent them from venturing out. The percentage of elderly people in Germany who feel unsafe in road traffic rose from 27% in 1975 to nearly 40% in 1984, and almost half of all elderly people said they rarely dare to go out onto the streets anymore because traffic at certain times is so heavy (Wittenberg, 1986). A European study replicating the respective questions revealed that the figures for people feeling completely or partly helpless in traffic amounted to 45% in the West German city and 65% in the East German city under study in 1995 (Mollenkopf, Marcellini, Ruoppila & Tacken, 2004).

2.4.2.3 Traffic accidents

More than 2.3 million road traffic accidents occurred in Germany in 2000. In 16.3% of the cases (382,949 accidents), personal injury was involved. The number of accidents with personal injury has remained relatively constant in the last twenty years. The rise in the number of vehicles has been accompanied by measures to increase safety on the roads, including expansion of the road system, mandatory use of seat belts and other safety technology used in vehicles.

The total number of persons killed in traffic accidents each year in Germany has declined. Whereas more than 21,300 persons died in traffic accidents in western and eastern Germany in 1970, the number of people killed on German roads in 2000 was 7,503 (Table 2.12), of whom 24.3% died in accidents within metropolitan areas. In 2000, 64% of all traffic accidents that resulted in personal injury occurred within metropolitan areas and 36% outside such areas. A total of 988 pedestrians and 655 cyclist were killed, but most of the traffic fatalities in 2000 (4,398 people) were passengers in cars. Among the dead in 2000 were 240 children aged 14 years or below and 1,296 persons over 64 years old. Of the 504,074 people injured in 2000, 36,340 were 65 years old or more (Statistisches Bundesamt, 2001).

Table 2.12: Elderly (65+) victims by type of accidents in 2000

	Victims	Injured	Dead
Eastern Germany	89,231	87,329	1,902
Western Germany	422,346	416,745	5,601
Total	511,577	504,074	7,503
65+ total	37,636	36,340	1,296
	Victims (%)	Injured (%)	Dead (%)
Eastern Germany	17.4	17	0.4
Western Germany	82.6	81.5	1.1
Total	100.0	98.5	1.5
65+ percentage of total victims	7.4	7.1	0.3
65+ percentage of victims 65+	100.0	96.6	3.4

Note. Statistisches Bundesamt [Federal Statistical Office of Germany], Wiesbaden 2001

Since June of 1990, the risk of being killed in a traffic accident has been clearly higher in eastern Germany than in the western part of the country because of the rapid increase of car ownership after reunification. In western Germany, there have been 8.2 traffic fatalities per 100,000 inhabitants, whereas the figure in eastern Germany is 13.6 (Statistisches Bundesamt, 2001; IRTAD, 2000). The differences are not as great among senior citizens but continue to be higher in the new Länder than in the old. Among persons 65 years or older, the risk of being involved in a traffic accident is above average (11.5) in western Germany, but it too is even higher (15) in eastern Germany.

Very old pedestrians have a higher-than-average rate of injury or death in traffic accidents. In 1991, the figure for men aged 65 to74 years was 4.5 serious accidents per 10,000 inhabitants (6.1 for women of that age bracket), and the pedestrians' risk of being involved in an accident rose sharply to 10.0 for men aged 75 year or more (10.6 for women of that age bracket). These figures on accident risk were Germany's second highest, exceeded only by those for children aged 6 to 9 years (Hautzinger, Tassaux-Becker, & Hamacher, 1996).

To reduce high accident rates among the older persons, the Deutsche Verkehrswacht (German Traffic Patrol) together with the Deutscher Verkehrssicherheitsrat (German Council for Traffic Safety, DVR) have developed special programmes such as 'Elderly active drivers', 'Travel by bus and tram' or 'Elderly pedestrians' which aim at securing the mobility of people in their immediate environments (Emsbach, 2001).

2.4.3   Hungary

During the long years of socialism Hungarians had to rely largely on public transportation. It was simply very difficult to obtain a passenger car. Even as late as 1989, only 120,674 new cars were sold in the domestic market, of which 27% were Dacias, 24% Ladas, 17% Trabants, and 13% Wartburgs. In addition to new cars made in the socialist countries, private persons imported a further 68,065 cars, mainly second-hand Western cars (mostly Fords, Opels, and Volkswagens; KSH - Központi Statisztikai Hivatal [Hungarian Central Statistical Office], 1991).

As a result, railway and bus transport played an important role in long-distance travel. In 1980, 287 million railway passengers travelled 13,714 million km. This figure declined substantially towards the end of the nineties, particularly following the systemic change. By 1990 rail traffic had decreased to just 211 million railway passengers who travelled 11,403 million kilometres. Within long-distance passenger transport, bus travel declined slightly in the mid-nineties, but had increased considerably by the end of the century. The number of bus passengers was 513 million in 1990, 494 million in 1995 and 544 million in 1999. The number of passenger kilometres covered by long-distance buses amounted to 10,237 million in 1990, 9,556 million in 1995, and 11,262 million in 1999 (KSH, 1991, 1998, 2000).

Traffic also changed with the end of socialism. The rate of car ownership rose from the 16.8% in 1989 to 18.8% by 1990, and this growth has continued steadily: in 1995, 21.9% of the populace owned a car, and in 1999 22.4%. The structure of the stock of passenger cars also changed with a strong shift towards Western makes (KSH, 2000). The car became important mainly for the younger generation. With the privatisation of the economy, firms began to give importance to their image. Many firms provided company cars for employees, replacing them at least every three years. All this affected the elderly much less since there was a cheaper and often more convenient solution available for them. The former government announced free public travel using every type of public transport for the over-65-year-olds. Pensioners younger than 65 were allowed to travel for half-price.

Up to the mid-90s, persons over 70 years could use local and long-distance transport free of charge. With the approach of the 1998 elections, the Socialist government reduced the age limit to 65 years, and this has remained in force. This means that all pensioners over the age of 65 years are automatically entitled, upon presentation of their pension card, to unlimited travel within Hungary. They are required to pay only for seat reservations on Intercity trains and on those long-distance bus services where reservations are compulsory. Since petrol prices are rising steadily, even pensioners who have a car take advantage of this opportunity. The mobility of the elderly in Hungary by means other than the car is thus ensured by current welfare policy and by the good public transport network.

Although the number of persons using the railway has declined, the average distance of journeys has increased: from 47.8 km in 1980 to 54.1 km in 1990 (KSH, 1991). In the larger towns, there are trams and trolleybuses and in Budapest, also an underground. However, there are also large towns, including Pécs, where buses are the only form of public transport. Between 1990 and 1998, the number of settlements with local bus traffic fell from 203 to 110. This is almost certainly related to the rapid increase in the number of cars. Between 1996 and 1999, the number of cars registered increased by 34% (KSH, 1998; KSH, 2000).

Together with the spread of motor vehicles in Hungary, the traditional vehicle, the bicycle, continues to be important not only for travel purposes but also for transporting persons and goods, especially on the Great Plain, the Little Plain, the region south of Lake Balaton and in other flat areas.

2.4.3.1 Driver licences regulation

Driving licences may be obtained by persons over the age of 18 years who have an identity card or passport. A prior medical examination, covering eyesight, hearing and nervous system functioning, is required. After the medical examination, candidates must attend a course on technical matters, the highway code and a course on first-aid (highway code 30 hours, first-aid ten hours). Candidates must then take a test in both subjects. After passing the tests, a course on driving routine follows (10 hours). This is followed by another examination covering driving routine and technical matters. (There are two technical tests: one on theory, the other on practice). It is only after successfully passing these tests that candidates can take part in practical driving instruction (30 hours). This is followed by another test. If the candidate passes this test, he or she is issued a driving licence which remains valid for ten years, after which the medical examination must be repeated. Persons over 80 must undergo a medical examination every two years.

2.4.3.2 Traffic accidents

The number of road accidents is presently declining despite the rising trend in the number of cars. Compared to the 27,801 accidents in 1990, there were only 19,817 in 1995 and 18,923 in 1999 (KSH, 2000). This reduction can be attributed to the stricter rules applying to drivers, to fines imposed on those using a bicycle without lights, etc. This has given rise to a positive trend, since fewer people have been killed and injured in accidents. The number of road accident deaths has fallen from 2,432 in 1990 to 1,589 in 1995 and 1,306 in 1999, meaning that the number has been almost halved in ten years. Over the same period, the number of persons injured in traffic accidents has fallen from 36,996 in 1990 to 25,886 in 1995, to only 24,670 in 1999 (KSH, 2000).

The proportion of persons over 60 years killed in accidents has remained largely the same: 25.5% in 1990, 22% in 1995 and 24.8% in 1999, while there has been a slight rise in the 25-60 years age group: 51.5% (1990), 55.6% (1995), 56.5% (1999). The same trend was found in the proportion of persons over 60 injured in road accidents: 10.9% in 1990, 11% in

1995, and 11% again in 1999. The corresponding figures for those aged 25-60 years were 48.6%, 49% and 52% (KSH, 2000).

The fact that fewer elderly persons have been killed or injured in road accidents is related to several reasons, including: a) access to public transport as mentioned above, is free and used by the majority of pensioners, b) many elders give up driving after retirement, c) the elderly are cautious in traffic, d) vehicles have been modernised (e.g. buses with low floors), e) for the reasons already indicated, many of the very old may not have ever owned a car while gainfully employed and for financial reasons, were not able to buy one as pensioners, so they do not take part in traffic as drivers.

Table 2.13: Involvement of persons 65 years and older in accidents, outcome of the accidents in 2000 (N)

		48 hours after accident				30 days after accident		
		Dead	serious	Light	Total	dead	serious	light
Driver	65 +	62	401	432	895	88	380	427
	Total Pop.	519	4161	7678	12358	581	4138	7639
Passenger	65 +	17	163	354	534	26	158	350
	Total Pop.	244	1988	5350	7582	273	1987	5322
Pedestrian	65 +	69	406	270	745	95	385	265
	Total Pop.	285	1571	2102	3958	346	1528	2084
Total (N)	65 +	148	970	1056	2174	209	923	1042
	Total Pop.	1048	7720	15130	23898	1200	7653	15045

Note. KSH. Közlekedési balesetek 2000 [Traffic accidents 2000], 2001a.

The indicators for the population 65 years and over are much worse than for those 60 years and over. Their risk is related to the deterioration of their general state of health. The 65+ age group represents 14.6% of the total population but 17.4% (209 out of 1,200) of those killed in accidents (Table 2.13). If we assume that they generally take part in traffic less often (i.e., they spend more time at home), the risk is even more striking. The proportion of deaths among the elderly 48 hours after the accident is lower than 30 days after the accident. This shows that their chances of survival after accidents are lower since their bodies do not heal so readily, and complications are more likely to arise, e.g., hip fracture, pneumonia, bed sores, embolisms, etc. The chance of injuries is especially high in accidents involving pedestrians; persons 65 years and over are the victims of 18.8% of such accidents, and more than one quarter of the serious injuries and deaths (30 days after the accident) are from this age group (Authors' calculations based on Table 2.13).

Table 2.14: Share of the 65+ age group in selected accident outcome subcategories, as percentage of the full population concerned in 2000

	48 hours after accident				30 days after accident		
	dead	serious	light	Total	Dead	serious	light
Driver	11.9	9.6	5.6	**7.2**	15.1	9.2	5.6
Passenger	7.0	8.2	6.6	**7.0**	9.5	8.0	6.6
Pedestrian	24.2	25.8	12.8	**18.8**	27.5	25.2	12.7
Total	14.1	12.6	7.0	**9.1**	17.4	12.1	6.9

Note. Authors' calculations based on Table 2.13

2.4.4 Italy

The transportation situation in Italy is characterised by a substantial unbalance in the dynamics of transportation. This is due to two structural elements which hinder the government's response to the increasing mobility demands of society. The first is the geography and history of the country and its distribution of settlements, the second the fragmentariness of competencies at different levels (national, regional, local) in defining transportation policy.

From the 70's on, the demand for mobility, i.e., the transportation of people and goods over short, medium and long distances, has grown very quickly. Over the last few years, this demand has grown faster than the GDP (Gross Domestic Product) as in the majority of the other EU countries. In particular, the growth in passenger traffic is due to an increasing short period mobility for vacation, pursuing cultural interests, and shopping, or simply commuting to work and study reasons.

This new demand has concentrated in large measure on road traffic, despite the fact that a variety of other transportation networks are valid alternatives. At a policy level, the main reason has been lack of planning the supply of the whole infrastructure system; instead, the road network has simply been expanded to serve increasing road traffic. From the users' perspective the agility, flexibility and control of the road vehicle and the lack or difficulty in utilising other means of transport have stimulated the demand for this kind of transport. Presently in Italy, cars constitute 80% of road traffic.

Though new infrastructure, created over the last 20 years, has been programmed to extend the national road network to 23,000 km and to create more efficient connections among different road systems and other transport networks, the present transportation system is still inadequate, partly because extensions have stimulated even more traffic (Table 2.15). Highway traffic has increased from 15 billion kilometres covered by vehicles in 1980 to 60 billion covered in 1995 to 66 billion in 1998. Heavy traffic often creates a situation of crisis along the main extra-urban roads and also inside the cities. A survey of Ministry of Transport showed that 7,500 out of 8,000 intersections were dangerous and the general state of repair was mediocre, especially in the southern part of Italy (Ministero dei Trasporti [Ministry of Transport], 1999).

Table 2.15: Passenger traffic

Years	(passenger-km) in millions
1985	480.799
1994	746.262
1998	868.916

Note. Ministero dei Trasporti [Ministry of Transport], 1999

Table 2.16: Means of transport of passengers. Years 1980-1994 (%)

Years	By road		Total	By rail	Other	Total
	Private car	Group transport				
1980	76.1	13.5	89.6	9.3	1.1	100.0
1994	81.9	10.5	92.4	6.4	1.2	100.0

Note. ISTAT (Istituto Nazionale di Statistica [Statistical National Institute]), Italian Statistical Yearbook, 1994

Comparing data between 1998 and 1994 (Table 2.16), we see that the car is by far the most common means of transport used by Italians. Moreover, the trend increased between 1980 and 1994. Table 2.17 shows that for trips away from home, including overnight ones, the car was still the means most often used in 2000, even if in 1998 there appeared to be a slight but steady reduction in journeys by car, which was used more for work trips and short vacations. Compared to the previous year, it was found that people going on work trips used the aeroplane much more than before (ISTAT, 2000a).

Table 2.17: Trips by type and by main means of transport used – Year 2000 (%)

Means	Holiday	Work	Total trips
Plane	9.7	34.1	13.2
Train	10.9	17.7	11.9
Ship	3.3	0.8	2.9
Car	67.8	39.7	63.7
Coach	6.1	3.8	5.8
Camper	1.6	0.7	1.5
Other	0.6	3.2	1.0
Total	**100.0**	**100.0**	**100.0**

Note. ISTAT (Istituto Nazionale di Statistica [Statistical National Institute]) 2000a,
I Viaggi in Italia e all'estero nel 2000 [Trips in Italy and abroad in 2000]

2.4.4.1 Driver licences regulation

The new legislation concerning driver licences has been in use since 1994. Driving licences of type A and B (motorcycles and cars, respectively) are valid for 10 years until 50 years of age, 5 years until 70 years of age, and 3 years after 70 years of age. At these ages, the individual must pass a psycho-physical fitness examination in order to renew the licence.

2.4.4.2 Traffic accidents

In large and middle sized towns, city traffic is characterised by heavy car traffic. The infra-urban presence of harbours, railway stations, and airports, as well as a high volume of persons commuting to work and school, congests the traffic system as well. Projects for bypassing traffic around cities, regulating traffic in the city centre, and improving the public transport system are often unfeasible or poorly executed, due to the fragmentation of competencies among different institutions and the lack of a general policy. The consequence has been an increasing risk of accidents, especially in urban areas. In 2000, 74.6% of all accidents occurred in urban areas and 25.4% in extra-urban areas. To control the rising number of accidents, new regulations were introduced since the 80s until the reform of the rules of the road (1993) which set new speed limits, provided safety measures, instituted procedures for monitoring the acquisition of driving licences and vehicle maintenance, and modernised traffic signals. These measures kept the number of accidents constant, which is actually a reduction in accident risk given increasing traffic flow (ISTAT 1997, 1999, 2000c).

Pedestrians are the weakest subjects in the urban area: 93% of accidents involving pedestrians in 2000 occurred inside urban areas. Pedestrians are the weakest subjects also considering the seriousness of accidents. In 2000, 5% of pedestrian accidents resulted in death. It is very important to underline that elderly persons (65+) run a higher risk of death; in fact they constitute 53% of victims (ISTAT, 2000c).

Table 2.18: Risk of accidents in Italy

Years	Number of accidents	accidents /10.000 vehicles	accidents /100.000 inhabitants
1980	163,770	68.4	290.0
1995	182,761	49.6	318.0
2000	211,941	52,1	366,4

Note. ISTAT (Istituto Nazionale di Statistica [Statistical National Institute]) - Statistiche degli incidenti stradali [Statistics of road accidents], 1997,1999, 2000c

Table 2.19: Elderly (65+) victims by type of accidents (percentage values respectively on the total of dead and injured people)

Years	As car drivers		as passengers		as pedestrians	
	Dead	Injured	Dead	Injured	Dead	Injured
1985	15.9	4.6	11.2	4.8	45.9	20.6
1995	17.4	6.3	14.7	6.9	51.0	28.1
1997	18.4	3.3	29.7	7,4	57.6	27.0
2000	17.2	6.3	12.5	6.5	52.9	29.7

Note. ISTAT (Istituto Nazionale di Statistica [Statistical National Institute] - Statistiche degli incidenti stradali [Statistics of road accidents]), 1997, 1999, 2000c

2.4.4.3 Improvements in public transport

In recent years, both state- and city-owned enterprises have instituted a policy of improving the number and quality of public transport services in order to relieve the congestion of traffic and improve the quality of life in the city. Projects involved the reorganisation of networks, an increase in the number of buses and trains and of their stops.

More low-floor buses have been put into service. As for trains, the situation has improved with the introduction of the Eurostar, which has considerably reduced travel times between the larger cities. However, service to the peripheral and mountain areas have been neglected and, compared to a few years ago, are now poorly serviced and they are difficult to get to. The effects of these improvements are still now limited to an increased level of satisfaction expressed by the users, but there has not been an increase of urban and extra-urban demand has remained stable.

The level of satisfaction is generally lower regarding urban transportation services (buses, trolley buses, tram) than with train and coach services. In particular, from 1993 on, the satisfaction with coach services has remained fairly stable, while two distinct attitudes can be found regarding urban transport and trains. Where the train is concerned, satisfaction has steadily decreased over the last 6-7 years, and therefore the improvement found in the last year has been an opposing trend (improvement mainly regards satisfaction with the frequency of service, punctuality, cleanliness of coaches and price of tickets). Regarding opinion on urban transport, the trend is one of steady growth in satisfaction. Data for 2000 are higher than those for 1993. So if the urban service generally presents lower levels of satisfaction (tiring waits at bus stops and the price of tickets are the least satisfying aspects, only 37.5% of users are satisfied with the former and 46.7% with the latter), it is also true that users have observed steady improvements in service quality (ISTAT, 2000b).

2.4.5   The Netherlands

First, let us review some general figures about the infrastructure in the Netherlands. In 1999, the total railnet consisted of 2808 km of track. The total length of paved roads was 117,430 km, of which 19,000 km were cycle paths. The intensity of the traffic on these roads has increased 76% on the highways and 34% on other roads since 1986 (CBS [Central Bureau of Statistics], 2000b).

The number of cars has increased between 1980 and 2000 from 5.1 to 6.3 million. This means an increase from 0.8 to 0.9 cars per household in the same period. Between 1980 and 1999, the total kilometres per day per person older than 12 years increased to 35.3. The total amount of travelled kilometres was 187 billion in 1999. Of these kilometres, 76% were travelled by cars, 12% by using public transport and 7% by bicycles. 81% of the populace owned a bicycle in 1999.

The car is an important means of transport. The number of cars was 6.3 million in 2000, which means that at least one in every three persons had a car. Three quarters of all households had at least one car. These cars are not only parked, but in total 142 billion km were covered by these cars in that year. The average person travelled 18.6 km a day by car as a driver and 7.2 km as a passenger. This means that 75% of the total travel distance per day of 32.2 km was covered by cars. The bicycle plays a more dominant role in ownership. With nearly 13 million bicycles in the Netherlands, almost every Dutch person owns a bicycle. The average person cycles a distance of 2.4 km a day, which means that 8% of all kilometres travelled are covered by bicycle. 12% of the total kilometres travelled are covered by public transport. The share of elderly travelling by public transport is low. Most trips involve commutes to work. Among elderly persons, public transport is just as popular among females (11%) as among males (11%).

On average, people made 3.1 trips a day. By trip we mean going from home to a place for a purpose; going by bicycle and then by bus to a shop, for example, is one shopping trip. Car drivers and car passengers made 1.5 trips a day, whereas bicyclists made 0.8 trips a day. Only 0.15 trips a day were made by public transport (CBS, 2000c).

2.4.5.1   Driver licences regulation

Driving licences are valid for a period of ten years. Every ten years one has to renew the licence. After the age of 70, a medical examination is needed and a new period of validity will be fixed. The driving licence is an important condition for using a car. In 1999, 86% of all men and 69% of all women possessed a driving licence, compared to 83% of all males and 43% of all females aged 65-74 years (CBS, 2000c)

2.4.5.2   Elderly persons and the traffic system

There are large differences between older males and older females in car ownership and possession of a driver's licence. Among males, these figures are 73% and 73%, respectively for those aged 65-74 years and 53% and 61% for those over 75 years. Among females, these figures are 2% and 43% for the 65-74 year olds and 12% and 18% for the over 75 year olds (1999) (CBS, 2000c). These figures also show a cohort effect: the younger generation more often has a driving licence and more often owns a car than the older generation.

The level of participation in traffic shows the percentage of people making at least one trip a day. This is 71% of those aged 65-74 years and 53% for those over 75 years. Females participate less often than males. Older people in more than one person households travel more kilometres a day than older people in single person households. People older than 18 years travel on average 36 km per day. Elders living in single person households travel 11 km compared to 17 km travelled by those living in larger households. This can totally be explained by the kilometres travelled as car passenger.

The use of different transport modes is a relevant aspect of elderly persons' mobility. Table 2.22 shows how the trips of men and women 65 and older were distributed by transport mode in the 1999 National Travel Survey (CBS, 2000c). The figures show that women make fewer trips than men. These differences can be found in cycle trips and car driver trips. The next Table shows that the number of trips made by women is generally lower and the distances covered are shorter, compared to men. This difference can mainly be explained by the much longer distances travelled by car. The general conclusion is that women aged 65 years and older make fewer trips than men and that these trips are mostly shorter (CBS, 2000c).

Table 2.20: The average number of trips a day made by men and women of 65 -74 and 75+ years using various modes of transportation in 1999

Trips made by mode	Males		Females	
	65 – 74	75+	65 - 74	75+
Car	1.22	0.69	0.36	0.15
Car passenger	0.5	0.13	0.53	0.30
Public transport	0.08	0.07	0.12	0.09
Bicycle	0.68	0.41	0.55	0.20
Walking	0.63	0.56	0.61	0.50
Other	0.05	0.05	0.04	0.10
Total	2.81	1.94	2.23	1.34

Note. CBS, The mobility of Dutch Population, 2000c

2.4.5.3   Problems and impairments

So far a few aspects of the travel behaviour of active people in the Netherlands have been described. The data of the Dutch National Travel Survey (NTS) also clearly shows that the higher the age the lower the number of trips. In the NTS, as many as 47% of those aged 75 and older mentioned no trips on the interview day, while this figure was 13% for those aged 40-50 years. This stresses that differences in outdoor mobility are related to the age of people (CBS, 2000c).

In the 65-74 year age group, women make relatively fewer trips (2.23) than males (2.81). The most striking differences exist between females and males in the use of the car in this age group: males make 1.25 trips per day as car drivers, and 0.41 as passengers, whereas females make 0.36 trips per day as car drivers and 0.53 as passengers. Car drivers make more trips than passengers. A relationship between these findings seems evident. Men, more often possessors of a driving licence, are the car users who make most trips.

Single persons travel less than married people. Several reasons can plausibly explain this fact: the partner, if a car driver, offers an opportunity to become mobile, people like to travel in the company of others, the partner can be helpful in organising the trip, and travelling together can lend one a greater feeling of security.

The over-representation of the people with lower education in the group making no trips combined with the under-representation of car owners in this group suggests that low education goes together with low income and lower chances of having a car. But another simple explanation is that the older generation (who are naturally less mobile) received less education.

Elderly persons are not the most dangerous group of people who cause accidents. Young drivers cause most car accidents. Compared to other adults, elders are more often victims of traffic accidents as pedestrians or cyclists (Table 2.21). In the oldest age group the proportion of car accidents is slightly lower than in the age group of 70-79. Most people have by then stopped driving a car and are most endangered by their slow movements.

Table 2.21: Number of accident victims, by age group

Males and Females	0-14	15-19	20-29	30-39	40-49	50-59	60-69	70-79	≥80	Total
Pedestrian	15	4	12	6	7	10	16	23	21	114
Bicycle	35	22	10	10	15	27	29	40	29	217
Moped	1	35	9	11	4	7	8	14	6	95
Bike	2	2	34	26	8	6	1	-	1	80
Car	20	50	159	77	66	45	41	54	30	542
Truck	-	-	2	1	2	2	1	1	-	9
Other vehicle	1	1	12	9	2	5	4	5	3	42
Unknown	-	1	-	-	1	-	3	1	-	6
Total	**74**	**115**	**238**	**140**	**105**	**102**	**103**	**138**	**90**	**1105**

Note. CBS: Niet-natuurlijke dood in Nederland [Non-natural deaths in the Netherlands], 1996-1998, 2000a

2.5   Conclusions

It is clear that the ageing of society will lead to profound demographic changes in developed countries, and especially in the European Union. This will require extensive re-organization of society, whether in the domain of public services, welfare policy or in private supply. The data and trends shown are a challenge also for the welfare systems of the countries under investigation. Making changes to existing pension systems - although this is one of the basic elements to handling the problem - is not by itself sufficient. By the same token, it would be a mistake to concentrate exclusively on the resources inherent in family relations. The care structure available to older people must be formed of interlinked elements, offering not only the existing forms of health and social services. It must also take into account the mobility of the elderly, especially their out-of-home mobility. The various countries have set out on the path of expanding the links in services for the elderly. Innovative services are being introduced in a few countries (such as Germany and Italy), which, when incorporated into the legislation, will have a direct or indirect influence on out-of-home mobility. The analyses of the present study aim to expand knowledge in this area.

The demographic revolution will have future consequences also for the transportation system and on guaranteeing mobility for the older age groups. These two factors will have to undergo changes bearing in mind the present situation and some possible tendencies:

- The number of potential elderly users will grow in quantity, as the demographic composition of the population changes;
- elderly traffic participants will be qualitatively different from previous generations: they will work longer, more often live alone, have a higher level of education and a certain number, still a minority but on the increase, could have reduced mobility or be disabled due to physical disability, cognitive impairment, or sensory disorders (such as vision or hearing impairment);
- the majority of the elderly will probably require greater mobility than at present; they will need to work, travel and maintain interpersonal contacts, especially in the south European countries;
- many elderly people will consider outdoor mobility to be very important for their quality of life. Loss of mobility with age does not necessarily indicate a decrease of desired mobility nor is it due to irremediable health problems; rather, it is often due to obstacles and hindrances in the environment and in the transport system;
- there will be more elderly people with driving licences and who own cars. In particular, the increase will be proportionally higher among women;
- elderly persons are victims of serious traffic accidents and have a poor time with the present chaotic traffic conditions;
- transport and the means of transport for elderly people in Hungary are influenced by political decisions and welfare policy.

Coming back to a wider outlook, we can say that certainly a new balance is necessary between demand and supply, through a reorganization of the offer and transport policies in relation to current changes and to the needs expressed by older people.

- The car will still be widely used by the older population, so that car industries will have to design cars that meet the real needs of older people and their gradually declining performance.
- Closely connected to this greater presence of elderly car drivers, there is the problem of traffic safety, which can be increased with new technological aids, both in the car itself and in the infrastructures. Often elderly drivers adopt compensatory behaviour probably to compensate for their slower reactions, avoiding long journeys or motorways (see Chapter 5, Transport and Behaviour); in this direction the new technologies such as telematics can give a lot of support.
- Improvement of public transport could counterbalance the use of the car, above all in the Mediterranean countries to better meet the needs of elders with reduced mobility, which we presently see to be a minority. It can be assumed that the current 'ageing of ageing' will increase the number of people with reduced psycho-physical performance, who today are often only potential users or excluded ones.
- Improvement of public transport must target all means of transport, including trains and planes (design, technological solutions, more public transport programmes, user involvement in research (see e.g., COST, http://www.cordis.lu/cost-transport/ home.html).
- Greater accessibility and diffusion of accessible transport (e.g., low-floor buses) must be considered. Flexibility in transport is very important and can be carried out

by adapting the existing system or with door-to-door solutions, which respond to the needs of the elderly people with reduced capacity or who live in isolated areas.

- Infrastructures must also be modified, improving the connectivity and integration between means of transport and traffic safety, especially for pedestrians.

These are the trends which we foresee; at the same time we must introduce a new methodological scheme to face the problems of the elderly people from the market perspective, i.e., in terms of supply and demand. Elderly people are not an undifferentiated group and therefore their needs vary, so mobility and transport have to be analysed in relation to many important variables, such as gender, age, income, level of education, degree of disability (personal aspects) and even the country and residential area (environmental aspects). In fact, transportation opportunities vary greatly, not only between the north and south European countries, but also within the same country or city. In this case, the offer conditions the need and perception of the need.

To conclude we can say that age reduces mobility and the use of transport, but public transport can be improved, and the current system and existing offer creates quite a substantial obstacle to elder mobility.

References

Bartal, A. (1998). *Elméleti kihívások és gyakoribb válaszok a nonprofit szektorban* [Theoretical challenges and common responses in the nonprofit sector]. Budapest: PhD thesis, manuscript.

Bundesanstalt für Strassenwesen (BASt) [Federal Highway Research Institute] (Eds.) (1999). *Verkehrs- und Unfalldaten. Kurzzusammenstellung der Entwicklung in der Bundesrepublik Deutschland* [Road Traffic and Accident Data. Brief Overview, Germany]. Bergisch Gladbach: BASt.

CBS (Central Bureau of Statistics) (2000a). *Niet-natuurlijke dood in Nederland* [Non-natural deaths in the Netherlands] 1996 - 1998. Voorburg.

CBS (2000b). *Statistical Yearbook*. Voorburg.

CBS (2000c). *The mobility of Dutch Population*. Voorburg.

COST (European Cooperation in the Field of Scientific and Technical Research). http://www.cordis.lu/cost-transport/home.html.

Deacon, B., & Szalai, J. (Eds.) (1990). *Social policy in the new Eastern Europe. What future for the welfare state?* USA, Hong Kong, Singapore, Sydney: Avebury, Aldershot-Brookfield.

ECMT (European Conference of Ministers of Transport) (2000). *Transport and Aging of the population*. Round table 112. Paris: OECD Publication Service.

Emsbach, M. (2001). Aktivierende Verkehrssicherheitsarbeit mit älteren Menschen [Activating Training of Older People with Respect to Traffic Safety]. In A. Flade & M. Limbourg (Eds.), *Mobilität älterer Menschen* [Mobility in Older People] (pp. 273-284). Opladen: Leske + Budrich.

Esping-Andersen, G. (1990). *The three worlds of welfare capitalism*. Oxford: Policy Press.

Esping-Andersen, G. (1999). *Social foundations of post-industrial economies*. Oxford: University Press.

European Foundation on Social Quality (2001). Amsterdam: Annual Report 2000.

EUROSTAT (1996). *Facts through figures*. Luxembourg: Office for Official Publications of the European Communities.

EUROSTAT (1997). *Demographic Statistics*. Luxembourg: Office for Official Publications of the European Communities.

EUROSTAT (1999). *Demographic Statistics*. Luxembourg: Office for Official Publications of the European Communities.

EUROSTAT (2000a). *First Demographic Estimates for 2000*. (Catalogue number: CA-NK-00-016-EN-I). Luxembourg: European Communities.

EUROSTAT (2000b). *Labour Force Survey*. Luxembourg: Office for Official Publications of the European Communities.

EUROSTAT (2000c). *The Social Situation in the European Union*. Luxembourg: European Communities, Eurostat.

EUROSTAT (2001a). *Disability and social participation in Europe*. Luxembourg: Office for Official Publications of the European Communities.

EUROSTAT (2001b). *Eurostat Yearbook: the statistical guide to Europe*. Luxembourg: Office for Official Publications of the European Communities.

EUROSTAT (2001c). *Panorama of transport*. Luxembourg: Office for Official Publications of the European Communities.

Fargion, V. (2001). *Lessons from recent changes in the Italian welfare state*. Paper presented at the International seminar "Welfare states and Southern-Eastern Europe. Lessons from History and other Regions" (pp. 13-15). Konjic-Bosnia-Herzegovina.

Ferge, Z. (1990). The fourth road. The future of the Hungarian social policy. In B. Deacon & J. Szalai (Eds.), *Social policy in the new Eastern Europe, what future for the welfare state?* (pp. 103 - 121). USA, Hong Kong, Singapore, Sydney: Avebury, Aldershot-Brookfield.

Ferge, Z., & Lévai, K. (Eds.) (1991). *A jóléti állam [The welfare state]*. Budapest: T-Twins Kiadó.

Ferrucci L., Guralnik J. M., Jylha M., Heikkinen E., Salani B., Bandinelli S., & Baroni A. (1996). Patterns of physical functioning and need for support in Italy as compared to five European countries. *Gerontologist 36, 393.*

Gennrich, R. (1994). Einigung bei der Pflegeversicherung [Agreement at care insurance]. *Kuratorium Deutsche Altershilfe, Pressedienst,* Vol. 2, 4, 5.

Grabher, G. (1995). The elegance of incoherence: economic transformation in East Germany and Hungary. In E.J. Dittrich, G. Schmidt, & R. Withley (eds.), *Industrial transformation in Europe* (pp. 33-53). London: Sage.

Guillemard, A.-M. (2001). *The advent of a flexible life course and the reconfiguration of welfare*. Paper presented at Cost A 13 Conference, Aalborg, November 2, manuscript.

Gyulavári, T. (2000). *Az Európai Únió szociális dimenziója* [Social dimension of the European Union]. Budapest: Szociális és Családügyi Minisztérium.

Hablicsek, L. (2000). A népesség öregedése, A holland-magyar összehasonlító vizsgálat margójára [Ageing of the population. Note on the Dutch-Hungarian comparative study]. In E. Daróczi & Z. Spéder (Eds.), *A korfa tetején, Az idősek helyzete Magyarországon* [At the top of the age-tree. Situation of the elderly in Hungary] (pp. 153-175.). Budapest: KSH Népességtudományi Kutatóintézet.

Harrington, T. L., Heys, W. J. M., Koster, W. G., & Westra, J. (2000). Housing. In T. L. Harrington & M. K. Harrington (Eds.), *Gerontechnology why and how* (pp. 59-83). Eindhoven: Herman Bouma Foundation for Gerontechnology.

Hautzinger, H., Tassaux-Becker, B., & Hamacher, R. (1996). *Verkehrsmobilität in Deutschland zu Beginn der 90er Jahre* [Traffic Mobility in Germany at the Beginning of the Nineties]. Band 5: Verkehrsunfallrisiko in Deutschland [Accident Risks in Germany]. In Bundesanstalt für Straßenwesen (Eds.), *Berichte der Bundesanstalt für Straßenwesen - Mensch und Sicherheit, Heft M 58* [Reports of the Federal Highway Research Institute - Person and Safety, vol. M 58]. Bergisch Gladbach: BAST.

IRTAD (2000). *International Road Traffic and Accident Database.* http://www.bast.de/htdocs/fachthemen/irtad//english/englisch.html.

IRTAD (2001). *International Road Traffic and Accident Database (OECD).* March.

ISTAT (Italian Statistical National Institute) (1994). Italian Statistical Yearbook. Rome: ISTAT.

ISTAT (1997). *Gli incidenti stradali negli anni '90* [Road accidents in the 90's]. Rome: ISTAT.

ISTAT (1999). *Statistica degli incidenti stradali* [Statistics of road accidents]. Rome: ISTAT.

ISTAT (2000a). *I viaggi in Italia e all'estero nel 2000* [Travelling in Italy and abroad in 2000]. Rome: ISTAT.

ISTAT (2000b). *Rapporto annuale* [Annual report]. Rome: ISTAT.

ISTAT (2000c). *Statistica degli incidenti stradali* [Statistics of road accidents]. Rome: ISTAT.

KSH (Központi Statisztikai Hivatal) [Hungarian Central Statistical Office] (1989). *Magyar statisztikai zsebköny 1988* [Statistical Pocket-Book of Hungary 1988]. Budapest: KSH.

KSH (1991). *Magyar statisztikai zsebköny 1990* [Statistical Pocket-Book of Hungary 1990]. Budapest: KSH.

KSH (1995). *Magyar Statisztikai Zsebkönyv 1994* [Statistical pocket-book of Hungary 1994] (p. 42). Budapest: KSH.

KSH (1996). *Magyar Statisztikai Zsebkönyv 1995* [Statistical Pocket-book of Hungary 1995] (p. 97, 98). Budapest: KSH.

KSH (1998). *Magyar statisztikai zsebköny 1997* [Statistical Pocket-Book of Hungary 1997]. Budapest: KSH.

KSH (2000). *Magyar Statisztikai Zsebkönyv 1999* [Statistical Pocket-book of Hungary 1999]. Budapest: KSH.

KSH (2001). *Demographical Yearbook 2000.* Budapest: KSH.

KSH (2001a). *Közlekedési balesetek 2000* [Traffic accidents 2000]. Budapest: KSH.

KSH (2001b). *Statistical Yearbook of Hungary 2000.* Budapest: KSH.

Kuratorium Deutsche Altershilfe (KDA) (1991). Angst vor Mieterhöhungen [Afraid of increasing rents]. *KDA Pressedienst*, Vol.1, 7.

Marcellini, F., Gagliardi, C., Spazzafumo, L., & Leonardi, F. (1997). Keeping the elderly mobile. Findings from Italy. In H. Mollenkopf & F. Marcellini (Eds.), *The Outdoor Mobility of Older People - Technological Support and Future Possibilities* (pp. 21-31). Luxembourg: Office for Official Publications of the European Communities.

Mengani, M., & Gagliardi, C. (1993). Family carers of older people in Italy: urban and rural area. In *Carers talking: interviews with family carers of older, dependent people in EC* (pp. 50-60). Dublin: European Foundation.

Ministero dei Trasporti e della Navigazione [Ministry of Transport and Navigation] (1999). *Conto Nazionale dei trasporti anno 1999* [Italian National Transport Statement year 1999], Servizio Sistemi informativi e Statistica, Sistema Statistico Nazionale [Service of Information Systems and Statistics, National Statistics System].

Mollenkopf, H., & Flaschenträger, P. (1997). Keeping the elderly mobile. Findings from Germany. In H. Mollenkopf & F. Marcellini (Eds.), *The outdoor mobility of older people. Technological support and future possibilities* (pp. 45-67). Luxembourg, Brussels: Office for Official Publications of the European Communities.

Mollenkopf, H., & Flaschenträger, P. (2001). *Erhaltung von Mobilität im Alter* [Maintaining mobility in old age]. Stuttgart, Berlin, Köln: Kohlhammer.

Mollenkopf, H., Marcellini, F., Ruoppila, I., Flaschenträger, P., Gagliardi, C. & Spazzafumo, L. (1997). Outdoor Mobility and Social Relationships of Elderly People. *Archives of Gerontology and Geriatrics, 24,* pp. 295 - 310.

Mollenkopf, H., Marcellini, F., Ruoppila, I., & Tacken, M. (Eds.)(2004). *Ageing and Outdoor Mobility. A European Study.* Amsterdam: IOS Press.

OECD (1996). *Caring for frail elderly people. Policies in evolution.* Paris: OECD.

Olsson Hort, S. (1993). Models and countries - the Swedish social policy model in perspective. In *Social Security in Sweden and Other European Countries - Three Essay* (pp. 51-59). Stockholm: ESO, 51.

Pestoff, V. A. (1995). Citizens as Co-producers of Social Services in Europe - from the Welfare State to the Welfare Mix. In *Reforming social services in Central and Eastern Europe - an eleven nation overview* (pp. 29-117). Krakow: Krakow Academy of Economics.

Road Accidents in Finland (1993). *Transport and Tourism 1994: 13.* Helsinki: Statistics Finland.

Road Accidents in Finland (1995). *Transport and Tourism 1996: 15.* Helsinki: Statistics Finland.

Road Traffic Accidents (2000). *Transport and Tourism 2001: 13.* Helsinki: Statistics Finland.

Salamon, L. M., & Anheier, H. K. (1995). *Szektor születik* [A sector is born]. Budapest: Nonprofit Kutató Csoport.

Salamon, L. M., & Anheier, H. K. (1996). *Social Origins of Civil Society: Explaining the Nonprofit Sector Cross-Nationally.* Working Papers of the John Hopkins Comparative Nonprofit Project, No. 22. Baltimore: The John Hopkins University.

Scheepers, P., Grotenhuis, M. T., & Gelissen, J. (2002). Welfare state and dimensions of social capital. *European Societies*, Volume 4, No. 2, pp. 185-207.

Seibel, W. (1992). *Funktionaler Dilettantismus, Erfolgreich scheiternde Organisationen im "Dritten Sektor" zwischen Markt und Staat* [Funktional Dilettantism, successfully breaking up organisations in the third sector between market and the state]. Baden-Baden: Nomos Verlagsgesellschaft.

Statistical Yearbook of Finland 2001. Helsinki: Statistics Finland.

Statistisches Bundesamt [Federal Statistical Office of Germany] (Eds.) (2000). *Datenreport 1999* [Data Report 1999]. Bonn: Bundeszentrale für politische Bildung.

Statistisches Bundesamt [Federal Statistical Office of Germany] (2001). *Statistisches Jahrbuch 2001* [Statistical Yearbook 2001]. Wiesbaden: Statistisches Bundesamt.

Széman, Z. (1995). *A banki szektor munkaerőpolitikája és az idősek* [Manpower policy of the banking sector and the elderly] (pp. 3-11). Esély.

Széman, Z. (1999). *Two towns: social alternatives in a time of change.* Budapest: British Know How Fund for Hungary & MTA Szociológiai Kutató Intézet.

Széman, Z., & Harsányi, L. (2000). *Caught in the Net in Hungary and Eastern Europe.* Budapest: Nonprofit Research Group & Institute of Sociology of the Hungarian Academy of Sciences.

Tardos, K. (1993). *Feláldozott egészség (Munkások, munkakörülmények, betegségek)* [Sacrificed health / Workers, working conditions, disease]. Budapest: candidate's thesis, manuscript.

U. S. Department of Commerce (1993). *Aging in Eastern Europe and the Former Soviet Union.* Washington DC: U.S. Department of Commerce.

United Nations publication (2002). *Population Ageing 2002.* New York: Population Division, Department of Economic and Social Affairs.

Vaarama, M., Törmä S., Laaksonen, S., & Voutilainen, P. (1999). *Omaishoitajien tuen tarve ja palveluseteleillä tilapäishoito* [The support needs of self-sufficient persons and the provision of temporary care]. Helsinki: Sosiaali-ja Terveysministeriö, STAKES.

Van Lamoen, E., & Tacken, M. (2001). *The MOBILATE Survey: enhancing outdoor mobility in later life. The findings of the Dutch project in Maastricht and Margraten.* Delft: Spatial Planning Department of Delft University of Technology.

Vogel, J. (1998). *Three Types of European Society.* Available from: http://www.nnn.se/n-model/ europe3/europe3.htm

Wittenberg, R. (1986). Einstellung zum Autobesitz und Unsicherheitsgefühle älterer Menschen im Straßenverkehr [Older People's Attitudes Towards Owning a Car and Feeling Unsafe in Traffic]. *Zeitschrift für Gerontologie*, 19, pp. 400-409.

Whelan, Ch. T., Fahey, T., & Maître, B. (2004). Economic Exclusion, Social Exclusion and Social Integration in an Enlarged European Union. *Paper presented at the CHANGEQUAL NETWORK WORKSHOP, Stockholm, 24-25 November.*

World Bank (1995). *Hungary: structure reforms for sustainable growth.* Washington D.C.: World Bank.

Chapter 3
Methodology

Stephan Baas, Fiorella Marcellini, Heidrun Mollenkopf, Frank Oswald,
Isto Ruoppila, Zsuzsa Széman, Mart Tacken, and Hans-Werner Wahl

3.1 Methods and research instruments

The scientific goals of the MOBILATE study made a comprehensive set of different research instruments necessary. One scientific goal was to deliver reliable and valid mobility-related data on older persons and their social-physical and technical environment. In order to reach this goal a set of reliable and valid instruments had to be developed to measure the characteristics, experiences, attitudes and coping strategies of older people as well as environmental characteristics related to their out-of-home mobility. Therefore the research design combined different types of methods: structured face-to-face interviews with standardised questionnaires, including self-rating scales and trustworthy psychological tests, and a diary in which the respondents wrote down the circumstances of the trips they undertook during two days. Another goal of the study was the emphasis of the international comparison and it was agreed that each country would ask the questions in the manner determined mutually.

The instruments were tested in each participating country and each regional area (urban and non-urban) in two phases. After a first pretest the instruments were further focused since they exceeded the planned duration of approximately 90 minutes per interview. In a second pretest, a total of 55 pretest interviews were carried out both in urban and rural areas. After analysing the results of this pretest, the Survey instruments were elaborated into a final version. The instruments were worked out in an English master version, which was obligatory for all participating countries and had been translated into the particular languages (Dutch, Finnish, German, Hungarian and Italian) by experienced translators.

3.1.1 The MOBILATE Survey Questionnaire

The two main aspects characterising the mobility of older people, i.e. the individual personal background and the environmental background, were established in the questionnaire including questions on basic person characteristics, psychological constructs being relevant for out-of-home mobility, aspects of the social environment, and the aspects of the physical environment. The questionnaire was constructed so that it covered all the most important components, which can influence out-of-home mobility:

- State of health
- traffic behaviour
- social networks

- housing and neighbourhood conditions
- availability and use of services
- leisure-time activities, and
- statistical background data.

Each theme included questions in relation to possible impediments and restrictions to out-of-home mobility as well as questions as to how it would be possible to prevent or reduce these or to improve these conditions. When suited, the themes contained a corresponding question regarding the subjects' satisfaction with it.

The questionnaire was in part based on methods used in previous studies on elderly persons and their outdoor mobility (Mollenkopf, Marcellini, & Ruoppila, 1998; Mollenkopf, Marcellini, Ruoppila, & Tacken, 2004). In part the questions on daily activities, services, leisure-time activities, social relationships and socio-demographic situation have been used in previous studies, such as the Finnish Evergreen-project (Heikkinen, 1998), the German Welfare Survey (Zapf & Habich, 1996) and the Nordic Research on Ageing Study (Avlund, Kreiner, & Schultz-Larsen, 1993). The statements relating to the traffic situation have been used in a German study (Wittenberg, 1986). Questions on sight and hearing ability have also been adopted from previous studies (Gillman, Simmel, & Simon, 1986; Holland & Rabbit, 1992). The questions on satisfaction were in part adopted from the German Welfare Survey and Socio-economic Panel (Glatzer & Zapf, 1984; Zapf & Habich, 1996). Also the standard demography of ZUMA (Centre for Survey Research and Methodology, Mannheim) was used.

Psychological measurements

Psychological constructs and indicators of environmental-relevant competencies, a substantial part of this project, are aimed to explain individual differences in outdoor mobility patterns, as well as to address the personal resources of older individuals which help them to cope successfully with challenges to their outdoor mobility.

The following well-established instruments were included in the questionnaire:

1. *Locus-of-Control Scale* (Kunzmann 1999; Smith, Marsiske, & Maier 1996): If individuals perceive events as highly contingent upon their own behaviour, an internal locus of control is assumed. If they perceive events not being related on their own actions, but on powerful others, luck, chance or fate, one may consider them as having an external locus of control. Control beliefs may influence out-of-home mobility in a variety of ways. For example, the experience of being in control over one's life circumstances may motivate one to maintain the highest possible level of outdoor mobility. Also, high internal control beliefs may help overcome adverse environmental conditions which would otherwise severely restrict out-of-home mobility.

2. *Positive and Negative Affect Scale (PANAS)* (Watson, Clark, & Telegen, 1988): Staying mobile in old age can be viewed as the result of several objective and subjective preconditions; however, it may also be seen as a precondition of subjective well-being or life satisfaction itself. To further strengthen this idea of well-being as an outcome of out-of-home mobility, an affect-oriented scale on emotional well-being was used.

3. *Tenacious Goal Pursuit - Flexible Goal Adjustment (TEN-FLEX)* (Brandstädter & Renner, 1990): To examine dispositional forms of coping, assimilative versus

accommodative tendencies in coping with age-related loss and everyday problems were distinguished. From an environmental and mobility perspective these two complementary strategies can be expected to be of critical importance. Whereas assimilation involves active modification of the environment due to life goals, accommodation involves the adjustment of personal goals due to differences in external resources and the functional capacity. Out-of-home mobility probably can be an important behavioral expression of these personal tendencies.

4. *Working memory/Digit Symbol Test* (Oswald & Fleischmann, 1995): There are good reasons to assume that out-of-home mobility draws strongly upon cognitive resources. Cognitive functioning supports basic daily functioning inside and outside the home and is important for way-finding and orientation as well. It is also critical for the use of automatic ticket machines or tellers.

5. A *visual acuity screening* (Sachsenweger, 1987) was carried out, because visual orientation as a proxy for objective visual functioning is a basic precondition for mobility.

3.1.2   The MOBILATE Diary of out-of-home mobility

Subsequent to the interviews, the respondents completed a specially designed diary (see Annex), which comprehensively described the details of the journeys they went on over a two-day period. The days reported in the diary were the day before and the day after the interview. So the interviewer could fill in one day together with the respondent and answer to questions if necessary. To get a representative overview of everyday journeys, it was important to cover all the days of a week. For that reason, the interviews were conducted on every day of the week, even on the weekend. The diary of out-of-home mobility included questions relating to the number, duration, destinations, and activities of the trips made as well as the transport means used, travel companions, and circumstances making the trip pleasant or unpleasant.

3.2   The research areas

One goal of the MOBILATE study was to describe and explain the mobility of older individuals living in various European regions. Essentially, the focus of this study was on how the personal and environmental resources impact on the out-of-home mobility of elders. Particular emphasis was placed on the contrast between rural and urban regions: it was presumed that environmental resources (and hence, outdoor mobility) differ greatly between rural and urban regions. For example, the disparity in the availability of public transportation, or in the presence of shops and services that are necessary for everyday life, might differentially impact on the mobility of elders from each area. Moreover, rural/urban comparisons in various European countries were intended for analysis, since national characteristics go beyond the rural/urban differentiation and play a decisive role in the availability of resources that promote or hinder mobility. Comparing different European regions is difficult, because of different situations, like for example the climatic conditions. Therefore, the goal of the MOBILATE study was not to recruit representative samples from six European regions or to impose a strict common standard when selecting suitable cities and rural areas, but rather, to select cities and regions which are characteristic for each participating country (Finland, eastern Germany, western Germany, Italy, Hungary and the Netherlands). Had the MOBILATE study attempted to make generally valid statements regarding elder mobility using representative samples drawn from each of the participating countries, the survey would have had to be conducted in approximately 150 communities in Germany alone.

The cities selected for the study were middle-sized industrial cities with diversified settlement structures, i.e., densely settled inner-city areas, more sparsely populated peripheral areas, and older and newer types of suburban settlements. All cities should have comparable cultural infrastructures including cultural facilities, adult education centres, sport facilities et cetera. All cities have diversified public transportation, as well as regional trains and buses. Hence, people can reach the surrounding countryside, e.g. for recreation and leisure facilities. Also a rail connection and national roads should be available in all cities.

In view of the diverging national conditions of the countries with respect to spatial extension, settlement structure, and population density, no common criteria in terms of identical standards were applied for selecting rural areas because what "rural" means differs greatly between the countries participating in the study. In Finland, for instance, population density outside urban areas is generally low and distances between rural settlements are large, while in the Netherlands the number of inhabitants per square km is the highest in Europe. Instead, inside rural regions of each country, villages or areas were chosen which are characteristic for the respective country. The areas selected should, for example, not have the same number of inhabitants per square km, but a typical population density in the country in question.

3.2.1   Finland

As urban area the city of Jyväskylä was selected; the interviews in the rural areas were conducted in the municipalities of Karstula, Kivijärvi and Nilsiä.

3.2.1.1   Urban area: Jyväskylä

Jyväskylä, the bustling centre of business and culture in the middle of Finland, was incorporated as town in 1837 and covers an area of 136.85 km^2. Jyväskylä landscape is known for its high-forested hills and mountains. In the beginning of the year 2001 there were 79,134 inhabitants in the city according to the civil register and there has been a tendency of more people moving into the city than moving out from it. The proportion of the 55+ years old inhabitants was 22% of the total population in 2000. 28% of 55+ years old inhabitants were men. In year 2000 there were altogether 1,507 (1.9%) foreigners living in Jyväskylä.

Jyväskylä can easily be reached by land and air, it takes only 35 minutes by plane and about 3 hours by car or train to travel the distance of 272 km from Helsinki. Inside the city itself, the public transportation is widely in use by the citizens both in the form of the traditional buses with low-floors as well as the modernised service-buses with more individualised service-routes offered especially for the elderly and handicapped persons. In order to develop the possibilities for special transport, the so called service-bus was first time taken for use in Jyväskylä in 1996 and due to the wide positive feedback given by its first passengers it is now an everyday means in traveling inside the city area of Jyväskylä and its vicinity. The service-bus is a smaller bus with only 22 cm high floor from the ground and the floor inside the bus is flat without any steps. There are three buses running with 15-25 standard seats and three fastening places reserved for the wheelchairs in each of them.

Service-buses have firm timetables and constant routes with possibility of asking for departure routes by the passengers. By phoning in advance a passenger can also order the bus to come and fetch him/her from the home-door and the passenger has an additional possibility to ask the bus-driver to let him/her off in certain places in the city. This type of bus can be stopped anywhere and not only in the marked bus stops. The cost (about 2.2 €) of this service is just the same as in the traditional buses in the city. The other flexible service was offered by the city of Jyväskylä, starting from the beginning of the year 2000, in the form of two City-buses, which run inside the city according to the wishes told by the passengers on the phone beforehand by collecting the passengers from different addresses to the city. There are two City-buses with 10-12 seats and one wheelchair place in both of them. The cost (3.4 €) of the ticket is slightly more expensive than regular one-way ticket of the traditional bus and the ticket must be paid in cash. There is, however, a possibility to buy a day-ticket for a reasonable price of 6.7 €.

The average income/year in 1998 was 16,114 € in Jyväskylä whereas in whole Finland it was slightly higher (16,450 €). Even if the number of the workplaces increased in year 2000, unemployment also bothered Jyväskylä due to the growing number of population especially in the work-force (15-64 years old citizens), as in the beginning of the year 2000 the proportion of the unemployed persons was 17% of the total work force, whereas in whole Finland 12% of the population were unemployed during the same period of time.

Jyväskylä took part in a comparative study in 2000 with some other cities in Finland studying the fall-accidents on the sidewalks, and was noted widely in the comparisons between different cities for the good safety of its residential areas. The citizens actively used the new nature and exercise opportunities. In addition to the open exercise services available to everyone, there were also some special exercise services provided weekly for the handicapped persons, citizens with long-term illnesses and aging population.

3.2.1.2 Rural area: Karstula, Kivijärvi and Nilsiä

Karstula is located 100 km to the northwest from Jyväskylä and covers an area of 960 km^2. The number of residents is 5,300 from which two thirds are living in the centre. The number of the population over 55years old at the end of 1996 was 1,609, 30% of the whole population in the municipality. The number of cars is 2,604. There is one vehicle almost to every two residents. From the beginning of the 19th century agriculture was the main source of livelihood. Nowadays, still 25% of population earn their living from agriculture, 50% from services, 25% from industry and construction-work. The municipality is not a rich one: 66% of population has low income (< 13,455 €/year), 27% middle income (13,455 - 23,546 €/year) and 7% high income (> 23,546 €/year). The most serious problem is unemployment, especially long-standing unemployment. Some good but still not quite sufficient results have been achieved by various alterations. The net emigration is also a problem. Karstula has a common hospital with a neighbour municipality (35 beds and 4 doctors). Karstula is situated along the bus routes from Jyväskylä to cities situated in the western coast, having good transport services to Sweden. There is also a special transportation line running once a week inside Karstula. The purpose of this is to pick up people straight from their home and bring them back to their home doors. This special transportation system is ideal, for instance, for the elderly and disabled persons.

Kivijärvi's location is 121 km to the northwest from Jyväskylä and covers an area of 476 km^2. The number of residents is 1,628. The number of cars is 682, which means almost one vehicle to every two residents. Nowadays economic structure is the following one: agriculture- and forestry economy 30%, breeding 15%, services 50%, unknown 5%. The economical structure has changed so that from the beginning of the 19th century agriculture was the main source of living, but has reduced to these days. Like Karstula, the municipality of Kivijärvi is not a rich one: 75% of population has low income (< 13,455 €/year), 20% middle income (13,455 - 23,546 €/year) and 5% high income (> 23,546 €/year). The most serious problems are unemployment and net emigration. Those actions which could reduce unemployment and net emigration in Kivijärvi are in focus. There is one doctor and 15 hospital beds in Kivijärvi. Kivijärvi situates along the bus routes from Jyväskylä to the western coast cities having good transport services to Sweden. Besides the constant Kivijärvi's bus lines there are so called line taxi routes. Four different routes will be driven once a week and the fifth route will be driven two times a week. Users of these routes pay the same price for this type of transportation as they would pay for common bus tickets.

Nilsiä became as its own decision, which is now possible, a city in 1998. The location is 199 km to the northeast from Jyväskylä. It covers an area of 848 km^2, and has got 7,030 residents. Population over 55years old is 32% of the whole population. The number of cars is 3,150, which is about one vehicle for close to every two residents. Nowadays its economic structure is the following one: agriculture and forestry 26%, breeding 16 % and services 54%. The economical structure has changed so that from the beginning of the 19th century agriculture was the main source of living, but has reduced to these days. During the last decades and years new entrepreneurial activity has speeded up the development of Nilsiä. 66% of population has low income (< 13,455 €/year), 25% middle income (13,455 - 23,546 €/year) and 9% high income (> 23,546 €/year). In Nilsiä there are five doctors and 65 hospital beds. Besides the constant bus lines available in Nilsiä, there are some special service lines driven in this rural area. This transportation has to be ordered beforehand on the phone. There are good connections via bus routes from Nilsiä to Kuopio from where good railway and flight connections to other large Finnish cities are available. The distance between Nilsiä and Kuopio, also a university city, is 55 km.

3.2.2   Germany

In Germany, history has brought about rather different social and environmental conditions that affect mobility in eastern and western Germany. There are considerable differences in the living conditions and degree of mechanisation, in the basic infrastructure and the transportation facilities necessary for commuting around cities and townships.

The cities selected for the study were Chemnitz (Saxony), in the eastern and Mannheim (Baden-Württemberg), in the western part of the country, the rural areas were the district of Vogelsberg (Hesse) in western Germany and the district of Jerichow (Saxony-Anhalt) in eastern Germany.

3.2.2.1   Urban areas: Chemnitz (eastern Germany) and Mannheim (western Germany)

Chemnitz

The city lies in an area of rolling hills at the foot of the Erzgebirge on the southeast border of the Federal Republic of Germany. The surrounding countryside is dotted with farms and forests. Chemnitz is the largest urban centre in the Chemnitz/Zwickau region and boasts approximately 1 million inhabitants: its population density of 600 persons per km^2 makes the region the most densely populated area in eastern Germany (after Berlin).

The city of Chemnitz was largely destroyed in the Second World War. But because of the proliferation of production machinery at the beginning of the 19th century in this area Chemnitz was one of the leading industrial cities in Saxony, and it has retained its importance for the former GDR, eastern Europe, and even western Europe, well into the 1990s. Since reunification, the region has been plagued with unemployment.

The important infrastructure facilities - such as the city auditorium, the employment office, the technical university, the post office, the city library, and the department of health - have been placed in the city centre. There is also a public sport's facility, an indoor public swimming pool, and a theatre or opera house, as well as schools and other buildings for the city's administration.

The public transportation network consists of tram and bus lines which are mainly operated by the Chemnitz Public Transit Authority (CVAG). Several lines are also run by private bus companies. The train station lies in the middle of Chemnitz. The tram network, which comprises a total 54.2 km of track, consists of four lines serving the western, southern, and eastern portions of the city. For trains, the standard German rail fares and reductions apply to persons over 60 years of age. With the 'Senior Ticket', which is valid for one year and could be purchased for 66.47/132.94 Euro (1./2. Class) in 2000, fare prices are reduced by 50%. With the exception of several smaller runways for gliders and non-commercial traffic, the Chemnitz region does not have an airport. Trans-regional traffic (national or international) is served chiefly by airports in Leipzig-Halle (90 km away) and Dresden-Klotzsche (80 km away).

Mannheim

The city of Mannheim lies in the southwest of the Federal Republic of Germany, in the so-called Rhine-Neckar triangle. Separated from Ludwigshafen only by the Rhine, it is the seventh largest conurbation in the country with 1.9 million inhabitants and a work-force of 700,000 strong. To the west of Mannheim runs the Neckar valley, northwest of the Odenwald, a large forest. In and around Mannheim are various industries specialising in chemistry, pharmacy, machinery production, electronics, food production, the manufacture of lubricants and cellulose, and construction.

During the Second World War, Mannheim was largely destroyed. Portions of the city were rebuilt according to original plans: the layout was finely detailed with a baroque residence at the foot of the circle. The downtown area is severely restricted by the Neckar (to the north), the Rhine (to the southwest), and the harbour (to the northwest). The inner city features a variety of small shops, department stores, banks, theatres, schools, and central administrative offices. In the very centre, there are pedestrian zones. The university, national theatre, concert and opera house can be found in districts at the outer edge of the downtown area.

Due to its position on the Rhine and Neckar - which made Mannheim an important traffic hub in the last century - transportation in and around the city is generally good. The city of Mannheim (as well as Ludwigshafen) is served by a dense traffic net consisting of five national highways and four national roads. Mannheim lies within the Rhine-Neckar Traffic Association's (VRN) service area, which covers ca. 5,700 km^2 with a unified system of fares and more than 450 lines. The public transportation network in the city itself is chiefly operated by the Mannheim Public Transit Authority (MVV). In addition, there are two private enterprises providing regional trains as well as one providing buses. All of the city routes operated by the MVG stop in the city centre. The major means of transportation in Mannheim is the network of trams. (The bus lines exist primarily to bring commuters to city districts that are not served by the city rail system.) The northern and western sections of the city are particularly well served by tramlines. As of 1999, 50 of the 86 trams in the MVG terminal had low flooring covering 90% of the seating area. Of the remaining 36 trams, 23 eight-jointed engines had minimal low flooring (25% of the seating area), and 13 six-jointed cars had no low flooring whatsoever. 35 of the 45 buses in operation in 1999 had low flooring (no steps until one reaches the passenger seats; the seats themselves rest upon steps. In 2000, the Senior Ticket for persons over 60 who live in the service area, cost 239.28 € (per year).

3.2.2.2   Rural areas: District of Jerichow and District of Vogelsberg

District of Jerichow

The district of Jerichow, a very plain area, belongs to the north-east of Saxony-Anhalt, one of the five so called 'Laender' of the former German Democratic Republic (GDR). With 101,200 inhabitants in an area of 1,337 square kilometres it is comparatively sparsely populated. The town of Burg with 23,797 inhabitants is the largest in the area. Located 150 km to the west of Berlin, it does not belong to the catchment's area of the capital. As such it does not benefit from the economical development of Berlin. The district of Jerichow is close to the motorway A2, which connects Berlin with western Germany and which is an important traffic junction. Compared to the western German rural district of Vogelsberg less inhabitants own a car (515 cars per 1,000 inhabitants in 1999), while the rate of traffic accidents is amazingly high. After reunification a lot of eastern German inhabitants bought cars, while this had been very difficult in the former GDR. Thus, a lot of car drivers in eastern Germany are not used to the increasing volume of traffic. In addition, bad road conditions, especially in eastern German rural areas, might be possible explanations for this high rate of traffic accidents. As regards further means of transportation, public transportation by bus is available. However, buses run very seldom and do not reach every village within the district of Jerichow. In addition, the district of Jerichow is connected to two rail road lines.

Important industries are in the region of Genthin: a shipyard, a factory for wash powder and a crisp bread plant. After reunification, new areas of trade were started in this region, which should help bring manufacturing industries to this part of Germany. Despite the rural character of this region, most of the economic activity takes place in the service sector. Only 4.2 of the engaged inhabitants work in agriculture, forestry and fisheries (1998). Due to big economic changes after the unification of the two parts of Germany, the rate of unemployment was very high (18.1% in December 2000), even compared to a very high general unemployment rate in eastern Germany (17.2 in December 2000). Compared to the Federal Republic of Germany less inhabitants of the district of Jerichow live in one-person-households. As well, a smaller proportion of inhabitants in this district are aged 65 years or older.

District of Vogelsberg

The district of Vogelsberg is a very hilly area and located in the middle of the state of Hesse in the centre of Germany. With 119,000 inhabitants in an area of 1,459 square kilometres it is similarly sparsely populated as the chosen eastern German region. This area includes 180 towns and villages. Alsfeld is the biggest town with 18,029 inhabitants. Sparsely populated and being close to the border of the former GDR, it was supported by the western German government before reunification (i.e., until 1990). After this the help was stopped. Subsequently, the European Community and the state of Hesse have been supporting the district of Vogelsberg with public funds.

The main industries in this area are textile and electronic. As over the last few years the textile industry lost work places due to industrialization, the administration of the district of Vogelsberg is taking measures to win new industries. This can also be seen when distributing engaged persons to economic sectors: only 1.4% (1998) of engaged inhabitants/person in the district of Vogelsberg work in agriculture, forestry or fisheries, which is a very low rate compared to other rural areas in western Germany. Moreover, most of the farms (approx. 62%) provide supplemental income, i.e., the owners have other, full-time employment. Tourism is a significant draw here; the nature reserve areas have made the district of Vogelsberg a known holiday area. As a result of the economic changes in this district, the rate of unemployment is about the same as in the Federal Republic of Germany.

The district of Vogelsberg is very close to four motorways, which connect this district with all directions of Germany. Bus lines as a part of public transportation are less available: each village is attached to this public transportation, but like in the eastern German rural area the buses run very seldom. Some of the more dispersed villages are not easily accessible by public transport. Moreover, the district is connected to only one rail road line, which stops only in few places within the district of Vogelsberg.

Cars seem to be a very common means of transportation, as can be seen in the high rate of inhabitants owning a car (588 cars per 1,000 inhabitants, compared to 508 cars per 1,000 inhabitants in the Federal Republic of Germany [FRG], all Figures in 1999). Compared to the FRG (15.8% in 1997) a bigger amount of inhabitants (18.2 in 1997) are aged 65 years and older. In addition, the size of an average household is bigger than in the eastern German rural area under investigation.

3.2.3 Hungary

The Hungarian project was carried out in Pècs (urban region) and in Jászladány (rural area). In both settlements, the researchers had good relations with the local authority and with the members of parliament for the district, who also helped to obtain the data and who supported the research.

3.2.3.1 Urban area: Pécs

With its 180,000 inhabitants Pécs is the biggest town in South-west Hungary, seat of Baranya County. Proportion of males is 46.7%. Proportion of females over 55 in the permanent population is 15.9%, proportion of women over 55 within the female population is 29.8%. Proportion of men over 60 in the permanent population is 7.9%, proportion of men over 60 within the male population 17.0%. It has an agglomeration with a population of one million. Pécs has a history reaching back 2000 years. It is a major university town and has an excellent education system. Therefore there is a large well trained and educated labour force on the labour market. Pécs is also an economic centre of the region launching innovative technologies. Mining had a long history but nowadays it is a declining branch. The main branches at present are the construction and electrical industries, there are lively trade, service industry and tourism. It has a lot of services, cultural facilities, sights. The town lies at the foot of the Mecsek Mountains where the gentle hills and valleys provide excellent sites for construction, excursions - in the neighbourhood there are good spas - and pleasant life. Houses generally have basic or high comfort. The town has a public transport bus system and an excellent intercity connection with the capital.

3.2.3.2   Rural area: Jászladány

Jászladány, the chosen non-urban area, is on the Great Hungarian Plain which covers an area of 50,800 km^2, representing 54.6% of the territory of Hungary. The number of residents is 6,179. Proportion of women over 55 years in the permanent population is 17.4%. Proportion of women over 55 within the female population is 33.9%, proportion of men over 60 within the permanent population 9.1%. Proportion of men over 60 within the male population is 18.7%. Together the proportion of the population over 60 is 24.8% which means a rather high ageing trend.

The way of life in Jászladány and the resulting mobility are also characteristic of many other settlements on the Great Plain. The economic and social history of the village can be summarised as follows: as a result of the regulation of the rivers in the 19th century there was a substantial increase in the area of land suitable for cultivation, and animal husbandry (cattle, sheep, horses) was also important. From the second half of the 19th century, due to the ever smaller size of land holdings, a large stratum of landless itinerant navvies emerged. In the 20th century, those entering employment in industry from the 1930s had to take jobs in other settlements. Mobility with long periods spent commuting became a characteristic way of life for part of the population. Following the systemic change in the 1990s and especially from 1997 economic development of the village speeded up.

The public administrative area of the settlement is 92.73 km^2. This is relatively high and the settlement also covers a large area. Population density per 1 km^2 in Hungary in 1998 was 108.9, in the county (Jasz-Nagykun-Szolnok) 75, and 66 in the village. Jászladány is sufficiently remote from the county seat, other towns and settlements (20 - 40 km) to prevent it from merging into a single agglomeration, but the relative proximity of the towns could favour mobility of the elderly. There are 23 hospitality industry units, 65 retail trade shops, 214 operating businesses, and 3 doctors in the village, which represents a rather good service network. However, there is no public sewage network, although 89% of the homes are connected to water supply. There are bus and train services in the village.

3.2.4   Italy

As a typical Italian urban region the city of Ancona was selected, the villages Mondavio, Montefelcino and Orciano were chosen as rural areas of investigation. The urban area and the rural areas studied are representative of many other Italian situations. In fact, there are some differences in the living, social and environmental conditions between rural and urban areas in Italy, which can affect the mobility of elderly people.

3.2.4.1   Urban area: Ancona

The Italian research was carried out in Ancona, a middle sized town in Central Italy (Marche Region) located on the Adriatic See (south of Venice). It is of ancient Greek origin, and the etymology of the name - 'ancon' is the Greek word for elbow - is related to its particular geographical position, where the coastline juts out like a bent elbow. Historically it has been considered a port open to East, and the city has grown around this natural port. The port was the heart of the Roman town and later on Ancona was a marine Republic. Still now it preserves its traditional marine and mercantile economy.

Regarding its territory it is a seismic zone and subject to landslides, characteristics that have had an influence also on the recent development of the town. The hilly country has influenced the urban structure of the town to this very day, the development of the transportation system, the use of transport means (for example, it is not possible to move by a bicycle) and the mobility of persons and goods which is mostly by vehicle.

The urban structure of the historical centre of Ancona was developed mainly after the unification of Italy (1860). The two main streets were created during the period from 1860 to 1930 and with them the new directrix of expansion of the town. This period also signs the characteristic separation of the town into two parts: the official, administrative one represented by the centre with the new planned directrix and a suburban area which remained separated determining the so-called two centres of Ancona. The Second World War caused considerable damage to the buildings and to the life of the historical centre, where the majority of people living there were older people. Even if a lot of houses were rebuilt, some buildings have still not been completely restored. The modern structure of the town was developed during the '70s and '80s away from the centre with residential and popular new districts located in the suburbs and in the villages to the north and south of the town. Due to an earthquake in 1972 the urban planning changed and lower houses were built consisting of three or four floors with a lift, while the older buildings were mostly higher and without lifts.

Ancona is served by two railway lines: the first is the north-south line which connects Ancona to Milano and Lecce, the second is the east-west line which links Ancona to Rome and other cities on the west coast of Italy. There are two railway stations: the main one is the Central Station, which is adjacent to the Bus Station, and the second and much smaller one is the Maritime Station which is inside the harbour. The bus system is constituted by an inter-urban and an urban network. With regards to the inter-urban one, there are three lines: the first one connects Ancona to the towns in the north-west area, the second links Ancona to the southern area and the third reaches the hinterland. This service is provided by a public company (COTRAN) and some private companies (ANAC, etc.). Concerning the urban network, it is constituted by 18 main lines and 17 secondary ones. This service is provided by a public company (ATMA): the number of daily trips is 1,700 (12,000 km). From 7:30 a.m. to 7:30 p.m. the buses run frequently while at early and later hours the buses run more seldom. During the night (from 1:00 to 4:30 a.m.) the bus service is substituted by taxis. The cost of a single bus trip (one hour) is about 0.7 Euro. With regards to the bus system, there are cheaper season tickets for older citizens (65 years and over) and disadvantaged people (about 25% cheaper). Furthermore the service is free for people with more than 80% of disability. Regarding the railway system, there is a special card (Silvercard) with which elders obtain a reduction of 20%. This facility is granted to people aged 60 years and over.

For the disabled elderly, there is a special taxi system allowing them to reach health and public services and to participate in social activities. This service is active also at night and during the holidays: the users have to pay only 5% of effective cost. Ancona is also served by the national air network, thanks to the airport located in the adjacent town of Falconara.

3.2.4.2   Rural areas: Municipalities of Mondavio, Montefelcino and Orciano

The chosen rural area consists of three small municipalities, prevalently agricultural and with limited industrial development (areas considered depressed and included in objective 2 of the

EU in the three-year period 1998-2000), not connected by railway lines and by important thoroughfares such as motorways or speedways. These villages, in the province of Pesaro, and about 50 kilometres from Ancona are Mondavio, Montefelcino and Orciano.

The municipality of *Mondavio* covers an area of 29.4 km² and has got 3,790 residents (50.3% male, 33% of all residents aged 55 year and older). The nearest hospital is 19 km away, the distance to the next important thoroughfares varies between 20 km (motorway) and 13 km (speedway).

In the municipality of *Montefelcino* (size 38.69 km²) about 50.2% of the 2,533 residents are males, about 35.5 of all respondents are aged 55 years or older. The distance to the nearest hospital is about 8 km, the next motorway can be reached in 30 km, the next speedway in 10 km.

The municipality of *Orciano* covers an area of about 23,78 km² and has got 2,274 inhabitants. About 49.4% of all respondents are male, again one third of all respondents are aged 55 years or older (35%). The next available hospital is 19 km away, the next motorway about 20 km, the nearest speedway about 15 km.

3.2.5   The Netherlands

The Dutch areas included in the project were located in the middle-sized city of Maastricht and environment (municipality of Margraten), which is located in the South-East of the Netherlands. The municipality of Margraten consists of some larger villages and a lot smaller villages, besides some groups of houses. This rural area is comparable with many Dutch rural areas. The main reason for this choice was the possibility to use the available knowledge in the research group on the local demand responsive transport system (Tailor made public transport: VoM). The trip data of the VoM-system were available to the Dutch researchers, who formerly worked out a geographical analysis on the origins and destinations of trips in relation to selected characteristics of the areas. Therefore the integration of this transport service to the MOBILATE project offered the opportunity to get important evaluative data on the VoM system and makes the Dutch part of the project more application oriented.

3.2.5.1   Urban area: Maastricht

Maastricht is a middle-sized city in the southern part of the Netherlands near to the border with Belgium and Germany. This municipality consists of the town of Maastricht and four former villages: Amby, Heer, Borgharen and Itteren. The last two villages have a more rural character and they are left out of the sample of Maastricht. The whole municipality had 122,087 inhabitants in January 2000. The population density is 2,165/km². The river Maas divides the city in two parts. This division is enforced by the highway, which also separates the eastern part of the city.

Maastricht is a tourist city, which attracts many tourists for the old inner city and for the many cafes and restaurants. The city has an image of a hedonic lifestyle. The dominant life style is the catholic way of life without the strict regulations. This lifestyle can be found back in social life and in the many associations for all kinds of leisure activities. The location near two other countries gives the city also an international character. In the past the labour force consisted of people with a low level of education: pottery, rubber industry, paper. This has changed in the last decades. The new university and the academic hospital have resulted in many new jobs on a higher educational level.

The public transport system is based on buses. They connect the different urban areas with the inner city. This line and time schedule based system is completed by a demand responsive system. This system (called VoM) has been started in 1994 as a transport facility for handicapped people and elderly people, but since a few years the system is accessible for everybody who wants to make a trip with the origin or destination in Maastricht. The main railway station gives, besides the connection with the rest of the Netherlands, also a connection to Aachen and Liege.

3.2.5.2   Rural (non-urban) area: Margraten

The municipality of Margraten is located in the southern part of the Netherlands near the border with Belgium. It is a hilly area.

This municipality consists of two larger villages and 19 small villages, hamlets, groups of houses with an own geographical name. The whole municipality has 13,740 inhabitants of which 51% are male. The surface is 57.7km^2. The number of dwellings is 5,128, which results in an average occupation of 2.6 persons/house. The population density is 240 persons/km^2 and the housing density is 89 houses/km^2. These villages vary in scale. Some have their own church, school and shops, but many of them have no public facilities. A café is a part of life. Many of the associations have a local café as place for meeting and activities. Music bands and choirs are part of the local community. The majority of people belong to the Roman Catholic Church.

The main source of income is agriculture and since some decades tourism is at least a second one. This means that some of these villages have more facilities than they would have only related to their population size. The public transport is served by a bus system. A small local bus complements this system for the smaller communities, which are not located near the routes of the bus connection.

3.3   Fieldwork and sample

One main objective of the MOBILATE study was the gathering of reliable and valid data about the actual out-of-home mobility of men and women aged 55 years and older in urban and rural regions in six European regions, especially about the out-of-home mobility of the oldest old. In order to be able to have a sufficient amount of respondents in both genders, in urban and rural regions and in older age groups, the sample was disproportionately stratified by

- age (55-74 and 75+ years),
- gender (50% males and 50% females),
- region (Finland, eastern Germany, western Germany, Hungary, Italy and The Netherlands), and
- living area (urban and rural (non-urban) areas).

This disproportional stratification accounted for 48 subcategories/strata for elderly people. For statistical and theoretical reasons, men and older persons are over-represented in the MOBILATE Survey. It enables one to conduct differentiated analyses of older men and of very old people who would otherwise be represented insufficiently in the actual population. Thus, the samples allow conclusions to be drawn regarding the situation of older adults as well as of very old men and women in different urban and rural areas. For each cell, at least

75 respondents were planned in order to analyse and compare the out-of-home mobility of different subgroups, which means 600 respondents in each participating country (300 respondents in the urban and 300 respondents in the rural areas each).

In contrast to the procedure described above, in the Netherlands about one third of the respondents to be interviewed in the urban area of Maastricht, were chosen from the users of the transport on demand system in Maastricht (VoM). In opposite to the main MOBILATE sample, these 100 persons with a pass for the VoM-transport in Maastricht have been approached from a list of all VoM pass holders aged 65 years and older (for the realised sample see Table 3.1).

3.3.1   Fieldwork

Different efforts were undertaken in order to reach the planned sample size in all participating countries, which took into regard the different national characteristics. In Finland, the sample was drawn from the Jyväskylä's civil register centre. During summer 2000 all possible participants of the Finnish survey were contacted with a first introduction letter followed by a second letter including the actual times for the interviews. The Finnish sub-sample was conducted by 25 female interviewers (most of them being psychology students) of the Department of Psychology in the University of Jyväskylä.

The German sub-samples in the urban areas of Chemnitz and Mannheim were drawn from the population registers of the Municipality Registration Offices. The interviews in the rural districts of Jerichow and Vogelsberg were collected in a random route procedure and took place in villages having less than 5,000 inhabitants. Inside the eastern Germany rural area, interviews were conducted in altogether 58 different villages in the district of Jerichow, while in the western German rural area (District of Vogelsberg) interviews took place in 39 different villages. Altogether 113 interviewers of German subcontractor USUMA (Berlin) conducted the German sub-sample. In the first phase of the fieldwork, the subjects were contacted by a letter from the research institute USUMA. This letter was accompanied by a recommendation of the respective municipalities to encourage persons to participate. Additional information concerning the study was also given beforehand through local newspapers.

In Hungary, the respective sub-sample was selected on the basis of the data of the population registry. The Italian sub-sample was also extracted from the official registers of the municipalities of Ancona (urban area) and Mondavio, Orciano and Montefelciano (rural areas). The Italian survey was conducted by six interviewers with a degree in psychology, trained by Italian subcontractor CSRSS (Centro Studi Ricerche Scienze Sociali - The Study Centre on Research in Social Sciences). The subjects were contacted by a letter signed by the mayors of the respective municipalities and by the general manager of INRCA, an institute which is well known in the chosen areas. This letter was accompanied by a recommendation to encourage people to participate. Additional information concerning the study was also given beforehand through local newspapers. As a gift, INRCA gave the interviewees a short leaflet with advice on improving mobility in older age, written by a physiotherapist and sociologist.

In the Netherlands, a sample of 100 pass holders of the VoM-transport was the start of the selection. This was done in order to have a relevant part of the sample consisting of people who were entitled to use this special transport system and who were registered as such. As already described and in opposite to the main MOBILATE sample, these 100 VoM-users were taken from all VoM-pass-holders aged 65 year and older. All other respondents in the city of Maastricht and the rural area of Margraten were drawn from the general administration with the help of the local authorities. The research office (Research & Marketing) got a list of addresses of all people selected by the demographical offices of the respective municipalities. The interviewers, who made appointments for the interviews, approached the respondents till the number of people in each stratum was reached or till the original sample was exhausted.

All respondents were interviewed during the end of September till January 2001. As an important prerequisite for the MOBILATE study all respondents lived in private households when being interviewed. In order to carry out the Survey before winter, in Finland fieldwork started already in August 2000. Hence, it was possible to carry out the interviews before winter started in all participating countries, which is a very important factor when studying the out-of-home mobility, especially among the ageing population.

Before the fieldwork started, all interviewers received careful and detailed instruction from the research institutes and were further supervised by the principal researchers. Within these instructions, special emphasis was given to the psychological tests, the physical measurement (hand grip strength test in Finland) as well as the trip diary.

All these efforts as described above were successful: With the exception of the Netherlands, each subgroup comprises at least 73 persons. In the Netherlands, the number of older respondents (aged 75 years and older) varied between 62 and 77 due to the different sampling structure. Altogether, out of 7,161 gross addresses (stratified by gender, age, region and living area) drawn from the particular population registers, 3,950 respondents were interviewed (Table 3.1).

Table 3.1: The realised MOBILATE sample

	Finland		Eastern Germany		Western Germany		Hungary		Italy		The Netherlands			All countries	
	Urban	Rural	Urban	Rural	Urban	Rural	Urban	Rural	Urban	Rural	Urban	VoM[1]	rural	Urban	rural
Male															
55-74	79	77	127	117	113	117	80	75	75	75	52	19	86	545	547
75+	78	75	76	73	75	74	74	76	75	75	48	14	67	440	440
Total	157	152	203	190	188	191	154	151	150	150	100	33	153	985	987
Female															
55-74	76	75	112	114	102	115	75	75	75	75	53	39	97	532	551
75+	76	74	74	75	78	77	76	74	75	75	50	27	64	456	439
Total	152	149	186	189	180	192	151	149	150	150	103	66	161	988	990
Total															
male + female	309	301	389	379	368	383	305	300	300	300	203	99	314	1973	1977
urban + rural areas	610		768		751		605		600		616			3950	

Note. MOBILATE Survey 2000
[1] Due to a different sampling procedure the users of the transport on system in the Dutch urban area (VoM) are aged 65 years and older

3.3.2   Drop-out

The goal of the MOBILATE study was to compare the out-of-home mobility of different subgroups of elderly people in six European regions: In each participating country, a number 600 persons was to be included (300 in each urban area and 300 in each rural area, disproportionally stratified by age and gender). Due to this restriction in the number of participants, a net response rate can only be interpreted under limitations: it was not our goal to reach as many participants as possible.

Of the net sample of eligible MOBILATE Survey participants (7,161 eligible respondents) drawn from the national population registers, about 55% of all possible participants were interviewed. In the rural areas, the net response rate was a little bit higher (58%) than in the urban areas (about 52%) (Table 3.2).

Table 3.2: Drop-out from the eligible sample

	All countries		Urban areas		Rural areas	
	N	%	N	%	N	%
Eligible sample	7161	100	3761	100	3400	100
systematic drop-out, from them						
refused: holiday, absent	329	4.6	193	5.1	136	4.0
refused: no time	443	6.2	244	6.5	199	5.9
refused: health reasons	371	5.2	222	5.9	149	4.4
refused: language problem	10	0.1	2	0.1	8	0.2
refused: person not reached	389	5.4	202	5.4	187	5.5
refused: interview refused	1620	22.6	891	23.7	729	21.4
no reason given	49	0.7	34	0.9	15	0.4
	3211	44.8	1788	47.6	1423	41.8
Realised interviews	3950	55.2	1973	52.4	1977	58.2

Note. MOBILATE Survey 2000

The main reasons for not participating in the study were

- refusal of the interview (22.6% for all countries),
- problems arranging an interview due to time constraints (6.2% of all countries), and
- problems reaching the participant (5.4% of all countries).

As stated earlier, elderly people are sometimes difficult to reach. When comparing the net response rate of 55% of the eligible net sample in the MOBILATE study with other studies investigated on older people, the quality of the study appears very good. This can moreover be seen in the fact that only between 4.4% of the possible participants in the rural areas and 5.9% of those in the urban areas denied the interview due to health reasons or problems, a very low rate for refusal in such surveys, where health reasons are an important reason for refusal. Because of the low drop-out due to health reasons, the MOBILATE sample should not show a strong bias or distortion towards very healthy respondents which is a common problem in surveys and leads to the misprepresentation of the underlying population.

Most of the drop-out analyses described above can be confirmed by taking a closer look inside the different European regions. With the exception of the Finnish urban area, the most often cited reasons for dropping out of the study were refusing without giving detailed reasons, having no time or being unreachable. In the Finnish city, a considerably greater percentage of the eligible participants (13%) refused due to health reasons or problems.

In some regions under investigation, fewer eligible participants were necessary in order to reach the planned sample size. This is especially true for the rural areas in Finland, Hungary and Italy. As a result, in these areas, the net response rate is very high compared to all other regions (between 67% in the rural Finnish area and 81% in the respective Italian area). On the other hand, huge efforts had to be taken in the rural Dutch area: from an eligible sample of 853 possible participants only about 37% participated in the study, while about 57% refused the interview.

3.3.3   Weighting the data

The disproportional sampling procedure can be counterbalanced by weighting the data. Due to stratification, older individuals in the sample, especially older men, are overrepresented in terms of the actual age and gender structure of the population. In sections of this report, however, descriptive results (such as frequencies or means) are not presented for each individual gender or age group, which would have required presenting statistics for 48 different demographic categories. The nonstratified presentation of these results, without weighting the data, would have produced distortions, such as in the description of satisfaction with various areas of life, since the proportion of older persons in the sample is clearly higher than in the respective populations of the countries participating in the study. Essentially, any reported characteristic with a relationship to age or gender - and this would include almost every characteristic investigated in the sample - would misrepresent the corresponding population of persons aged 55 years and older. By means of the weighting procedure, the sample scores are weighted according to the demographics of the general population; hence, the profile of scores obtained in the sample, after weighting, affords a more accurate representation of the population's profile. For example, if there are twice as many men aged 75 or older in the sample as in the general population, each of the scores observed in the study receives a weight of 0.5.

In order to make accurate statements regarding various MOBILATE subgroups, all of the respondents were assigned an individual transformation weight based upon official population statistics regarding age and gender. By means of this transformation weight, it became possible to present descriptive results, differentiated in terms of country and urban/rural region, without further differentiation in terms of age and sex. In the following Table, the samples are compared in terms of their underlying national population statistics: the results show that a satisfactory estimation of the actual population characteristics could be achieved by weighting the individual demographic subgroups present in the MOBILATE sample (Table 3.3).

Table 3.3: Actual proportion of strata, actual proportion in population, proportion of strata after weighting the strata (in %)

	Finland			Eastern Germany			Western Germany			Hungary			Italy			The Netherlands		
	Sample	FIN	Weighted sample	Sample	GER (E)	Weighted sample	Sample	GER (W)	Weighted sample	Sample	HUN	Weighted sample	Sample	IT	Weighted sample	Sample	NL	Weighted sample
Urban																		
male																		
55-74	25.6	32.1	32.0	32.6	34.8	34.6	30.7	36.2	36.1	26.2	33.5	33.4	25.0	31.1	31.1	23.5	34.8	34.8
75+	25.2	7.4	7.4	19.5	6.4	6.4	20.4	7.6	7.6	24.3	7.0	6.9	25.0	10.8	10.7	20.5	9.2	9.3
female																		
55-74	24.6	42.0	42.1	28.8	41.5	41.8	27.7	38.6	38.6	24.6	44.5	44.6	25.0	39.0	39.1	30.5	38.8	38.4
75+	24.6	18.5	18.4	19.0	17.3	17.2	21.2	17.7	17.7	24.9	15.0	15.1	25.0	19.1	19.1	25.5	17.5	17.5
Rural																		
male																		
55-74	25.6	35.9	35.9	30.9	36.5	36.7	30.5	36.0	36.0	25.0	30.5	30.4	25.0	33.8	34.0	27.4	41.3	41.3
75+	24.9	8.7	8.6	19.3	5.6	5.5	19.3	8.8	8.9	25.3	9.5	9.4	25.0	11.1	11.0	24.3	7.6	7.6
female																		
55-74	24.9	37.5	37.5	30.1	42.5	42.5	30.0	37.7	37.9	25.0	42.0	42.5	25.0	35.7	35.7	30.9	39.5	39.7
75+	24.6	17.9	17.9	19.8	15.4	15.3	20.1	17.5	17.2	24.7	18.0	17.7	25.0	19.4	19.3	20.4	11.6	11.4

Note. MOBILATE Survey 2000

Using the following equation, the transformation weights could be calculated according to the following sample (men aged 75 or older from the urban region of Italy):

Weight = proportion in urban Italian region/proportion in sample = 10.8/25 =0.43.

When results are presented according to the stratified sampling procedure, data have not been weighted. Moreover, data employed in analyses that are not merely descriptive, i.e., examine relationships between variables, such as correlations or regressions, have not been weighted.

3.4   Basic description of the samples

In the following the main demographic facts of the respondents such as age, marital status, education, employment, financial situation, and health status are presented in order to have a first glance at the older persons who participated in the study.

3.4.1   Mean age

In order to get a first impression whether the disproportional stratification of the sample has brought comparable sub-groups, the age means of the different strata were analysed. As can be seen in Table 3.4, within most strata (e.g., young male respondents in the urban areas under investigation), the average age of the respondents does not differ significantly. The biggest difference can be found among the younger female respondents in the urban areas under investigation. Younger female respondents in the corresponding Dutch sub-group are significantly older than all other respondents of the respective sub-groups. This might be due to the different sampling procedure in the Netherlands, where about one third of the respondents to be interviewed in the urban area, were chosen from the users of the transport on demand system in Maastricht (VoM). In opposite to the main Survey sample, these 100 persons with a pass for the VoM-transport have been approached from a list of all VoM pass holders aged 65 years and older, while in all other strata the younger respondents taken from the municipality registers were aged 55 to 74 years.

Moreover, the following significant differences were found between the average ages by testing interactions, but cannot be explained by any sampling procedure:

- The Finnish younger women in the urban area are partly younger than respective women in other regions, especially when compared with western Germany and Hungary.
- The older male respondents in the eastern German and the Hungarian rural areas are on average younger when compared against the other respective respondents.
- Older female respondents in the Hungarian rural area are a little younger than respective respondents in Hungary and Italy.

These differences should be kept in mind when analysing the data because they might influence the results.

As background information on age the life expectancy figures from each participating country were obtained. In Table 3.5 the years to be remained can be seen, measured mainly from the years of 1995 and 2000 (or close) of the 60 and 80-years old citizens (in the Netherlands 60.5 and 80.5 years old citizens). The figures refer to the periodic life-tables and are therefore based on cross-sectional data.

Table 3.4: Mean of age, differentiated by strata (mean)

	Finland		Eastern Germany		Western Germany		Hungary		Italy		The Netherlands	
	Mean	SD	Mean	SD	Mean	SD	Mean	SD	Mean	SD	Mean	SD
Urban												
Male												
55-74	62.5	5.9	64.3	5.5	64.5	5	64.2	5.2	64.6	5.8	64.4	6.1
75+	79.6	3.7	80.3	4.9	79.6	4.1	79.2	4.4	80.7	5	79.2	3.7
Female												
55-74***[1]	62.9	6.1	64.2	5.5	65	5.1	65.1	5.8	64.3	5.2	67.8	5
75+	81.2	4.5	80.9	5.4	80.8	4.7	80.1	4.1	80.5	4.5	80.4	4.6
Rural												
Male												
55-74	64	5.8	65.4	5.5	65.4	5.2	65.4	6	65.7	5.9	64.5	6
75+*[2]	79.7	4.8	78.4	4	80.1	5.3	78.4	3.7	80.4	4.4	79.8	4.5
Female												
55-74	64.7	5.2	64.9	5.4	64.8	5.2	65.5	5.5	63.8	5.3	64.1	6
75+*[3]	80.8	4.8	79.5	4.4	79.8	4.5	78.4	3.2	80.7	5.3	79.4	4.9

Note. MOBILATE 2000-Survey, N=3950, interactions significant *=$p<0.05$, **=$p<0.01$, *** $p<=0.001$ between
[1] Netherlands - all other countries; Finland-Western Germany; Finland-Hungary
[2] Eastern Germany-Western Germany; Eastern Germany-Italy; Western Germany-Hungary; Hungary-Italy
[3] Finland-Hungary; Hungary-Italy

Table 3.5: The life-expectancy in the participant countries

Life-expectancy in years remained (age+years to have)	1995 or close to this year				2000 or close to this year			
	60 years old		80 years old		60 years old		80 years old	
	male	female	male	female	male	female	male	female
Finland[1]	18.1/[a]17.7	22./22.	6./6.	7.9/7.7	19.2/18.7	23.7/23.4	6.6	8.2/8.1
Eastern Germany[2]	17.3	21.9	6.	7.6	18.3	22.7	6.5	8.1
Western Germany[2]	18.5	22.9	6.	8.1	19.2	23.4	7.0	8.4
Hungary[3]	14.8	19.5	not av.	not av.	15.0	19.8	not av.	not av.
Italy[4]	19.2	23.7	6.	8.4	19.7	24.3	7.0	8.8
The Netherlands[5]	18.1	22.8	6.	8.1.	18.8	23.0	6.3	8.1

Note. MOBILATE Survey 2000.
[a] The first numbers refer to the exact years of data (e.g. year 1995 and 2000 in Finland and in the Netherlands and 1995 and 1998 in Hungary and Italy) and the latter numbers to the period of years of measurement (e.g. in Finland 1) years 1991-1995 and 1996-2000; in Eastern and Western Germany 2) years 1994-1996 and 1997-1999)
[1] Statistics Finland, [2] Federal Statistic Office Germany, [3] KSH, 2000, [4] ISTAT, 2000, [5] CBS, 2001

The average in the expected years increased between the years of 1995 and 2000 in all participant countries. The highest life-expectancy was found in Italy, followed by western Germany, Finland, the Netherlands, eastern Germany and last Hungary. The good life-style (healthy food based on Mediterranean diet with less alcohol and fat animal consumption than in the Northern European countries) combined with socio-cultural aspects (i.e., warm and strong integration with family and friends, and family care in favour of older persons when they are ill or disabled) might partly explain the high life-expectancy in Italy. On the other hand, the rather low level of standard of living compared to the other participant countries might be the reason for the low life-expectancy in Hungary.

3.4.2   Marital status

The marital status of the respondents is strongly linked with age and gender. Most of the younger men and women were still married, whereas the situation changes with increasing age. While the majority of older men were still married, an overwhelming amount of older women was already widowed. A difference can be found among older men in the western German city: In opposite to all other regions studied about every second man in this area was already widowed and only 44% of the respective respondents were still married. Some differences were found between urban and rural areas. While the proportion of married persons did not differ systematically between urban and rural areas, in some European regions (eastern and western Germany, Hungary and Italy) younger women were married more often in the countryside than in the cities.

The biggest difference was found regarding the proportion of divorced: persons living in the urban areas were more often divorced than those living in the rural areas. Finnish and Hungarian urbanites were most often divorced compared to all other areas, while in Italy (and this is partly true for the Dutch rural area) due to the strong catholic tradition hardly any respondent was divorced. The most diversified pattern regarding people being never married or living separated from their partners was found in the Dutch sub-sample.

3.4.3   Education

Further important socio-demographic variables include the level of education and professional training, because they might be relevant for one's out-of-home mobility. National education systems and structures and the reached levels of schooling differ widely in the European regions and are not easily comparable between the national samples. However, the length of one's full-time education, including school, occupational training and university affords a sufficient impression of a person's education (Table 3.6).

In the *Finnish* regions, urban respondents reported a longer education (between 7.5 and 11.8 years of full-time education on average) than those living in the rural area (between 5.0 and 8.7 years). Especially older women in the rural area reported a very low amount of full-time education (about 5 years on average). Generally, men and younger persons reported a longer full-time education than women and older respondents.

Comparing both parts of *Germany*, men in the eastern German city had the longest education (about 13 years on average), although men in the other areas had a good education as well (between 10 and 13 years on average). Conversely, women reported in general a lower level of education in both parts of Germany - with the exception of younger women in the eastern German city. They had about as much education as men of the same age in this area.

Also in *Hungary* the education of men was better than that of women, when measured in years of full-time education. Younger persons and those living in the Hungarian city attended school for a longer time than older people and those living in the Hungarian countryside. The biggest difference was found between the Hungarian urban and rural areas: Urban elders had spent between 9 and 12 years of full-time education on average, while people in the rural area had spent between 6 (older women) and 9 (younger men) on such education.

Table 3.6: Years of education (mean)

	Finland		Eastern Germany		Western Germany		Hungary		Italy		The Netherlands	
	Mean	Std.	Mean	Std.	Mean	Std.	Mean	Std.	Mean	Std.	Mean	Std.
Urban												
Male												
55-74	11.8	4.8	12.8	2.8	12.7	2.6	12.1	3.6	10.8	5.2	10.8	3.4
75+	8.0	3.7	13.4	3.0	11.2	2.8	11.8	4.2	7.7	4.1	10.5	3.9
Female												
55-74	11.1	4.4	12.6	2.8	11.6	2.5	11.0	4.0	7.8	4.3	10.0	3.4
75+	7.5	4.2	10.8	2.5	10.3	2.87	9.1	3.8	5.0	3.0	9.2	3.2
Rural												
Male												
55-74	7.7	2.8	11.8	2.9	10.8	2.6	8.7	3.0	6.6	4.2	10.7	3.2
75+	5.3	2.4	11.3	2.8	10.2	2.8	7.0	3.0	5.2	3.7	10.7	4.7
Female												
55-74	8.7	3.3	10.3	2.2	9.6	2.0	8.4	3.8	5.1	2.6	10.2	3.1
75+	5.0	1.8	9.3	1.9	8.7	2.2	6.4	2.1	3.6	2.4	9.8	3.2

Note. MOBILATE 2000-Survey, N = 3929

The level of education in the *Italian* regions can best be compared with the Hungarian situation. In general and like in the Hungarian regions studied, the level of education when measured in years of full-time education is very low compared to other regions. Elders who live in the Italian urban area reported higher levels of education than those living in the rural area. The older age groups reported lower levels of education than the younger ones, and again the difference between male and female respondents was even greater in the countryside where women had an average length of about four years of education, which is the lowest in the complete MOBILATE-sample.

The smallest differences between age-groups, urban vs. rural areas, and men's and women's level of education revealed in the *Dutch* areas. Although younger elders reported more years of full-time education than older respondents, men reached a higher level of education than women, and those living in the Dutch urban area of investigation spent more years on full-time education on average than those living in the respective non-urban area, the differences were much smaller than in all other European regions under investigation.

In general, as regards the amount of full-time education, the following characteristics were found in all regions under research:

- Elders living in the urban areas were better educated than those living in the rural areas (with the exception of the Netherlands due to the suburban character of the Dutch rural area). This was especially true for the Finnish, Hungarian and Italian regions: In Hungary, up to 59% of the respondents living in the rural area had not completed the elementary school, while in the Hungarian city this was the case for only about 26%.

- Men reported more years of full-time education than women. The biggest difference between male and female respondents was found in Italy.

- Younger elders attended school, occupational training and university for a longer period of time than people aged 75 years or older.
- Women in the rural areas were most disadvantaged: they reported the lowest education measured in years of full-time education. Women in the Italian countryside reported the lowest amount of full-time education of all respondents in the MOBILATE sample (about 4 years).

In addition, the following differences between the regions under research appeared: Eastern Germans reported the highest education measured in years of full-time education. Moreover, younger women in the eastern German urban area reported almost as much education as their male contemporaries. They were also more skilled than western German women, especially when comparing the level of occupational training. Dutch elders, and older Dutch women in particular, were also well educated. As in the Netherlands, only small differences between the urban and rural regions, male or female respondents and those being younger or older revealed with respect to education in the eastern and western German regions.

On the other side, Italian elders were those being most deprived as regards full-time education: With the exception of younger urban men, Italian respondents in all sub-groups reported the lowest level of education. This low level of education of older Italians depends on the low social and economic conditions which existed in Italy in the past. Schooling was obligatory only for the first three or five years of primary school. This was especially diffused in the rural areas where manual abilities to work in the fields were more necessary than cultural skills. Especially older women, who had worse social opportunities and economic positions in the rural society compared to men, have due to these reasons the lowest level of education.

3.4.4   Occupation and status of employment

Occupation is a further important characteristic of the social circumstances older people live in. Although it can be assumed that most of the study participants were already retired due to the sample stratification, the occupation practised before might have strong effects especially to their financial situation. Due to the different structures of labour market and professions in the European regions under research, the current or last profession of the respondents will be described on the background of the respective national terminology.

Among the *Finnish* elders living in the countryside, the majority reported to be farmers. About 50% of the older and almost one third of the younger respondents were farmers. Besides, younger men often had worked or still worked as a skilled worker, while women reported lower qualified jobs (unskilled worker). In the Finnish city, men most often worked or still work in upper white collar professions or as skilled workers, while women reported again professions with a lower level of qualification. About 19% of the older Finnish women living in the rural areas and 15% of those living in the urban area were housewives.

Also in the *western German* rural area, about one third of the women reported being a housewife. In the western German city, 26% of the older compared to only 14% of the younger women were housewives. If women in the western German regions had an occupation, they most frequently worked as entry or midlevel employees, with some older women working as untrained help. The situation is different in *eastern Germany*: A maximum of 5% of the eastern German women reported being a housewife. Their most frequent occupation was an entry level or midlevel employee, and similar to western Germany, some older women worked as untrained help. But unlike West German women, between 11% and 16% of the East German women also worked as trained help, skilled workers or craftsmen.

In line with their better education, men in both eastern and western Germany reported occupations which generally require higher qualifications: One half of the younger men and 32% of the older men in the rural area of western Germany worked or still work as skilled labourers or craftsmen. Also a high proportion had occupations such as academic professionals, freelancers, or civil officials. The structure of occupations among East German men is not that different from the western German situation: Most of them, especially younger men, worked or still work as skilled labourers or craftsmen. Similar to the western German rural area, a number of the eastern German men worked as academic professionals or as freelancers. The biggest difference between eastern and western Germany can be seen in the fact that in the eastern German countryside only up to 7% of the men reported to be farmers whereas 15% of the younger and 30% of the older men in the rural area of western Germany were farmers.

The level of schooling is reflected by occupation, as can especially be seen in the *Hungarian* regions studied. The low level of schooling of Hungarian elders means an unfavourable position on the labour market: a high proportion of unskilled workers (which are poorly paid) were found among both men and women. The proportion of such work was already higher among women than among men, and especially in the rural area under investigation. Up to two thirds of those respondents - independent from gender - in this area worked or still work as unskilled workers in industry or agriculture, while in the urban area more women (up to 46%) than men (up to 22%) reported such occupation. In the Hungarian city, a considerable amount of men worked or still work as skilled workers or as midlevel employees.

The differences between age-groups and genders described above with respect to occupational status revealed also in the *Italian* regions. There were especially big differences between the occupations of men and women, as Italian women were often housewives or carried out less qualified jobs.

The small differences, as regards the level of education in the *Dutch sample*, could not be found in the current or last occupation of the respective respondents. Especially between men and women there were big differences as regards labour market participation: Most of the Dutch men worked (or still work) in blue collar jobs, while most of the Dutch women were housewives. In addition, much more men worked or still work as higher employees when compared with women. However, and due to the suburban character of the Dutch rural area studied, there were only small regional differences.

In opposite to an analysis based on the sample stratification it may be more interesting to examine the status of employment by the respective retirement age in each country (Table 3.7): Among the respondents who had reached retirement age, only some 8% of the male respondents in the Hungarian city still worked, all other respondents reported to be retired. The reasons for this are complex: pensions in Hungary were (and still are) low which means that work done while on pension was important for a livelihood in old age. The proportion of the labour force employed as pensioners within the total number of employees was still quite high in 1992 (6.1%; KSH [Központi Statisztikai Hivatal], 1993). Then, as a consequence of the more limited opportunities on the labour market following the systemic change, it fell to 3.1% by 2000 (Kardos, Szabó, Széman, & Talyigás, 2002). Today it is mainly pensioners with a high level of qualifications who are able to find a job on the labour market. Since Pécs is a big city and university centre, and in the sample the level of schooling of the Hungarian urban population including the women is much higher than in the rural area, it is obviously easier for them to find work, even with the more limited demand for labour.

This picture completely changes when having a look on those older adults who have not yet reached the retirement age in each country: Men living in urban areas most often worked in Finland, Italy and the Netherlands (about 40%, mostly in full-time jobs). Also in western Germany and Hungary over one fourth of the respective respondents still worked. The employment rate of men in the eastern German city was the lowest (22%). About 10% were unemployed due to a generally high unemployment in eastern Germany. Women living in the urban areas worked less often - with the exception of Finland: As a result of a low gender-related segregation of the labour market, every second female respondent in the Finnish city still worked, mostly at a full-time job. In the other cities, women worked less often.

The status of employment is different in the countryside: Again, men in the Finnish rural area who had not reached the retirement age worked most often (about 60%, both in full-time and part-time jobs). In addition, Finnish women in this area reported the highest rate of employment (about 27%) compared with all women living in rural areas. Only in the western German rural area worked men more than in the urban area. In eastern Germany, again a considerable proportion of men were unemployed. Conversely, in Hungary and Italy only few elders still worked although they had not reached the national retirement age. None of the Hungarian rural women below the official retirement age of 62 years was still working when surveyed within the MOBILATE study.

In addition to their status of employment and independent from being retired or still at a full-time or part-time job, the respondents were asked if they pursue some additional work like other paid jobs, voluntary work or if they care for a relative. In Finland, up to 40% of the younger respondents pursued voluntary work or care for a relative (especially women). Men in the rural areas more often held regular second jobs or had occasional paid work, whereas in both parts of Germany and Hungary such activities were less common. In West Germany only few younger respondents reported some voluntary work or caring for a relative (up to 7%), and in East Germany the respective rates were even lower (up to 3%). In Hungary, additional activities seem to be much more concentrated on earning additional income: up to 15% of the younger men in the urban area and 23% of the respective women had additional income, mostly by a second paid job or occasional work. In addition, some younger men in the Hungarian city worked voluntarily, while women in this area cared for a relative or a child.

Additional activities are much more common in Italy and the Netherlands: Up to 50% of the younger urban elders and 30% of those living in the rural areas reported such activities. They mostly cared for a relative (32% of the younger women living in urban areas did so). In addition, especially men reported to pursue voluntary work. Due to the catholic tradition and almost independent from gender, voluntary work has got an important meaning in the Netherlands: up to 28% of the younger respondents in the regions studied in this country were engaged in voluntary work.

Table 3.7: Status of employment by retirement age (%)

Below retirement age?	Finland[1] Urban		Finland[1] Rural		Eastern Germany[2] Urban		Eastern Germany[2] Rural		Western Germany[2] Urban		Western Germany[2] Rural		Hungary[3] Urban		Hungary[3] Rural		Italy[4] Urban		Italy[4] Rural		The Netherlands[1] Urban		The Netherlands[1] Rural	
	yes	no	yes	no	yes	no	yes	no	yes	no	yes	no	yes	no	yes	no	yes	no	yes	no	yes	no	yes	no
Full-time job																								
Men	39	0	31	0	22	0	17	0	27	0	35	0	30	7	19	2	41	1	9	0	38	1	19	0
Women	42	0	27	0	10	0	12	0	8	0	15	0	11	2	0	1	17	1	9	1	0	2	9	0
Part-time job																								
Men	6	0	4	0	0	0	3	0	0	0	0	0	0	3	0	1	3	1	0	1	6	1	9	1
Women	8	0	2	0	5	0	2	0	2	0	6	0	7	2	0	0	4	1	5	0	26	0	26	1
Not regularly or less employed																								
Men	0	0	3	0	3	0	2	0	0	0	0	0	0	1	0	0	0	0	0	1	0	1	0	0
Women	0	0	0	0	2	0	0	0	0	1	4	0	7	1	9	0	0	0	0	0	0	0	2	0
Unemployed																								
Men	12	0		0	10	0	13	0	4	0	2	0	6	0	4	0	0	0	0	0	3	0	5	0
Women	4	0	7	0	15	0	16	0	2	0	0	0	0	0	0	0	0	0	0	0	0	0	0	0
Housewife/housemen																								
Men	0	0	0	0	0	0	2	0	0	3	0	0	3	0	0	0	0	0	0	0	3	0	5	3
Women	0	2	2	0	2	0	0	0	11	1	15	1	4	3	0	3	39	14	36	2	22	36	42	54
Retired																								
Men	44	100	58	100	66	100	64	100	69	97	64	100	61	90	77	98	57	98	91	98	50	97	63	96
Women	46	98	62	100	68	100	70	100	77	98	62	99	71	93	91	96	39	84	50	97	52	62	22	45

Note. MOBILATE 2000-Survey, N = 3912; [1] Retirement age 65 years (2000); [2] Retirement age women 64 years/men 65 years (2000); [3] Retirement age 62 years (2000); [4] Retirement age women 60 years/men 65 years (2000); In Italy the retirement age depends on different job categories; In this Table the average estimated retirement age is shown.

3.4.5   Financial situation

The most important socio-demographic characteristic, as regards an indispensably prerequisite for one's out-of-home mobility, might be the personal income. When comparing the income per person[1] in all regions under investigation, huge differences became visible, especially between the Hungarian conditions and all other regions (Table 3.8). The highest average income per person was reported by persons living in both parts of Germany and the Netherlands (between 700 and over 1000 Euro per person), while the average income in the Hungarian sample reached a maximum of only 142 Euro. Despite costs of living are different in the countries involved in the study, it can be stated that a lot of Hungarian people are disadvantaged as regards their personal income. Also Italian respondents reported a lower personal income when compared to the other regions (mean average income differs between 447 and 685 Euro).

Table 3.8:   Income per person in EURO (mean)

	Finland		Eastern Germany		Western Germany		Hungary		Italy		The Netherlands	
	Mean	Std.	Mean	Std.	Mean	Std.	Mean	Std.	Mean	Std.	Mean	Std.
Urban												
Male												
55-74	952	321	852	194	945	393	142	67	685	385	987	384
75+	863	335	988	197	1003	412	131	48	594	312	825	297
Female												
55-74	944	398	955	318	1066	507	133	56	598	297	897	344
75+	752	269	983	266	1022	513	111	43	447	178	1035	405
N (%)	*298*	*96.4*	*334*	*85.9*	*308*	*83.7*	*265*	*86.9*	*240*	*80.0*	*198*	*65.5*
Missing (n; %)	*11*	*3.6*	*55*	*14.1*	*60*	*16.3*	*40*	*13.1*	*60*	*20.0*	*104*	*34.4*
Rural												
Male												
55-74	656	278	717	217	814	327	99	27	486	197	850	305
75+	605	277	739	182	707	274	110	36	492	236	989	640
Female												
55-74	691	367	732	226	774	341	116	37	454	173	925	386
75+	577	228	715	235	753	240	113	33	501	216	873	449
N (%)	*277*	*92.0*	*323*	*85.2*	*322*	*84.1*	*285*	*95.0*	*263*	*87.7*	*218*	*69.4*
Missing (n; %)	*24*	*8.0*	*56*	*14.8*	*61*	*15.9*	*15*	*5.0*	*37*	*12.3*	*96*	*30.6*

Note. MOBILATE Survey 2000; N = 3922

Independent of these differences, the following patterns were found regarding income: The greatest variety of income seems to exist in Finland (577 to 952 Euro). This is due to the reason that elders living in the urban area, the younger and the male respondents reported a higher income than those living in the rural areas, older or female respondents. A similar pattern, but less strong, was found in the Italian regions. In all other regions under investigation, this structure did not reveal. Although in both parts of Germany elders living in

---

[1] The respondents were asked to give the categorical income of their household. By dividing the centre of this non-metric information by the size of each household, we generated a pseudo-metric income per person.

the urban areas reported a higher income than their rural contemporaries, there were no systematic differences between female and male respondents.

Moreover, older men in the urban areas reported a higher income than the respective younger men. A possible explanation might be the fact that some younger men's main source of income was unemployment benefits, which is probably lower when compared to a pension. No systematic differences between the urban and rural regions, between female and male respondents and younger and older ones at all can be stated for the Dutch sample, which indicated the smallest range of income (873 to 1,035 Euro).[2]

The main source of income of a person's household is of course linked with his or her status of employment: Most of the older people got their main income from a pension after having retired from the labour market. Compared to the older respondents, more younger elders households' main source of income came from a full-time job. In addition, and also most probably linked with their status of employment, some younger respondents got their main income either from a pension due to early retirement or from unemployment benefits.

Table 3.9: Satisfaction with financial situation (mean) [1]

	Finland		Eastern Germany		Western Germany		Hungary		Italy		The Netherlands	
	Mean	Std.	Mean	Std.	Mean	Std.	Mean	Std.	Mean	Std.	Mean	Std.
Urban												
Male												
55-74	8.1	1.1	7.0	1.7	7.0	2.0	5.0	2.2	7.2	1.7	7.5	1.2
75+	8.2	1.9	7.4	1.6	6.3	2.3	5.5	2.5	6.9	1.9	7.5	1.5
Female												
55-74	7.8	1.7	6.7	1.9	7.5	2.4	4.6	2.6	6.7	2.1	7.1	1.7
75+	7.7	2.2	7.1	1.5	6.2	2.4	5.1	2.7	6.8	1.9	7.6	1.3
Rural												
Male												
55-74	7.5	2.3	6.5	2.4	7.7	1.8	4.1	2.4	5.4	2.6	7.6	1.1
75+	8.1	1.7	7.6	1.6	7.9	2.1	4.8	2.3	5.8	2.4	7.8	1.7
Female												
55-74	8.1	2.0	6.4	2.2	7.5	2.1	4.0	2.4	5.6	2.8	7.8	1.2
75+	8.0	1.7	7.0	2.1	7.4	1.8	4.6	2.4	5.4	2.3	7.6	1.3

Note. MOBILATE Survey 2000; N = 3922
[1] Self-evaluation rating on an 11-point rating scale, higher scores indicating higher satisfaction

Main sources of income differ in the Dutch sample: Up to two thirds of the older Dutch respondents got their main income from a basic pension. In the Netherlands each person aged 65 year or older is entitled to get a basic pension, independent from former income or having paid any contribution. In addition to this basic pension, it is possible to build up a private pension either as a private pension scheme or as an employer-sponsored pension scheme (up

---

[2] However, the income information about Dutch respondents should be interpreted with caution, because about one third of the Dutch respondents did not answer the question regarding their income. In general, questions about income are linked with high non-responses. In the MOBILATE study non-responses regarding income fluctuate between 4% (Finnish urban area) and 34% (Dutch urban area).

to 38% of the Dutch respondents get their main income from this 'private' pension). If one stops working for health reasons before having reached the retirement age of 65 years, a sick-benefit will be paid (9% of the younger male respondents in the Dutch urban area, 5% of the respective female respondents).

Besides all described differences regarding the amount and type of one's income, satisfaction with one's financial situation might be the best indicator for a person's financial situation. Besides the Dutch elders, those living in Finland seem to be the most satisfied as regards this aspect (Table 3.9), almost independent from their actual income. The above described differences between urban and rural regions or male and female respondents were not reflected in different satisfactions with financial situation. Only in the urban areas a slight tendency was found that younger respectively male respondents were somehow more satisfied when compared to older or female respondents. Also the Dutch elders, showing no systematic differences in their personal income, did not differ all too much in their evaluation of their financial situation: independent from any socio-demographic characteristics such as age, gender or living region most of them were more or less satisfied on average. On the other side, and what could be expected, Hungarian respondents were mostly dissatisfied with their financial situation. Especially younger Hungarians and those living in the Hungarian rural area were quite unsatisfied in this respect.

Also among the Italian elders, satisfaction with financial situation was lower compared to other regions under investigation. Especially respondents living in the Italian rural area showed low satisfaction. Satisfaction with financial situation also varied in both parts of Germany, but was mostly not linked with any socio-demographic characteristic like age, gender or living region, except in East Germany, where younger respondents and men were slightly more satisfied than older and female respondents.

3.4.6   Health status

For a further understanding of older people's personal characteristics which are important prerequisites for out-of-home mobility we give also some insight in their health. The health related aspects displayed in Table 3.10 include objective functional capacity (activities of daily living, ADL) on the one hand and subjective evaluations of one's health on the other. The latter include general satisfaction with health and self-evaluation of physical mobility (for further health indicators see Chapters 4 and 6).

Comparison of the different objective and subjective health aspects showed the following findings: As regards differences between urban and rural locations, there were no, or only slight, significant differences between these two types of areas. With respect to age, the individuals aged 55 to 74 years reported a better health and were able to perform a broader range of activities of daily living (ADL) compared to older persons (aged 75 years or older) in all areas, as was to be expected. Men slightly tended to be more satisfied when compared to women as regards the subjective aspects of health (general satisfaction with health and evaluation of physical mobility). This assessment was reinforced when analysing the objective aspects of health – the ability to perform activities of daily living: In all regions, women showed lower values in functional health than men.

Table 3.10: Different aspects of respondents' health (mean)

	Finland			Eastern Germany			Western Germany			Hungary			Italy			The Netherlands		
	(a) Satisfaction with health[1], (b) evaluation of physical mobility[2], (c) activities of daily living[3]																	
	(a)	(b)	(c)	(a)	(b)	(c)	(a)	(b)	(c)	(a)	(b)	(c)	(a)	(b)	(c)	(a)	(b)	(c)
Urban																		
Male																		
55-	7.4	3.7	28.8	6.6	3.7	26.7	6.8	3.7	26.8	6.1	3.3	25.5	7.2	4.0	28.6	6.9	3.9	27.4
75+	6.5	2.9	25.5	5.4	3.0	22.5	5.2	3.1	22.2	5.5	2.8	21.9	6.8	3.4	23.0	6.9	3.5	24.0
Female																		
55-	7.3	3.6	27.7	6.5	3.5	25.8	7.1	3.8	26.3	5.8	3.2	24.9	6.8	3.7	26.1	6.8	3.6	25.3
75+	6.6	3.0	22.4	4.8	2.7	20.5	5.2	2.9	20.9	4.9	2.6	19.8	6.6	3.1	21.0	6.9	3.3	21.8
Rural																		
Male																		
55-	7.1	3.3	28.4	6.3	3.6	27.1	6.7	3.5	26.7	4.7	2.8	23.7	7.4	3.9	26.5	7.4	3.9	27.8
75+	6.9	3.0	24.8	5.5	3.2	24.4	5.8	3.1	22.8	5.1	2.7	21.0	6.8	3.1	21.8	7.1	3.4	24.7
Female																		
55-	7.5	3.5	26.2	6.4	3.6	26.4	6.5	3.6	25.6	5.1	3.0	22.4	6.4	3.6	24.8	7.4	4.0	27.0
75+	6.9	2.7	21.4	5.3	2.9	21.6	5.3	2.8	20.7	4.5	2.3	19.0	6.4	2.8	18.5	6.9	3.4	23.9

Note. MOBILATE Survey 2000; N = 3950

[1] Self-evaluation rating on an 11-point rating scale, higher scores indicating higher satisfaction

[2] Self-evaluation of physical mobility on a 5-point scale from 1 (very poor) to 5 (very good)

[3] Sumscore of activities of daily living (ADL) ranging from 10 (no ADL possible) to 30 (all ADL possible)

When comparing elders in the different countries, all aspects of health showed consistent differences: Respondents in Finland and the Netherlands reported a better health as regards objective and subjective aspects of health when compared to other regions; respondents in Hungary who had revealed the lowest values in almost all health aspects and in all subgroups were very unsatisfied with their health – especially in the Hungarian rural region. Only in the Italian countryside results were inconsistent: Despite low functional health, older people in this region reported a relatively high satisfaction with their health in general.

3.5　Summary

An important prerequisite for comparing older adults out of six different European regions is basic demographic information such as age, marital status, education, employment or the individuals' financial situation and status of health. The disproportional stratification of the MOBILATE-sample has almost brought comparable sub-groups, as regards the age means of the different strata. One exception concerns younger women in the Dutch urban area who, due to the different sampling procedure in the Netherlands, are significantly older than all respondents of the respective sub-groups.

As expected, most of the younger elders (aged 55 to 74 years) were still married, whereas the situation changes with increasing age: While the majority of older men was still married, women were more often widowed. Only in the West German city was the situation different: about every second older man in this area was already widowed. Regarding differences between the European regions, the highest proportion of divorced respondents was found in Finland, while in Italy hardly any respondent was divorced.

Elders living in the urban areas under investigation were better educated than those living in the rural areas, with the exception of Dutch respondents. Moreover, men and younger respondents reported more years of education than women and those who belonged to the older age group. Respondents in eastern Germany reported the highest education. On the other side, Italian elders – older women in the Italian rural area, in particular - were those being most deprived as regards education.

Connected with the level of education a person's former or present occupation might have strong effects especially on the financial situation. Despite the fact that occupations cannot easily be compared due to the different structure of the respective labour markets and professions in Europe, occupations and therefore the socio-economic status of the respondents differed between the European regions under research, and between men and women. Except for the eastern German region, women reported generally occupations which require a lower level of qualification when compared to men.

Independent from profession, almost every older individual who had reached the respective retirement age in the different European regions was retired, except for some Hungarian respondents, who still worked due to the low pensions in Hungary. Of those who had not reached the retirement age, especially men were still working, mainly in full-time jobs (up to 60%). The highest employment rates for men was found both in the Finnish urban and rural areas, while the lowest employment rates were reported by men in the rural Italian and Hungarian areas. The highest unemployment rates were found among East German men. Women worked less often, except for the Dutch and especially the Finnish areas: Finnish women below the retirement age reported the highest employment rate when compared to all other female elders. In addition to being retired or still working in a full-time or part-time job some elders pursued additional work, especially in the Italian and Dutch regions: a lot of Italian elders reported to take care for a relative or to be engaged in voluntary work, and voluntary work is most common in the Netherlands.

Most of this socio-economic 'background-information' became apparent in the personal income: The lowest income was reported by older Hungarians, while elders living in both parts of Germany and the Netherlands reported the highest income. For this reason it is not amazing that the Hungarians were the most unsatisfied with their financial situation. Also Italian respondents had a comparatively low income.

And finally, objective and subjective health – a substantial preconditions for outdoor mobility – decreased with advancing age in all regions studied.

References

Avlund, K., Kreiner, S., & Shultz-Larsen, K. (1993). Construct validation and the Rasch model: Functional ability of healthy elderly people. *Scandinavian Journal of Social Medicine, 21*, 233-245.

Brandtstädter, J., & Renner, G. (1990). Tenacious Goal and Flexible Goal Adjustment (TEN-FLEX). *Psychology and Ageing, 5*, 58-67.

CBS (Central Bureau voor de Statistieken) (2001). *Statistical Yearbook*. Voorburg, Heerlen.

Gillman, A. E., Simmel, A., & Perlman Simon, E. (1986). Visual handicap in the aged: Self-reported visual disability and the quality of life of residents of public housing for the elderly. *Journal of Visual Impairment and Blindness, 80*, 588-590.

Glatzer, W., & Zapf, W. (Eds.) (1984). *Lebensqualität in der Bundesrepublik. Objektive Lebensbedingungen und subjektives Wohlbefinden* [Quality of Life in the Federal Republic of Germany. Objective Living Conditions and Subjective Well-being]. Frankfurt, New York: Campus.

Heikkinen, E. (1998). Background, design and methods of the Evergreen Project. *Journal of Aging and Physical Activity, 6*, 106-120.

Holland, C. A. & Rabbit, P. M. A. (1992). People's awareness of their age-related sensory and cognitive deficits and the implications for road safety. *Applied Cognitive Psychology, 6*, 217-231.

ISTAT (Italian Statistical National Institute) (2000). *Annuario Statistico Italiano 1999* [Annual Statistics Italy 1999]. Rome: ISTAT.

Kardos, A., Szabó, L., Széman, Z., & Talyigás, K. (2002). *Új időspolitikai elképzelések. A kormányzati idősügyi nemzeti cselekvési programmhoz* [New ideas for policy on the elderly. Contribution to the national programme of action, governmental policy on the elderly]. Budapest: manuscript.

KSH (2000). *Magyar Statisztikai Zsebkönyv 92* [Hungarian Statistical Pocket-book] (p. 25). Budapest: KSH.

KSH (Központi Statisztikai Hivatal) (1993). *Magyar Statisztikai Zsebkönyv 92* [Hungarian Statistical Pocket-book] (p. 23). Budapest: KSH.

Künemund, H. (2000). Datengrundlage und Methoden [Data and methods]. In M. Kohli & H. Künemund (Eds.), *Die zweite Lebenshälfte. Gesellschaftliche Lage und Partizipation im Spiegel des Alters-Survey* [The second half of life. Social conditions and participation as reflected in the Ageing Survey] (pp. 30-40). Opladen: Leske + Budrich.

Kunzmann, U. (1999). *Being and feeling in control. Two sources of older people's emotional well-being*. Berlin: Sigma.

Mollenkopf, H., Marcellini, F., & Ruoppila, I. (1998). The Outdoor Mobility of Elderly People - A Comparative Study in Three European Countries. In J. Graafmans, V. Taipale & N. Charness (Eds.), *Gerontechnology. A Sustainable Investment in the Future* (pp. 204-211). Amsterdam: IOS Press.

Mollenkopf, H., Marcellini, F., Ruoppila, I., & Tacken, M. (Eds.)(2004). *Ageing and Outdoor Mobility. A European Study*. Amsterdam: IOS Press.

Oswald, W. D., & Fleischmann, U. M. (1995). *Digit-Symbol-Substitution. Nürnberger-Alters-Inventar (NAI)* [The Nuremberg Age Inventory]. Göttingen: Hogrefe-Verlag.

Sachsenweger, M. (1987). *Nahsehproben und ergophthalmologische Sehtests* [Near Visual Acuity test]. Leipzig: Thieme.

Smith, J., Marsiske, M., & Maier, H. (1996). *Differences in control beliefs from age 70 to 05. Locus-of-control-scale*. Unpublished Manuscript. Berlin: Max Planck Institute for Human Development.

Statistics Finland (2001). *Statistical Yearbook of Finland 2001*. Keuruu: Otavan Kirjapaino OY.

Statistisches Bundesamt [Federal Statistic Office of Germany]. *Abgekürzte Sterbetafel 1994/96 und Abgekürzte Sterbetafel 1997/99* [Abbreviated mortality figures 1994/96 and 1997/99]. Wiesbaden: Statistisches Bundesamt

UNESCO (1997). *International Classification of Education: ISCED 1997*. [http:// unesdoc.unesco.org/images/0011/001113/111387eo.pdf].

Watson, D., Clark, L. A., & Telegen, A. (1988). Development and Validation of Brief Measures of Positive and Negative Affect: The PANAS Scales. *Journal of Personality and Social Psychology, 6*, 1063-1070.

Wittenberg, R. (1986). Einstellung zum Autobesitz und Unsicherheitsgefühle älterer Menschen im Strassenverkehr [Older People's Attitudes Towards Owning a Car and Feeling Unsafe in Traffic]. *Zeitschrift für Gerontologie 19*, 400-409.

Zapf, W., & Habich, R. (Eds.) (1996). *Wohlfahrtsentwicklung im vereinten Deutschland* [Welfare Development in Germany after Unification]. Berlin: Edition sigma.

Chapter 4
Physical Health and Mobility

Nina Hirsiaho and Isto Ruoppila

4.1   Introduction

Basic to the theme of outdoor mobility is that its resources on the individual, environmental and technological level are distributed differently among the EC- countries and among urban and non-urban regions in particular, as well as between age groups/cohorts and genders. Health may be the most important resource, or lack of it a risk factor on the individual level affecting on the outdoor mobility of ageing persons.

Health is the product of processes operating at many levels, including the biological, psychological, social and cultural. Distinction between disease (biological pathology) and functional health (experience of health problems) has been made by social and clinical scientists. Disease is categorized using diagnostic standards. Functional health is affected by social and cultural meanings as well as by physical or emotional discomfort. Ageing is often associated with changes by functional health. Some of them are gradual, others are abrupt. They bring dysfunction and functional decline, also often requiring participation in unfamiliar institutional and social structures while dealing with personal physical dysfunction (Leventhal, Idler, & Leventhal, 1999).

In epidemiological studies health has been assessed both by using self-ratings and objective measures as well as medical check-ups by general practitioners. Generally these different assessments correlate with each other, although the correlations are quite low. The subjective health and medically evaluated health only partly describe the same thing. It is still open, which kind of predictions can be best made by using self-ratings and objective assessments (Jylhä, 1994).

The very general findings, as regards ageing and disease, describe the increasing number of diseases with the ageing process although all the time the mortality is selecting more often those subjects having more and more serious diseases at the baseline than the subjects having better health-states (Guralnik, LaCroix, Abbott et al., 1993; Laukkanen, Leinonen, & Heikkinen, 1999; Sakari-Rantala, Heikkinen, & Ruoppila, 1995).

As regards the gender, the general trend in research results is that after the age of 75/80 years women have more diseases and impairments as well as disabilities than men, especially those which hinder, restrict or slow down their PADL (physical activities of daily life) and IADL (instrumental activities of daily life) activities as well as their outdoor mobility (Guralnik et al., 1993; Laukkanen, Heikkinen, Schroll, & Kauppinen, 1997; Laukkanen, Leinonen, & Heikkinen, 1999; Sakari-Rantala et al., 1995; Schroll, 1994). Sakari-Rantala et al. (1995, 1999) found, in the Finnish Evergreen project, the poor performance of women aged 75 years or older in different mobility tasks. Men suffer more often from fatal diseases compared to women, and women, on the contrast, from disabling diseases. Men have higher mortality than women, while among women disability not only continues for a longer time, but also increases in severity (Laukkanen, Sakari-Rantala, Kauppinen, & Heikkinen, 1997). In the studies by Sakari-Rantala and colleagues (1995, 1999), the 75+ years old women had the highest number of chronic diseases.

The more frequent widowhood of the older women when compared to men results to losing a close relationship as well as to diminished possibilities of receiving practical help in every day living, like in transport from home to friends and relatives, to leisure activities or to get necessary services. An additional factor decreasing the outdoor mobility possibilities of elderly women is their low level of income. Its effects become more prominent when there are no other persons bringing money into the household.

The urban vs. rural/non-urban differences in health are studied very little. But on the basis on the selective migration it is possible to suppose that the people living in urban areas are healthier, also because they usually have better health services in their nearhood. However, the reversed way of reasoning could be likewise used: people with worse health go to cities where more facilities and caring or nursing homes exist.

Self-ratings of health

The self-rated health has a long tradition in the study of health in later life. Different research traditions have contributed to our understanding of self-rated health. Quantitative surveys have tried to identify the antecedents of self-rated health like basic demographic variables, socio-economic status, social activities and relationships, also sometimes life satisfaction (Heikkinen et al., 1992, 1997; Laukkanen et al., 1997; Sakari-Rantala et al., 1999); studies of social comparison processes (e.g. own health compared to same-aged persons' health) in late life, and qualitative studies have explored the references and indicators, which individuals use in assessing the quality of their health (Jylhä, 1994). Individuals and social groups differ in the extent to which bodily experiences are attributed to disease, the extent to which symptoms are perceived as severe, and the extent to which symptoms are viewed as responsive to treatment (George, 2001). Compared to young and middle-aged persons, older adults see themselves as more susceptible to disease, view their symptoms as more severe, but are yet less afraid of being ill.

During the ageing process individuals are confronted with the challenges of discriminating changes that are part of the 'normal' ageing process from those that result from diseases or dysfunctions. There is strong evidence that many old adults 'normalize' at least some of their symptoms, attributing them to ageing rather than illness (Stoller, 1993; Stoller & Forster, 1994). Qualitative studies also reveal those difficulties, which the older persons face in deciding whether symptoms are caused by ageing or by disease (Abrums, 2000; Jylhä, 1994). Symptom attribution refers to the interpretation of specific bodily experiences. In contrast self-rated health refers to individuals' global assessments of their health.

The Women's Health and Aging Study (Jylhä, Guralnik, Balfour, & Fried, 2001) demonstrated that walking difficulty, and low walking speed besides age predict later lowered self-ratings of health showing that also the functioning capacity needed in everyday life and in different PADL and IADL activities is an important effector on self-assessed health.

As regards the self-rating of health the research focused first on the validity of self-rated health as a proxy for more objective indicators of health status, including physician assessment and chronic diseases. There are varying strong relationships between objective health measures and self-rated health (e.g. Jylhä, 1994; Jylhä, Guralnik, Ferrucci, Jokela, & Heikkinen, 1998; Kivinen, Halonen, Eronen, & Nissinen, 1998; Laukkanen, Leinonen, & Heikkinen, 1999; Sakari-Rantala et al., 1999). Self-ratings of health seem to be, at least in older age groups, and within reasonable interval, quite permanent as was shown by Leinonen, Heikkinen and Jylhä (1998). However, when these 75- and 80-years old subjects were asked about the possible change in their health status during the past five years, nearly half of them felt their health becoming worse. These two approaches measure quite another thing; in men they, surprisingly, did not have any significant association, but among women these ratings were associated but not strongly. The authors conclude that self-rated health seems to be age-adjusted; elderly people who say their health has become worse as they age actually self-rate their health as the same or better than five years earlier.

Leinonen, Heikkinen and Jylhä (1999) have analysed the structure of self-rated health among 75-year-old subjects. The path analysis models used showed that a smaller number of difficulties in performing the physical activities of daily living (PADL), fewer chronic diseases, and better maximal working capacity were associated with better self-rated health. In addition, among the women a smaller number of depressive symptoms, and among the men better cognitive capacity had a positive effect on self-rated health.

Leinonen, Heikkinen and Jylhä (2001 a,b) have shown that of 75-year-old subjects, among women, better health ratings at baseline, better functioning and higher maximal working capacity as well as a higher number of social contacts were important direct predictors of better health ratings at follow-up. Among men, better health ratings at baseline, either physical activity or a lower number of chronic conditions and better functioning were the most important direct predictors. These findings show that health ratings reflect multiple dimensions of health and functioning.

The 10-year longitudinal study of the subjects being 75-year old at the baseline demonstrated different indicators of health status, functioning and physical as well as social activity predicting the self-rated health; better over the first 5-year period than over the 10-year period (Leinonen, Heikkinen, & Jylhä, 2002). Likewise Manderbacka, Lahelma and Martikainen (1998) have shown that self-rated health forms a continuum from poor to good health in relations to risk factors (BMI, exercise, alcohol consumption) and ill health (long-standing diseases, limitations in mobility, short-term disability, somatic symptoms and psychological symptoms).

The vast majority of older adults describe their health as 'good' or 'excellent' (Heikkinen et al., 1997; Jylhä, 1994), especially when comparing themselves to their age peers (Jylhä, 1994; Smith, Shelley, & Dennerstein, 1994). Older people seem to believe that they are exceptions to the usual patterns of ageing and that their health is superior to that of most of their age peers perhaps of the same sex. Older adults have a strong preference for social rather than temporal comparisons (Robinson-Whelen & Kiecolt-Glaser, 1997). One function of social comparisons is to protect feelings of self-worth.

The association between self-rated health and gender is, in some extend, inconsistent across studies. In a few studies (e.g. Idler, 1993) older women report higher levels of self-rated health compared to others, whereas in most studies men, especially over 75 years old, are reporting higher levels (Heikkinen et al., 1997; Jylhä, 1994). Also the level of education is related to self-rated health; those having a higher level of education rate their health to be better than those who have less education (Heikkinen et al., 1997).

Health and physical mobility

With the ageing process motor control declines increasingly, including sensorimotor changes, generalized slowing, and decrements in balance and gait. It is well known that individuals of advanced age have structural and functional changes that accumulate over time and contribute to decrements and abnormalities in movement control (Laukkanen, Heikkinen, & Kauppinen, 1995; Schroll, Avlund, Era, Gause-Nilsson, & Davidson, 1997). The changes with increased age include neuroanatomical reductions, muscular changes, reduced proprioception, and decrements in sensor motor integration (Ketcham & Stelmach, 2001). Although all of these decrements result in slow uncoordinated movements, they do not accumulate in a linear manner.

Motor actions slow down with ageing and the interindividual differences increase which can be seen in the variances. The much-studied reaction time and movement time increase in different motor tasks. Also the kinematics analyses show differences between younger and older subjects. Older adults have lower force production and also the force production variability increases with age (Era & Rantanen, 1997; Häkkinen et al., 1996; Häkkinen et al., 1998; Rantanen & Avela, 1997; Smith & Brewer, 1995).

It has been assumed that reductions in central planning, proprioception, force production and regulation, and irregular muscle patterns in the elderly decrease the capability to control volitional actions (Era & Rantanen, 1997). This creates a greater need to use vision to guide and regulate movements (Gottlob & Madden, 1999; Seidler-Dobrin & Stelmach, 1998). The visual monitoring of an ongoing movement is thought to compensate for sensorimotor information loss during execution. The consequences of the increased reliance on vision are that movements are performed slower with more variability (Chaput & Proteau, 1996; Seidler-Dobrin & Stelmach, 1998).

Mobility is an extremely important concern in the elderly population. With decreasing mobility people become more dependent on others' help and their autonomy will get threatened. One big 'cause' of mobility problems and difficulties are the falls, which also come more fatal with ageing. Also the environmental factors, like snow and ice, contribute to the risk of falling producing injuries and temporary or permanent disabilities hindering mobility.

The ability to stabilize posture is not only important for upright stance, but also for performing different upper extremity movements needed in many activities in daily life. Gait changes in older adults include a decreased preferred speed of walking, shorter stride lengths, increased stride frequency, a wider stance, and longer support times (Baumann, 1994; Ho et al., 1997). Muscular strength, power, and force control are important components of walking stability, as well as flexibility and range of motion in gait deficits.

Mobility affects health

The relations between health and mobility have been discussed in the foregoing as health being an 'explaining' factor. In fact, mobility also affects on the health, especially different kinds of physical activities that require a many-sided use of the sensorimotor and motor systems. Long-term physical activities and physical training have beneficial effects on muscle and cardiovascular function in elderly people. Their effects seem to last into the age of 70 to 80 years. What seems to be a lasting effect of former training may be that these people have a physically more active lifestyle without actual training or it may be a confounding effect of primary constitutional factors.

Wagner and LaCroix (1992) and Buchner et al. (1992) review the experimental evidence that increasing activity reduces or eliminates functional decline. The results show that most of the decline associated with ageing is due to inactivity rather than the ageing process itself. However, the experimental evidence is limited by short follow-up intervals, highly selected samples of subjects and interventions largely involving vigorous activities. The intervention programs, like IVEG project (Frändin, Johanneson, & Grimby, 1992) demonstrate that those who were more physically active had fewer problems with energy, pain, emotions and physical mobility (Grimby, Grimby, Frändin, & Wiklund, 1992). However, it takes more time to remobilise and rehabilitate musculoskeletal components than the time needed to cause immobilization atrophy. Poorer adaptability to strain with increasing age makes sufficient time an even more important factor in rehabilitation of elderly people.

The possibilities to improve motor skills and the different components needed for different kind of motor performance can be found out also in very late age. The learning needs only more time and more training times. Maybe, the slower rate of motor learning is not only a result of a reduced plasticity of the elderly motor system, but also the result of the need to process different sources of sensory information independently (Chaput & Proteau, 1996). Fiatarone (1990) and Sipilä, Multanen, Kallinen, Era and Suominen (1996) have, among others, demonstrated that muscle strength training is possible in very advanced age. In a controlled trial of exercise with the residents of old people's homes, even very old residents could benefit from participation in regular seated exercise and improve their postural sway, flexibility, hand grip and functional ability as compared with controls.

Physical activities affect on muscle strength, which has been noted to predict mortality in initially healthy men (Laukkanen, Kauppinen & Heikkinen, 1998; Rantanen et al., 2000; Sihvonen, Rantanen, & Heikkinen, 1998) as well as old age disability (Rantanen et al., 1999). By physical activities in middle age it is possible to affect on the risk of all-cause mortality (Rantanen et al., 2000) and by strength training it is possible to decrease the risk of physical disability in old age (Rantanen et al., 1999). Leventhal, Rabin, Leventhal and Burns (2001) summarize that even moderate exercise by older persons maintains strength and physical functioning, prevents adverse sequel of myocardial infarction, increases life expectancy, enhances functioning and reduces morbidity in the final years of life. Even though exercise in the later years is clearly beneficial, e.g. merely walking about 2 km daily, it will be of greater benefit for those who have previously been sedentary.

Health, cognition and outdoor mobility

Already in 1960s the Finnish researcher Eeva Jalavisto and her co-workers demonstrated, albeit in a cross-sectional study, that the cognitive level of ageing persons is strongly related to their high age (Jalavisto, Lindqvist, & Makkonen, 1964). After that all the longitudinal studies, which have analysed the effect of the level of cognition, cognitive processing or information processing on life-expectancy, have indicated that high level cognitive processes predict the life-expectancy, and cognition is in most studies the strongest selective factor as regards the mortality between the baseline and follow-up assessments (Busse, 1993; Laursen, 1997; Mortensen & Kleven, 1993; Ruoppila & Suutama, 1997; Schaie 1993; Suutama & Ruoppila, 1999).

Besides that the cognitive level is affecting the health of persons, it is directly and via health affecting on the outdoor mobility of people. Outdoor mobility requires all the information processes, which are included into the cognition like perceptual processes, planning, and performing as well as evaluating all the time own performance in relation to the planned goal. Walking, cycling and driving a car require planning the route, visual perception and tactual perception to keep the static and dynamic balance when walking and cycling, or different coordinative functions when driving a car. The cognitive processes, which different transport modes require for their successful use, vary greatly; for the passenger in a car these requirements are minimal compared to the car driver. Walking and cycling in daylight is much less demanding cognitive processing than in dark, snow or ice. That is why it can be assumed that there is a strong association between the level of cognitive processes and different indicators of outdoor mobility. Especially, the significance of speed, both in cognitive processing and motor performances, has to be emphasized.

The generalized slowing hypothesis presented by Birren (1974) and later on by Salthouse (1985), suggests that all fundamental neural events behind the cognitive and motor processes become slower with advanced age. General slowing of movements has been shown in everyday tasks, like reaching and grasping (Bennett & Castiello, 1994; Carnahan, Vandervoot, & Swanson, 1998) and continuous movements (Wishart, Lee, Murdoch, & Hodges, 2000). It has generally been found out that within task difficulty, increasement of cognitive and motor requirements, older adults are slower, with increases in movement duration compared to the younger age groups (Ketcham & Stelmach, 2001).

Health, in its broad sense either objectively or subjectively assessed, is a strong resource factor of outdoor mobility. That is why, one of the aims of the MOBILATE project is to analyse the relationships between various aspects of health and indicators of outdoor mobility in different countries, localities, gender and age groups.

4.2   Health and mobility in the MOBILATE study

4.2.1   Research question and hypotheses

How are the various aspects of health associated with different outdoor mobility indicators? Because health is a strong explaining factor for interindividual differences in outdoor mobility, we assume that this can be seen with different indicators of outdoor mobility. The better the health, the more active the subjects are in their outdoor mobility. Especially we assume that those being healthier make more frequently journeys measured by the trip diary's means of journeys and can also make more often longer trips, lasting at least for one week, and furthermore use more different transport modes, and have a greater number of outdoor activities when compared to the less healthy ones. Similarly it is expected that the ones with better health are more often able to walk the distance of 2 km than the ones with poorer health. Additionally the Wittenberg (1986) statements of traffic will be analysed in this context with the assumption that those having weaker health status would also state more critical attitudes towards the present traffic behaviour than those with better health status. This is due to the greater pressure of the present traffic on the ones with weaker health than on those with better health.

4.2.2   Methods

The data used for the analyses in this chapter are based on the MOBILATE Survey 2000 interviews as well as on the trip diaries described in the Methodology chapter in this publication. The specific health variables are built up on the basis of the correlation and factor analyses using the Finnish MOBILATE Survey data. The Finnish data was decided to be used on the core of the factor analyses in this stage, as the reliabilities of the participant countries were high, indicating that the structure of the factors would remain rather same in each country. The factor analysis method used was 'principal axes factoring'. Oblique rotation (oblimin) was used to produce solutions where each of the variable loadings is distinguished more clearly to one factor compared to varimax rotation. Although the factors correlate with each other, the oblimin solutions proved to be clearer to be interpreted. The analysis of the health variables resulted to three interpretable factors. On the basis of them and after analysing the Cronbach's alphas of each of the variable to be used later on in the analyses, the following sum-variables of health were formed. The ADL variables are handled as continuous ones in the factor analysis. After deciding to combine some variables with the ADL variables, these other variables were rescaled to the same scale as the ADL variables.

Factor I '*Heavier ADL-activities and physical activity*' included the following questions:
- Have you been suffering from an ailment or chronic illness which impairs your mobility constantly, periodically or not at all? (constantly = 1; temporarily = 2; no problems = 3)
- Which of the following options best describes your physical activity? (hardly any = 1; light physical activity = 2; moderate activity or physical exercise, regularly and several times a week = 3)
- Can you carry heavy bags or luggage? (without difficulties = 3; with difficulties = 2; not possible = 1)
- Can you carry beverage crates (heavy boxes)? (without difficulties = 3; with difficulties = 2; not possible = 1)
- Can you do heavy housework, e.g. washing the windows? (without difficulties = 3; with difficulties = 2; not possible = 1)

The sum-scales of the ADL-functions have been converted according to the other health-variables when forming the sum-variable, so that the greater values refer to the better ADL-functioning. The theoretical range of the heavy ADL sum is 5-15. This sum variable describes health required for heavy and demanding activities of daily living. We call it as 'Heavy activities of daily life' (Heavy ADL). Its Cronbach's alpha in the whole sample was 0.86 (see Table 4.1).

Factor II '*Lighter ADL-activities*' included the following questions:
- Can you move around your house/apartment? (without difficulties = 3; with difficulties = 2; not possible = 1)
- Can you bend down? (without difficulties = 3; with difficulties = 2; not possible = 1)
- Can you climb stairs? (without difficulties = 3; with difficulties = 2; not possible= 1)
- Can you go outdoors? (without difficulties = 3; with difficulties = 2; not possible= 1)
- Can you go for shopping? (without difficulties = 3; with difficulties = 2; not possible = 1)

- Can you do light housework, e.g. do the dishes? (without difficulties = 3; with difficulties = 2; not possible = 1).

The theoretical range of the light ADL sum varies between 6 and 18. The higher the score, the less difficulties in these tasks. This sum variable describes the capability to take care of light activities of daily life. We call it as 'Light activities of daily life' (Light ADL). Its Cronbach's alpha in the whole sample was 0.91 (see Table 4.1).

Factor III '*Satisfaction with health*' included the following self-ratings:
- Satisfaction with health (0: very unsatisfied to 10: very satisfied)
- Self-evaluation of physical mobility (from 1 = very poor to 5 = very good = 5; variable was rescaled to 0 - 10; new scale = ((old scale –1) / 4)*10)

The theoretical range of this varies between 0 and 20. The higher the score, the more satisfied a person is with his/her health. This factor describes satisfaction with health and self-estimated mobility and can be called as satisfaction with health. Its Cronbach's alpha in the whole sample was 0.75 (see Table 4.1).

Other variables to be used describing health are visual acuity score: scores from 0.02 to 1.0 (Visual Acuity Screening by Sachsenweger, 1987) and the Digit Symbol Substitution Test score measuring visual-motor coordination: scores from 0 - 67 (Oswald & Fleischmann, 1986; Wechsler, 1981). The higher the score, the better the visual acuity and cognitive speed.

For the further variance models, the sum-score of health (including 3 factors together with the visual ability and cognitive speed) was formed to study the relationship, which health has both to outdoor mobility and to the leisure time activities. When correlating the five health variables with each other their intercorrelations were found to be high. Thus, the average score of each of them was calculated using standardized values (z-values) and these were summed up. To find out possible independent effects of individual health variables, the average score was controlled in the statistical model by using two step analysis strategy. First the variance analysis model was estimated by using only the average score of health variables and the residual score was saved as a variable. The next step was that the five health variables were analysed by using the residual score as a dependent variable. The reliability of the health-sum in the whole sample was high 0.80 (0.76 Finland; 0.82 both eastern and western Germany; 0.78 Hungary; 0.80 Italy and 0.74 the Netherlands).

The mean number of journeys per day from the trip diary was used as one indicator of outdoor mobility. Similarly the item 'Can you walk at least 2 km?' was used as another indicator of the outdoor mobility variable and it was handled as a continuous variable.

Also the sum-variable of the statements on traffic (Wittenberg, 1986) was used as third indicator in detecting the relation of health to outdoor mobility. The response choices for these 18 items were: not true = 1; partly true = 2; true = 3; do not know/do not use = 4. 'Do not know/do not use' -answers were handled as missing data in the analyses when forming the sum-score. The Cronbach's alpha of the Wittenberg statements was 0.86. The factor structure of these items was also analysed on the basis of the Finnish data. It resulted to three factors, which however correlated moderately with each other. Due to these intercorrelations it was decided to use only the arithmetical sum of these 18 items. Wittenberg's statements seem to assess a quite general acceptance vs. critical attitude towards the prevailing traffic.

Table 4.1: Reliability of the factors (Cronbach's Alphas) in general and separately in different countries

Reliability of the factors	Heavy ADL	Light ADL	Satisfaction with health	Sum of health	Traffic today
Generally	.86	.91	.75	.80	.86
FIN	.85	.88	.70	.76	.83
GER (E)	.88	.93	.79	.82	.89
GER (W)	.87	.93	.78	.82	.90
HUN	.86	.90	.71	.78	.88
IT	.85	.90	.65	.80	.72
NL	.85	.90	.72	.74	.77

Note. MOBILATE Survey 2000; Total N = 3837.
The first 4 factors relate to the health factors and the last one to the outdoor mobility.

The reliability of 'Heavy ADL' sum is very high in different countries varying between 0.85 and 0.88. Also the sum of 'Light ADL' is even more highly reliable (Cronbach's alphas 0.88 - 0.93). The reliability of the sum of satisfaction with health is satisfactory (0.65 - 0.79). Health-sum has also quite high reliabilities in different countries (0.74 - 0.82). The reliabilities of Wittenberg statements are very high in other countries (0.83 - 0.90) except in Italy and the Netherlands, which had the coefficients of 0.72 and 0.77.

4.2.3 Statistical analyses

The health-related analyses were made using the strata-based data. The aim was to analyse the effects of localities (country; region), gender and age. When analysing the health variables, age has been included into the models to demonstrate the strong relations of age to them. In the analyses on the health's relationship to the outdoor mobility, age is not included any more in the models as age is having such a strong impact to health, and health, on the other hand, defines these other domains in a large part. The statistical analyses methods used in this chapter consists also of variance analyses. Because of the large number of subjects, only effects significant at least at the level $p < .01$ were taken into account and interpreted.

In the univariate analysis of variance, the distributions of the residuals for observed variables were normal enough in most variables enabling us to count on the models' results ($p < .01$). However, there were two variables, namely holiday trips lasting at least for one week, and indoor activities that were skewed and were therefore transformed to the logarithmic scale before the actual analyses. In the figures, the predicted values of these two variables are changed from the logarithmic values back to the values based on the basic scales by using the exponential transformation. Models test the effect of each factor (e.g. age*gender -interaction) after all the other effects have been controlled. Firstly, all main and interaction effects are included into the model, after which the most complex, non-significant effects from the model will be excluded, one-by-one. The factor's own effect to the model will not be interpreted if this variable has an interaction, at the same time, with some other variable/-s.

When building ANOVA/ANCOVA models, we actually used GLM (generalised linear model) univariate procedure in SPSS when testing the effects. In that procedure the predictors could be categorical and/or continuous. In the first step we estimated the full model - e.g. all the main effects and interaction effects. Using sum of squares partition method means that all other effects in the model are controlled when testing some specific (main or interaction) effects.

The basic analysis demonstrates that age's relation to health variables is non-linear. Adding the second order polynomial term (quadratic AGE^2=age*age) to the model, the scatter plot of age and residual values shows no more dependence. After that we decided to include quadratic term of age into the models.

The model was built so that if the highest interaction term in the model was not statistically significant, it has been removed. If some interaction term was statistically significant, all the lower level effects were included in the model, despite their statistical significance. As an example: if gender*age interaction was significant, it meant that magnitude of age's effect was different in women than with men or that difference between men and women depended on age. So we additionally needed the basic effect of age and gender in the model. For example, when building the model of satisfaction with health, the highest possible interaction effect was COUNTRY*REGION*GENDER*AGE^2 which we leave outside of the model in the first step due to insignificance. After estimating the model, we found that there were three 3-way non-significant effects. The higher p-value is in COUNTRY*GENDER*AGE^2 effect. After estimating the model without the above mentioned two effects, we found that there were two 3-way non-significant effects and the higher p-value is in REGION*GENDER*AGE^2 effect. When continuing this stepwise modelling we came to the final results.

If some effects, e.g. effect related to differences between countries, were found, we decided to omit a more detailed analysis (pair wise comparisons) and interpreted the results roughly by pictures based on the predicted values. Predicted values are calculated using estimates of the model parameters. Using these predicted values instead of observed means is necessary in describing the models consisting of continuous predictors. In the final model of satisfaction with health there is e.g. country*age interaction effect. It means that the age's effect differs between countries. This effect is similar between urban women, urban men, rural women and rural men. That is because age and country interaction terms are not connected to the gender effect. Also we could describe the country*age effect using the picture made for rural women. In that manner we need three different pictures interpreting results of satisfaction with health.

Regression analyses were furthermore done to find out the best health explanators of different outdoor mobility indicators.

4.3   The relation between health and outdoor mobility

4.3.1   The relation between health and single outdoor mobility variables

Being able to walk at least 2 km

For interpreting Figure 4.1 concerning ability to walk at least 2 km, the code value 3 refers to ability to walk this distance without difficulties, value 2 to walk only with difficulties and value 1 not capable for that long walk. Gender's own effect as well as significant interactions of country*region and region*health-sum were seen when analysing the 2 km walking ability.

More men were able to walk the distance of 2 km's compared to women. The differences between urban and rural regions varied in different countries. In Hungary, both western and eastern Germany as well as in Finland the subjects in the urban regions were more often able to walk the distance of 2 km compared to the rural subjects, whereas in the

Netherlands this was opposite, which can be due to the suburban character of the rural Dutch area under investigation. No differences were found between Italian subjects in the urban and rural regions.

Similarly the effect of health-sum to the 2 km walking ability differed in different regions. Those having better health status were more often able to walk 2 km although in the rural regions the health-sum had the slightly more obvious relation to the ability to walk 2 km compared to the urban regions. In spite of the health-sum, the rural region's subjects were able to walk 2 km more often compared to the urban subjects. Could we perhaps assume that the rural subjects need to do more walking in reaching certain services or social contacts, or perhaps the nature itself in the rural regions would tempt the citizens to pursue more walking in their livinghood areas? It probably depends on acquired personal habits, since in both areas people are able to walk 2 km.

Figure 4.1: Being able to walk at least 2 km by country*location*gender

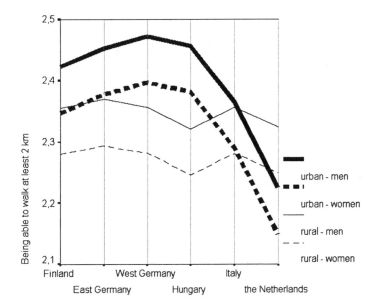

The mean number of journeys per day from the trip-diary

As regards the mean numbers of journeys related to health, significant interactions were found. The differences between urban and rural regions varied in different countries (Figure 4.2). In Finland, eastern Germany, Hungary and the Netherlands the subjects in the urban regions showed generally higher means of journeys per day compared to the rural subjects, whereas in western Germany and Italy this was opposite. In Italy, inhabitants of rural areas usually went out many times during day in order to carry out agricultural activities around the house, to have a chat with the neighbours, favoured by good weather conditions and short distances between the villages and the houses.

Also the gender's effect on the means of journeys per day differed in the participant countries. Especially in Italy, but also in the other countries, except in the Netherlands, men had higher means of journeys per day compared to women (Figure 4.2). This could, perhaps, be explained by the better health status of men, possibly by their more vivid outdoor leisure activity level compared to women or by men owning and driving cars more often than women.

Figure 4.2: The mean number of journeys per day by country*location*gender

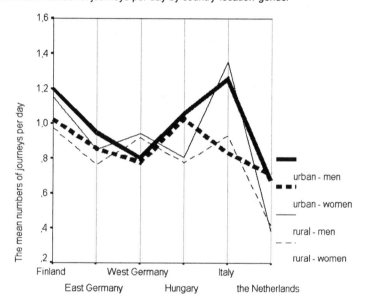

Similarly the effect of health-sum differed in the participant countries. In Figure 4.3 it can be noted that the health-sum had the most obvious relation to the means of journeys per day made in Finland and Italy, whereas the weakest relationship can be noted in the Netherlands and eastern Germany. In Figure 4.3 it is shown as an example how rural women differing in their health had made a variety amount of journeys per day in different participating countries. The values '+sd' and '-sd' in Figure 4.3 demonstrate the journeys made per day by the women with deviant health-sum. The middle in Figure 4.3 describes the amount of journeys per day made by those women having an average health-sum. Generally, the healthier people are, the higher the number of journeys per day.

Figure 4.3:   The mean number of journeys per day by country*health

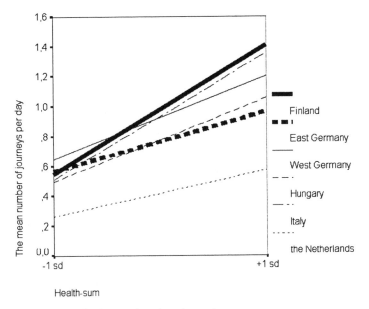

Health-sum

Note. The predicted values are based on the rural women

Traffic attitudes

One important factor for outdoor mobility are the attitudes and values of the subjects towards traffic in general and specially towards its different subject-groups like walkers, cyclists, car drivers and the public transport users. We can assume that there are cultural differences as well as health-related differences in these traffic attitudes. The findings show that health-sum and gender have significant own effects on the Wittenberg traffic statements as well as there is one significant interaction country*region. Generally, those who are healthier as well as men have more positive attitudes towards the present traffic. The country*region (Figure 4.4) interaction is based on the differences which can be found in Finland, eastern Germany and the Netherlands in the direction of the rural citizens being less critical than the urban ones. This could be a result of the less heavy traffic in the rural regions or, on the other hand, for example of the subjects not needing the public transportation because having mostly cars on their own etc. In Hungary an opposite result to the above mentioned countries was seen. One explanation to this could be the more limited private and public transportation possibilities in the rural regions of Hungary than in the other participant countries. In western Germany and Italy there were no urban-rural differences in the traffic attitudes.

Figure 4.4:   Predicted Wittenberg's statements on the traffic by country*location*gender

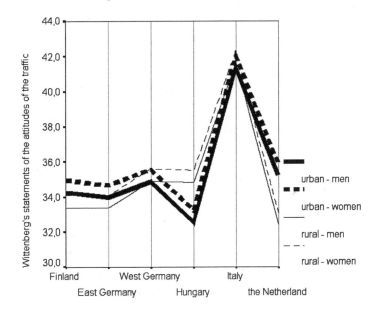

4.3.2   The relations between health and outdoor mobility indicators

The options of transport modes used

A significant 3-way country*region*health-sum interaction was found as regards the number
of transport modes used. In each country and region the subjects with better health used more
various transport modes. The effect of health was, however, different between countries and
the localities. Generally urban citizens had greater differences in using transport modes due to
their health. The greatest differences between subjects of better and poorer health both in
urban and rural localities were noted in Finland and the Netherlands, additionally the
difference between urban western Germans of different health status was high (Figure 4.5).
Health had the least effect on the use of various transport modes in Italy and Hungary.

Figure 4.5: Transport modes and sum of health by country*region*health

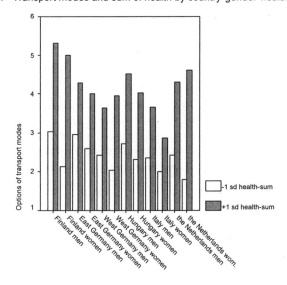

Note: Predicted values based on the women

Another 3-way interaction was that of country*gender*health-sum. In each country both men and women with better health used more different types of transport modes than those with poorer health, as could be expected (Figure 4.6). This was noted most clearly in Finland and the Netherlands, where health additionally affected more women than men in the use of different transport modes. The smallest effect that health had on the use of different transport modes was in Italy, where health was a more prevalent determinant on using the different transport modes among men than women.

Figure 4.6: Transport modes and sum of health by country*gender*health

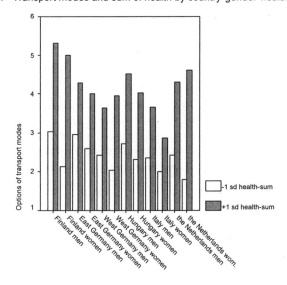

Note: Predicted values based on the rural region

There are more different transport modes to be used both by men and women in the urban than rural regions due to the bigger variety of transport options in the cities. Men generally use more different options of transport modes than women, which is even more evident in the rural regions.

The options of outdoor activities

The significant 3-way country*region*health-sum interaction was found as regards the number of outdoor activities. In all participant countries and every region those with better health took part in more different outdoor activities than the ones with poorer health (Figure 4.7). The clearest differences between regions were seen in Hungary and Italy, where the rural citizens with better health status had clearly more different outdoor activities than their urban fellows.

Figure 4.7:   Outdoor activities and sum of health by country*region*health

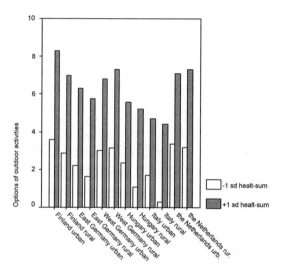

Note. Predicted values based on the women

Additionally a 2-way interaction of country*gender was noted. Men and women take part in outdoor activities in different ways in the participant countries (Figure 4.8). In Italy rural men had clearly more different outdoor activities they engage in than women, whereas in Finland and the Netherlands this was opposite. Both in western and eastern Germany as well as in Hungary there were not so big differences between genders.

Figure 4.8: Outdoor activities and sum of health by country*gender

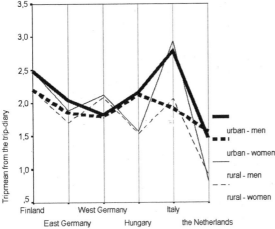

The means of trips lasting at least one week made since the beginning of 2000

Three significant 2-way interactions were found as regards the means of holiday trips lasting at least one week. Country*region interaction is illustrated in Figure 4.9. In Finland there were no differences between urban and rural citizens' mean numbers of trips, whereas in the Netherlands and Hungary the urban citizens had higher means for trips than their rural fellows. In western Germany this was reverse.

Similarly a 2-way interaction of country*gender was noted (Figure 4.9). In Hungary, the Netherlands, and western Germany women and men had about the same mean numbers for the trips lasting at least one week, whereas in Finland, eastern Germany and especially in Italy men did more trips than women.

Figure 4.9: Means of trips lasting at least one week by country*region, and country*gender

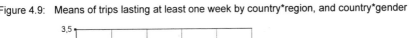

Additionally country*health-sum interaction was noted, as healthier subjects making generally more trips in each country. Figure 4.10 demonstrates health's greatest effect on the means of trips in Finland and Italy, whereas the mildest effects were noted in the Netherlands and eastern Germany.

Figure 4.10: Means of trips lasting at least one week by country*health-sum

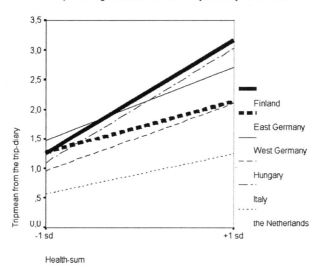

Note. Predicted values based on the rural women

4.4 Regression analyses of health variables explaining outdoor mobility indicators

4.4.1 Regression analyses of transport modes used

Regression analyses were used to find out which background variables as well as which health indicators were strongest related to different used outdoor mobility indicators. As background variables age, gender and urban vs. rural living region were chosen, which we have noted to be in relation to health as well as to outdoor mobility. We did the regression analyses by countries, controlling the chosen background variables. When analysing the tables, only results with significance level at least $p<.01$ are presented. The 'best' health explanators for the transport modes used differed in the participant countries, those being Digit Symbol Substitution Test score for Finland and Italy, self-evaluated physical mobility for eastern Germany and Hungary, satisfaction with health for western Germany, and LnADL (sum of ADL with logarithm-values) and self-rated physical mobility for Hungary and LnADL for the Netherlands. This makes it impossible just to choose one best explanator of health to the regression analyses of transport modes used (Table 4.2). The background variables explained differently the transport modes used across participant countries.

Table 4.2: Regression analyses of transport modes used

Country	Variable	Beta	t	p
Finland	Gender	-.109	-2.72	.007
	Region	-.178	-4.67	.000
	Visus	.137	3.31	.001
	Digit Symbol Substitution Test	.189	3.51	.000
Eastern Germany	Age	-.273	-7.23	.000
	Gender	-.098	-3.19	.001
	Region	-.098	-3.25	.001
	Physical mobility	.168	3.68	.000
	Visus	.112	3.20	.001
Western Germany	Age	-.172	-4.81	.000
	Region	-.403	-13.71	.000
	LnADL	.148	3.32	.001
	Satisfaction with health	.159	3.58	.000
	Digit Symbol Substitution Test	.126	3.82	.000
Hungary	Age	-.125	-2.85	.004
	Gender	-.149	-3.95	.000
	LnADL	.181	3.31	.001
	Physical mobility	.181	3.21	.001
	Digit Symbol Substitution Test	.172	3.94	.000
Italy	Gender	-.215	-6.42	.000
	Region	-.276	-8.08	.000
	Physical mobility	.130	3.02	.003
	Digit Symbol Substitution Test	.329	7.57	.000
The Netherlands	Age	-.137	-3.00	.003
	Region	-.186	-4.53	.000
	LnADL	.168	2.86	.004
	Satisfaction with health	.156	2.89	.004

Note. MOBILATE Survey 2000; Total N = 3936;
Due to sum of ADL being greatly skewed to right (maximum score got by 24%
subjects), the logarithm- values of ADL (LnADL) were used. The other variables are
accepted into the regression model in their original format.

4.4.2 Regression analyses of outdoor activities subjects take part in

The best health explanators for the outdoor activities subjects engage in differed in the
participant countries, them being Digit Symbol Substitution Test both for eastern and western
Germany, Hungary, and Italy, self-evaluated physical mobility for the Netherlands, and
LnADL for Finland (Table 4.3). This makes it impossible just to choose one best explanator
of health to the regression analyses of outdoor activities. There are, additionally, theoretical
reasons to select the Digit Symbol Substitution Test, which represents validly the cognitive
functioning, which is needed in varying degrees in different outdoor activities. The
background variables explained differently the outdoor activities subjects take part in across
the participant countries.

Table 4.3:   Regression analyses of outdoor activities

Country	Variable	Beta	t	p
Finland	Gender	.105	2.72	.007
	Region	-.139	-3.77	.000
	LnADL	.255	4.68	.000
	Visus	.117	2.91	.004
Eastern Germany	Region	-.106	-3.78	.000
	LnADL	.159	3.76	.000
	Satisfaction with health	.149	3.81	.000
	Physical mobility	.156	3.68	.000
	Visus	.162	4.97	.000
	Digit Symbol Substitution Test	.201	6.42	.000
Western Germany	Age	-.109	-2.97	.003
	LnADL	.148	3.22	.001
	Satisfaction with health	.180	3.95	.000
	Digit Symbol Substitution Test	.196	5.76	.000
Hungary	LnADL	.204	3.66	.000
	Physical mobility	.200	3.48	.001
	Digit Symbol Substitution Test	.226	5.05	.000
Italy	Age	-.166	-3.42	.001
	Gender	-.218	-5.73	.000
	Region	-.179	-4.60	.000
	Physical mobility	.134	2.73	.007
	Digit Symbol Substitution Test	.205	4.17	.000
The Netherlands	Physical mobility	.166	2.79	.005

Note. MOBILATE Survey 2000; Total N = 3936
Due to sum of ADL being greatly skewed to right (maximum score got by 24%
subjects), the logarithm- values of ADL (LnADL) were used. The other variables are
accepted into the regression model in their original format.

4.4.3   Regression analyses of means of trips from the trip-diary

The best health explanators for the means of trips differed in the participant countries, them
being Digit Symbol Substitution Test for Finland, eastern Germany, and Italy, and self-
evaluated physical mobility for Hungary (Table 4.4). The background variables explained
differently the tripmean across participant countries.

Table 4.4: Regression analyses of tripmean from the trip-diary

Country	Variable	Beta	t	p
Finland	Gender	-.120	-2.78	.006
	Digit Symbol Substitution Test	.250	4.30	.000
Eastern Germany	LnADL	.163	3.12	.002
	Digit Symbol Substitution Test	.164	4.22	.000
Western Germany	Age	-.136	-3.19	.001
Hungary	Region	-.233	-5.82	.000
	Physical mobility	.233	3.93	.000
	Digit Symbol Substitution Test	.179	3.90	.000
Italy	Gender	-.228	-5.89	.000
	Physical mobility	.151	3.03	.003
	Digit Symbol Substitution Test	.299	5.96	.000
The Netherlands	Region	-.207	-4.64	.000

Note. MOBILATE Survey 2000; Total N = 3936
Due to sum of ADL being greatly skewed to right (maximum score got by 24%
subjects), the logarithm- values of ADL (LnADL) were used. The other variables are
accepted into the regression model in their original format.

4.5   Discussion

The general theoretical model of the MOBILATE project has described out-of-home mobility
to be based on the interaction between an individual, his/her transport modes in usage and
his/her living environment. Of the individual's resources, health can be seen as the most
important one and its lack or weaknesses as risk factors causing difficulties and obstacles in
outdoor mobility. Health is also perhaps the most universal factor affecting on the outdoor
mobility generally at the same way independent of the country, region and gender. With
increasing age and decreasing health all transport modes were reduced and the outdoor
mobility decreased. This could similarily be found out in the regression analyses, in which,
regardless of the outdoor mobility indicator predicted, the health-related variables like
performance of the ADL or self-rated physical mobility explained the largest part of different
outdoor indicators' variance.

The obstacles and difficulties caused by health can, in different degree, be compensated
at the individual, transport mode and environmental level. At individual level many technical
aids can be used beginning from spectacles, artificial joints and limbs and ending to
motorized wheel-chairs with different aids. Likewise biological means, like different
medicines, can be used for improving the outdoor mobility in case of diseases restricting the
outdoor mobility. Other possible compensatory means concern social factors like travelling as
a passenger in a private car or using special public transport services arranged for people
having outdoor mobility obstacles and difficulties. The third level for using compensatory
measures is the living environment like the density of roadnet and different factors making the
usage of public transport easier or more difficult, e.g. different kinds of lifts and wheel-chair
ramps. To the environment belong additionally the geographical and climatical factors like
steep hills or snow and ice making the mobility in outdoors more difficult as well to young
age-groups. Because of the possibility to use very different compensatory mechanisms, the
health's effect on outdoor mobility is, in principle and practice, modifiable by these measures.

Additionally it has to be taken into account that the outdoor mobility affects on health and perhaps this is one very important preventive factor in keeping aged people healthy or at least slowing down the weakening of their health. One of the ways for facilitating this is to build a secure street network for walkers and cyclists.

Age is so many-sided variable that its explanatory value remains very diffuse. Age includes the biological, psychological and social changes, which the individual experiences; at the same time it includes both all the expectations other members in a society have to the ageing persons and the written legislation regarding the status of aged persons in a society. One of the first factors labelling a person 'old' is the retirement age and then all other regulations concerning the allowed participation of aged persons in different public and private organizations. Also the unwritten expectations concerning the 'acceptable' way of behaviour may very strongly affect the behaviour of the ageing persons. It has been said that due to age having so strong relations to many kinds of behaviour it, in fact, explains nothing; only the specific variables describing age-related changes are usable explanators when trying to find out what exactly in the ageing process is causing different changes in behaviour.

The regression analyses, including besides background variables also different health indicators broadly defined, showed that different socio-economic background and health indicators 'explain' different outdoor mobility indicators in different countries. This needs more analyses on the basis of existing MOBILATE data.

4.6   Conclusions

Along ageing, all indicators of health, as well as outdoor mobility show worse health status and less outdoor mobility among the older strata than among the younger ones as was assumed. The better health was related to the greater number of journeys made/day, especially in Finland and Italy. Similarly healthier people were more often able to walk the distance of 2 km compared to the less healthy subjects; this being even more the case in the rural than in the urban areas. Those being healthier also stated to be more satisfied with the present traffic than the ones with poorer health status. These results supported our hypotheses.

It was assumed that with men better self-rated health would remain in the 'advanced ages' compared to the women. With the ADL-functions, this could be noted from the age of about 60 years old till the age of about 83 years old, after which the opposite tendency could be seen. The gender difference could be seen in the ability to walk at least 2 km. A higher number of men than women in every country and region replied to this question positively. The means of trips were lower among women than men, especially in Finland and Italy. In other countries the gender differences in this respect were negligible. In Finland and Italy clearly more men than women had a driver's licence and therefore men were able to drive a car on their own which might explain this result. It is obviously more convenient and faster to do more trips with a car than either by bicycle or walking. Gender differences between the countries are strong and depend on attitudes and cultural patterns. In Italy the older women, especially in rural areas, have strong social roles inside the family as mothers, grandmothers or wives thus keeping them at home.

The urban-rural differences varied from country to country, although being quite small as regards health and outdoor mobility indicators. Perhaps the generally better medical care in urban areas compared to rural regions can be seen in the better health of the urban aged persons than among their counterparts in the rural regions. The urban-rural differences in transport modes and outdoor activities are related to the differences in supply of the different transport modes and outdoor activity possibilities. It is worthwhile to emphasize the clear urban-rural differences in the ability to walk 2 km, urban subjects showing a higher competence for that task. The urban-rural differences generally favoured the urban subjects compared to the rural ones as regards the health and outdoor mobility indicators. However, especially among the western German participants, regional differences remained generally negligible.

The country-based differences regarding different outdoor mobility indicators can, at least be partly explained by the population density and besides it by the density of the road and other traffic routes. These affect the distances and times to get services, to participate in outdoor activities and to meet relatives and friends. Of the MOBILATE countries, Finland and the Netherlands represent the both extremes. The supply of different transport modes and outdoor leisure activities have the greatest distances in Finland and the shortest in the Netherlands.

Although the MOBILATE Survey data are cross-sectional, we analysed how different health-variables are related to different outdoor mobility indicators. As regards the transport modes used, the strongest explanators differed in the participant countries. Digit Symbol Substitution Test and self-rated physical mobility "explained" the number of transport modes used in Hungary and Italy, visus and Digit Symbol Substitution Test in Finland, visus and self-rated physical mobility in eastern Germany, satisfaction with health and Digit Symbol Substitution Test in western Germany, and satisfaction with health in the Netherlands. However, the 'explanators' often differed only very little in regard to their beta-values. Besides, their "explaining" power remained very low. In most countries also age, gender, and region were significant 'explanators' of the transport modes used. For the outdoor activities especially the Digit Symbol Substitution Test and ADL were the variables 'explaining' it in most countries. Additionally, in most countries age, gender, and region were related to the outdoor activities indicator. It shall be mentioned that in the Netherlands only self-rated physical mobility related to outdoor activities significantly. Likewise these could explain only a very small part of variance of the number of outdoor activities. The variables 'explaining' the number of trips varied quite a lot being Digit Symbol Substitution Test in Finland, in addition ADL in eastern Germany, and in addition self-rated physical mobility in Italy as well as in Hungary. Besides age, gender and region were differently related to the means of trips. In western Germany only age and in the Netherlands only region were related to the means of trips. Altogether, the above mentioned variables "explained" a very small part of variance of the amount of trips based on the trip diaries. One explanation for the different findings of the regression analyses based on health indicators is their high interrelationships which cause random variation in the combinations, which in the regression analyses have resulted in varying 'explanators' of the different outdoor mobility indicators.

References

Abrums, M. (2000). "Jesus will fix it after awhile": Meanings and health. *Social Science and Medicine, 50*, 89-105.

Baumann, J. U. (1994). Gait changes in elderly people. *Orthopade, 23*, 6-9.

Bennett, K. M. B., & Castiello, U. (1994). Reach to grasp: Changes with age. *Journal of Gerontology, 49*(B), P1-P7.

Birren, J. E. (1974). Translations in gerontology - from lab to life. Psychophysiology and speed of response. *American Psychology, 29*, 808 - 815.

Buchner, D. M., Beresford, S. A., Larson, E. B., LaCroix, A. Z., & Wagner, E. H. (1992). Effects of exercise on functional status in older adults: interventional studies. *Annual Review of Public Health, 13*, 469-488.

Busse, E. W. (1993). Duke University longitudinal studies of aging. *Zeitschrift für Psychologie, 26*, 123-128.

Carnahan, H., Vandervoot, A. A., & Swanson, L. R. (1998). The influence of aging and target motion on the control of prehension. *Experimental Aging Research, 24*, 289-306.

Chaput, S., & Proteau, L. (1996). Modification with aging in the role played by vision and proprioception for movement control. *Experimental Aging Research, 22*, 1-21.

Era, P., & Rantanen, T. (1997). Changes in physical capacity and sensory/psychomotor functions from 75 to 80 years of age and from 80 to 85 years of age - A longitudinal study. *Scandinavian Journal of Social Medicine, Suppl, 53*, 25-43.

Fiatarone, M. A. (1990). Exercise in the oldest old. *Topics of Geriatric Rehabilitation, 5*, 63-77.

Frändin, K., Johanneson, K., & Grimby, G. (1992). Physical activity as part of an intervention program for elderly persons in Göteborg. *Scandinavian Journal of Medicine & Science in Sports, 2*, 218-224.

George, L. K. (2001). The social psychology of health. In R. H. Binstock, & L. K. George (Eds.), *Handbook of aging and the social sciences* (pp. 217-237). New York: Academic Press.

Gottlob, L. R., & Madden, D. J. (1999). Age differences in the strategic allocation of visual attention. *Journal of Gerontology, 54 B*, 165-172.

Grimby, G., Grimby, A., Frändin, K., & Wiklund, I. (1992). Physically fit and active elderly people have a higher quality of life. *Scandinavian Journal of Medicine & Science in Sports, 2*, 225-230.

Guralnik, J. M, LaCroix, A. Z., Abbott, R. D., Berkman, L. F., Satterfield, S., Evans, D. A., & Wallace, R. B. (1993). Maintaining mobility in late life. I. Demographic characteristics and chronic conditions. *American Journal of Epidemiology, 137*, 845-857

Häkkinen, K., Kallinen, M., Izquierdo, M., Jokelainen, K., Lassila, H., Mälkiä, E., Kraemer, W. J., Newton, R. U., & Alen, M. (1998). Changes in agonist-antagonist EMG, muscle CSA, and force during strength training in middle-aged and older people. *Journal of Applied Physiology, 84*, 1341-1349.

Häkkinen, K., Kraemer, W. J., Kallinen, M., Linnamo, V., Pastinen, U. M., & Newton, R. U. (1996). Bilateral and unilateral neuromuscular function and muscle cross-sectional area in middle-aged and elderly men and women. *Journal of Gerontology, 51 A*, B21-B29.

Heikkinen, E., Era, P., Jokela, J., Jylhä, M., Lyyra, A., & Pohjolainen, P. (1992). Socio-economic and life-style factors as modulators of health and functional capacity with age. In J. J. F. Schroots (Eds.), *Aging, health and competence* (pp. 65-86). Amsterdam: Elsevier Science Publishers.

Heikkinen, E., Leinonen, R., Berg, S., Schroll, M., & Steen, B. (1997). Levels and associates of self-rated health among 75-year-old people living in three Nordic localities. In E. Heikkinen, S. Berg, M. Schroll, B. Stehen, & A. Viidik (Eds.), *Facts, Research and Intervention in Geriatrics* (pp. 121-148). Paris: Serdi Publisher.

Ho, S.C., Woo, J., Yuen, Y. K., Sham, A., & Chan, S. G. (1997). Predictors of mobility decline: the Hong Kong old-old study. *Journal of Gerontology, 52 A*, M356-M362.

Idler, E. L. (1993). Age differences in self-assessments of health: Age changes, cohort differences, or survivorship? *Journal of Gerontology: Social Sciences, 48*, 289-300.

Jalavisto, E., Lindqvist, C., & Makkonen, T. (1964). Assessment of biological age. Mental and neural factors in longevity. *Annales Academiae Scientiarum Fennicae*. Series A. V. Medica 106/1. Helsinki.

Jylhä, M. (1994). Self-rated health revisited: Exploring survey interview episodes with elderly respondents. *Social Science and Medicine, 39*, 983-990.

Jylhä, M., Guralnik, J. M., Balfour, J., & Fried, L. P. (2001). Walking difficulty, walking speed, and age as predictors of self-rated health: The Women's Health and Aging Study. *The Journals of Gerontology. Biological Sciences and Medical Sciences, 56 A*, M609-M617.

Jylhä, M., Guralnik, J. M., Ferrucci, L., Jokela, J., & Heikkinen, E. (1998). Is self-rated health comparable across cultures and genders? *Journal of Gerontology: Social Sciences, 53 B*, 144-152.

Ketcham, C. J., & Stelmach, G. E. (2001). Age-related declines in motor control. In J. E. Birren, & K. W. Schaie (Eds.), *Handbook of the psychology of aging* (pp. 313-348). New York: Academic Press.

Kivinen, P., Halonen, P., Eronen, M., & Nissinen, A. (1998). Self-rated health, physician rated health and associated factors among elderly men: the Finnish cohorts of the Seven Countries Study. *Age and Ageing, 27*, 41-47.

Laukkanen, P., Heikkinen, E., & Kauppinen, M. (1995). Muscle strength and mobility as predictors of survival in 75-84 -year-old people. *Age Ageing, 24*, 468-473.

Laukkanen, P., Heikkinen, E., Schroll, M., & Kauppinen, M. (1997). A comparative study of factors related to carrying out physical activities of daily living (PADL) among 75-year-old men and women in two Nordic localities. *Aging. Clinical and Experimental Research, 9*, 258-267.

Laukkanen, P., Kauppinen, M., & Heikkinen, E. (1998). Physical activity as a predictor of health and disability in 75- and 80-year-old men and women: A five-year longitudinal study. *Journal of Aging and Physical Activity, 6*, 141-156.

Laukkanen, P., Leinonen, R., & Heikkinen, E. (1999). Health status among Finnish persons born 1904-23 in an eight-year follow-up study by the Evergreen project. In T. Suutama, I. Ruoppila, & P. Laukkanen (Eds.), *Changes in functional abilities among elderly people. Findings from an eight-year follow-up study by the Evergreen project* (pp. 133-170). Helsinki: The Social Insurance Institution, Finland, Studies in Social Security and Health, 42.

Laukkanen, P., Sakari-Rantala, R., Kauppinen, M., & Heikkinen, E. (1997). Morbidity and disability in 75- and 80-year-old men and women. A five-year follow-up. *Scandinavian Journal of Social Medicine, Suppl.* 53, 79-100.

Laursen, P. (1997). The impact of aging on cognitive functions. An 11 year follow-up study of four age cohorts. *Acta Neurologica Scandinavica, 96, Suppl. 172.*

Leinonen, R., Heikkinen, E., & Jylhä, M. (1998). Self-rated health and self-assessed change in health in elderly men and women. A five-year longitudinal study. *Social Science & Medicine, 46*, 591-597.

Leinonen, R., Heikkinen, E., & Jylhä, M. (1999). A path analysis model of self-rated health among older people. *Aging. Clinical and Experimental Research, 11*, 209-20.

Leinonen, R., Heikkinen, E., & Jylhä, M. (2001a). Predictors of decline in self-assessments of health among older people. A five-year longitudinal study. *Social Science & Medicine, 52*, 1329-1341.

Leinonen, R., Heikkinen, E., & Jylhä, M. (2001b). A pattern of long-term predictors of self-rated health among older people. *Aging. Clinical and Experimental Research, 13*, 454-464.

Leinonen, R., Heikkinen, E., & Jylhä, M. (2002). Changes in health, functional performance and activity predict changes in self-rated health: A 10-year follow-up study in older people. *Archives of Gerontology and Geriatrics, 35*, 79-92.

Leventhal, H., Rabin, C., Leventhal, E. A., & Burns, E. (2001). Health risk behaviours and aging. In J. E. Birren & K. W. Schaie (Eds.), *Handbook of the psychology of aging* (pp. 186-214). New York: Academic Press.

Manderbacka, K., Lahelma, E., & Martikainen, P. (1998). Examining the continuity of self-rated health. *International Journal of Epidemiology, 27*, 208-213.

Mortensen, E. L., & Kleven, M. (1993). A WAIS longitudinal study of cognitive development during the life span from ages 50 to 70. *Developmental Neuropsychology, 9*, 115-130.

Oswald, W. D., & Fleischmann, U. M. (1986). *Nürnberger-Alters-Inventar (NAI)*. Universität Erlangen-Nürnberg: Eigenverlag.

Rantanen, T., & Avela, J. (1997). Leg extension power and walking speed in very old people living independently. *Journal of Gerontology, 52 A*, M225 - M231.

Rantanen, T., Guralnik, J. M., Foley, M., Masaki, K., Leveille, S., Curb, J. D., & White, L. (1999). Midlife hand grip strength as a predictor of old age disability. *The Journal of the American Medical Association, 281*, 558-560.

Rantanen, T., Harris, T., Leveille, S. G., Visser, M., Foley, D., Masaki, K., Curb, D. J., & Guralnik, J. (2000). Muscle strength and body mass index as long-term predictors of mortality in initially healthy men. *Journal of Gerontology: Medical Sciences, 55 A*, M168 - M173.

Robinson-Whelen, S., & Kiecolt-Glaser, J. (1997). The importance of social versus temporal comparison appraisals among older adults. *Journal of Applied Social Psychology, 27,* 959-966.

Ruoppila, I. & Suutama, T. (1997). Cognitive functioning of 75- and 80-year-old people and changes during a 5-year follow-up. In E. Heikkinen, R-L. Heikkinen, & I. Ruoppila (Eds.), *Functional capacity and health of elderly people - the Evergreen project. Scandinavian Journal of Social Medicine, Suppl. 53,* 44-65.

Sachsenweger, M. (1987). *Nahsehproben* [Near Visual Acuity Test]. Stuttgart: Gustav Fischer.

Sakari-Rantala, R., Heikkinen, E., & Ruoppila, I. (1995). Difficulties in mobility among elderly people and their association with socioeconomic factors, dwelling environment and use of services. *Aging. Clinical and Experimental Research, 7,* 433-440.

Sakari-Rantala, R., Laukkanen, P., & Heikkinen, E. (1999). Self-assessed functional capacity of Finnish elderly people in an eight-year follow-up. In T. Suutama, I. Ruoppila, & P. Laukkanen (Eds.), *Changes in functional abilities among elderly people: Findings from an eight-year follow-up study by the Evergreen project* (pp. 171-197). Helsinki: The Social Insurance Institution, Finland, Studies in Social Security and Health, 42.

Salthouse, T. A. (1985). *A theory of cognitive aging.* Amsterdam: North-Holland.

Schaie, K. W. (1993). The Seattle Longitudinal Study: a thirty-five-year inquiry of adult intellectual development. *Zeitschrift für Gerontologie, 26,* 129-137.

Schroll, M. (1994). The main pathway to musculoskeletal disability. *Scandinavian Journal of Medicine & Science in Sports, 4,* 3-12.

Schroll, M., Avlund, K., Era, P., Gause-Nilsson, I. & Davidson, M. (1997). Chronic diseases and functional ability in three Nordic localities: Musculoskeletal diseases, functional limitations and lower limb function. In E. Heikkinen, S. Berg, M. Schroll, B. Steen & A. Viidik (Eds.), *Facts, Research and Intervention in Geriatrics* (pp. 149 - 168). Paris: Serdi Publisher.

Seidler-Dobrin, R. D., & Stelmach, G. E. (1998). Persistence in visual feedback control by the elderly. *Experimental Brain Research, 119,* 467-474.

Sihvonen, S., Rantanen, T., & Heikkinen, E. (1998). Physical activity and survival in elderly people: A five-year follow-up. *Journal of Aging and Physical Activity, 6,* 133-140.

Sipilä, S., Multanen, J., Kallinen, M., Era, P., & Suominen, H. (1996). Effects of strength and endurance training on isometric muscle strength and walking speed in elderly women. *Acta Physiologica Scandinavica, 156,* 457-464.

Smith, A. M. A., Shelley, J. M., & Dennerstein, L. (1994). Self-rated health: Biological continuum or social discontinuity? *Social Science and Medicine, 39,* 77-83.

Smith, G. A., & Brewer, N. (1995). Slowness and age: Speed-accuracy mechanisms. *Psychology and Aging, 10,* 238-247.

Stoller, E. P. (1993). Interpretations of symptoms by older people: A health diary study of illness behavior. *Journal of Aging and Health, 5,* 58-81.

Stoller, E. P., & Forster, L. E. (1994). The impact of symptom interpretation on physician utilization. *Journal of Aging and Health, 6,* 507-534.

Suutama, T., & Ruoppila, I. (1999). Test result and self-evaluation based changes in cognitive functioning in eight years among Finnish elderly persons. In T. Suutama, I. Ruoppila, & P. Laukkanen (Eds.), *Changes in functional abilities among elderly people. Findings from an eight-year follow-up study by the Evergreen project* (pp. 99-116). Helsinki: The Social Insurance Institution, Finland, Studies in Social Security and Health, 42.

Wagner, E. H., & LaCroix, A. Z. (1992). Effects of physical activity on health status in older adults: observational studies. *Annual Review of Public Health, 13*, 451-468.

Wechsler, D. (1981). *Wechsler Adult Intelligence Scale-Revised.* New York: The Psychological Corporation.

Wishart, L. R., Lee, T .D., Murdoch, J. E. & Hodges, N. J. (2000). Effects of aging on automatical and effortful processes in bimanual coordination. *Journal of Gerontology, 28*(S1), 56 - 60.

Wittenberg, R. (1986). Einstellung zum Autobesitz und Unsicherheitsgefühle älterer Menschen im Strassenverkehr [Older People's Attitudes Towards Owning a Car and Feeling Unsafe in Traffic]. *Zeitschrift für Gerontologie 19*, 400-409.

Enhancing Mobility in Later Life
H. Mollenkopf et al. (Eds.)
IOS Press, 2005

Chapter 5
Transport Behaviour and Realised Journeys and Trips

Mart Tacken and Ellemieke van Lamoen

5.1   Mobility and behaviour

5.1.1   Introduction

In Chapter 1, the basic significance of mobility has been explained. For transport planning and research mobility is commonly considered as trip-making: movements from an origin to a destination. In the first part of this chapter, a few background conditions for mobility are analysed and compared between countries. This analysis has been based on the information gathered by the questionnaire. Mobility, as a basic need, is dependent on the available means of transport. Therefore, the main topics in this chapter concern the availability and use of several means of transport. Why certain forms of transportation are chosen over others is a question of central importance. Accidents are part of life and they can be very decisive for the further mobility of people. However, older people often encounter impediments to their mobility. In a second part of this chapter the realized trip making is analyzed. Mode choice, temporal aspects, trip motives and comfort of trips get attention. The realized mobility of older people is mainly described in this section by analysing the trip diaries (additional detailed figures in tables and graphs can be found in Tacken & van Lamoen, 2002). A tailor-made mode of transportation that responds flexibly to user demand might help older people to cope with hindrances. What features of a demand-responsive transportation service are important, in the eyes of the elderly, and how did a group of elderly actually use this service in Maastricht?

Most of the explanations discussed in this chapter are very commonly accepted (Brög, Erl, & Glorius, 2000; Centre d'études sur les réseaux, les transports, l'urbanisme et les constructions publiques (CERTU), 2001; Chu, 1994; Leinbach & Watkins, 1994; Mollenkopf & Flaschenträger, 2001; Tacken, 1998). It is known that physical health declines with age. Older people have more physical deficiencies in walking, visual acuity, hearing, memory, etc. (Fozard, 2003). In the higher age groups, more women are surviving their male partners, which means that they are more often widowed and living alone. Older women of the present generation have less education, a lower income and less frequently own a car or possess a driving licence. These background variables explain some of the differences in mobility. Another focus of this chapter is on the international differences in social-cultural, economic and social life as well as differences in climate, geography, and urban development that affect mobility.

5.1.2   Satisfaction with mobility

Satisfaction with mobility can be a first indication of how people value this aspect of life. One might expect that satisfaction with mobility might be worse in rural areas, but this was not a general finding of the present study. In Italy the transport facilities were worse in the rural areas, which is evident in the satisfaction of respondents. This pattern of results was even stronger in Hungary. In Finland and western Germany, urban-rural differences were much smaller, while in the Netherlands and eastern Germany the relation was even reversed.

Table 5.1:   Satisfaction with mobility by country and area (means)

	Urban		Rural	
	Mean	Std Deviation	Mean	Std Deviation
Finland **	8.5	1.7	8.1	2.0
Eastern Germany	7.6	2.4	7.7	2.3
Western Germany	7.8	2.3	7.6	2.5
Hungary**	7.9	2.3	6.0	2.9
Italy**	8.1	2.4	7.0	2.4
The Netherlands**	7.5	2.0	7.8	1.6

Note. MOBILATE Survey 2000; N = 3950, weighted
** p<0.01 T-test, difference satisfaction with mobility between urban and rural areas.
11 point scale: 0 = very unsatisfied, 10 = very satisfied

We have to realise that the subject of inquiry in this analysis is satisfaction, which means that people evaluate their factual feelings with some unknown reference point. People in the city may expect more from some typical urban facilities and become disappointed when their own perception deviates from this reference point.

Table 5.2:   Satisfaction with mobility by country, area and age (means)

	Urban		Rural	
	age in 2 categories		age in 2 categories	
	55 - 74	75+	55 - 74	75+
Finland	8.8 **	7.7	8.3 **	7.5
Eastern Germany	8.1 **	6.0	7.8 **	7.1
Western Germany	8.1 **	6.9	7.8 **	6.9
Hungary	8.1	7.4	6.2	5.2
Italy	8.7 **	6.9	7.4 **	6.1
The Netherlands	7.7 **	7.0	7.9	7.3

Note. MOBILATE Survey 2000; N = 3950, weighted
** p<0.01 T-test, difference in satisfaction with mobility between age groups per country and area.
11 point scale: 0 = very unsatisfied, 10 = very satisfied

In looking at age as an explanatory variable, the same tendency can be seen. Older people were less satisfied in both urban and rural areas than younger people. Within a given age group, these differences were also evident, while in the Dutch sample, these differences were reversed: people in the rural region were more positive. The most negative reactions were found among women living in the countryside.

One might expect a relation between satisfaction with mobility and satisfaction with public transport. This correlation was in the expected direction, but it was not very high (R=0.316). The relationship was the same when controlled by region and country, which might indicate that the objective quality of public transportation is not a very decisive factor for satisfaction with mobility.

The physical mobility of people might be expected to have much more influence. For this purpose, the ten ADL activities that had been asked for were aggregated. This variable explained more satisfaction with mobility as evidenced by the correlation of 0.467. Satisfaction with mobility is strongly related to the ability to undertake basic activities.

5.1.3   Availability and use of a car as driver and passenger

Table 5.3:   Respondents who have a car available in their household by country and area (%)

	Urban	Rural	Total
Finland**	60	71	66
Eastern Germany	58	65	61
Western Germany **	58	69	64
Hungary**	37	17	27
Italy	82	83	83
The Netherlands**	53	69	61

Note. MOBILATE Survey 2000; N = 3950, weighted
** p<0.01, difference in availability of cars in the household between areas per country.

A comparison of car ownership in urban and rural areas shows that in all countries, car ownership was higher in the rural regions, except for Hungary (Table 5.3). In Hungary and Italy the percentage of people who have a car available diverges from the other three countries where the percentages are more or less the same. In Italy this percentage is rather high (83%), and in Hungary it is rather low (27%). Less frequent car ownership in the latter country may be due to the poor socio-economic situation in the Hungarian rural area.

Table 5.4:   Availability of a car in the household by area, gender and age (% available)

	Urban				Rural			
	55 - 74		75+		55 – 74		75+	
	male	female	male	female	male	female	male	female
Finland	87	58	59	19	91	76	56	28
Eastern Germany	72	62	42	16	75	59	51	51
Western Germany	76	61	37	12	79	78	57	30
Hungary	58	28	22	21	29	14	13	8
Italy	97	85	73	56	96	83	80	63
The Netherlands	74	47	48	24	76	75	58	28

Note. MOBILATE Survey 2000; N = 3950

In Table 5.4 the figures have been distinguished for age and gender. In the urban areas, older females frequently did not have a car available in the household. In rural areas, women tended to have cars more often. It is striking that in eastern Germany, there was no difference between the older men and women in the rural area. In Hungary, car ownership in the household was very low in the rural area, especially for women and older men.

We analysed also the availability of a car related to a few background variables (Table 5.5). A first condition is the size of the household. Not surprisingly, the larger the household the more likely people are to have a car. A second variable is age, differentiated into four groups (55-64, 65-74, 74-84, 85+). Several other variables go together with age: income, presence of a partner, possession of a driving licence, and gender. The type of locality (urban vs. rural) was also related to car availability; in rural areas, there is apparently a greater need for a car. Gender was another condition: women had a lower income and were less likely to possess a driving license. Moreover, their health may differ from men's, and handling a car requires good health. Health is also related to age, of course.

Table 5.5:   Coefficients of multiple regression of the availability of a car in the household

	B	S.E.	df	Sig.
ADL score[1]	.044	.011	1	.000
Self rated physical mobility	-.237	.053	1	.000
Age in 4 categories (55-64, 65-74, 75-84, 85+)	.344	.051	1	.000
Trip mean	-.175	.026	1	.000
Education in years	-.042	.011	1	.000
Household size	1.973	.090	1	.000
Sex (male=0)	.308	.083	1	.000
Urban-rural (urban=0)	-.321	.083	1	.000
Constant	-2.341	.289	1	.000

Note. MOBILATE Survey 2000; N = 3950
[1] 0 = no problems mentioned to 20 = ADL not possible

Table 5.6 gives an overview of how many respondents drive their cars or simply ride as a passenger. The passenger role was the most common. In both parts of Germany, the percentages of people who don't use a car were the highest. The relation between car use and public transport available has not been investigated here. In Italy people seem to be most dependent on the car. Hungary has been left out of this analysis because the Hungarian survey only assessed people who have a car in their household (instead of the people who say they drive themselves).

Table 5.6:   How people use their car in rural and urban areas (%)

	Finland		Eastern Germany		Western Germany		Italy		The Netherlands	
	urban	rural	urban	rural	urban	rural	urban	rural	urban	rural
I drive myself	37	21	31	28	36	36	48	45	44	38
I travel only as a passenger	47	48	35	44	33	43	40	43	46	55
I do both	9	28	8	13	10	16	10		9	4
I do not drive or ride a car at all	7	4	26	15	20	5	3	12	1	2
Total N =	*309*	*301*	*389*	*379*	*368*	*383*	*300*	*300*	*283*	*309*

Note. MOBILATE Survey 2000; N = 3320, weighted

In most countries, the percentage of people who drive was higher in the urban than in the rural areas. In Finland, Italy and the Netherlands, the percentage of people who do not drive at all was lower than in the other countries.

One might expect age, gender, ADL-score, and self-rated physical mobility to play a role in the use of a car. Gender played a major role: 60% of the men drove whereas only 14% of the women did so. The ADL-score was also an important indicator: 54% of people with a high ADL-score drove versus 15% of people with a low score. For self-rated physical mobility, these figures were: 47% of people with a very good mobility and 9% of people with a very bad mobility. For age these differences were: 41% (for young respondents) versus 14% (for older ones).

If they do in fact drive, respondents use their car rather often (between 56% in Germany and 84% in Italy). Women used the car less often and the youngest respondents more often. In Finland, Italy, western Germany and the Netherlands, almost two thirds of the respondents used their car daily or almost every day (Table 5.7). For eastern Germany, this percentage was approximately 50%, because many respondents used their car only once or twice a week. There was hardly any difference between the urban and rural areas in how often people used their car, with the exception of western Germany and Finland. In these two areas, people tended to drive less often in the rural area than in the urban area.

Table 5.7:   How often do people drive a car? (%)

		daily or almost every day	1 or 2 times a week	less often?	Total N
Finland	urban	72	21	8	141
	rural	66	25	9	147
Eastern Germany	urban	48	46	6	155
	rural	53	43	4	149
Western Germany	urban	62	37	1	172
	rural	56	41	4	198
Italy	urban	74	23	4	159
	rural	74	21	5	127
The Netherlands	urban	62	28	10	130
	rural	63	28	9	174

Note. MOBILATE Survey 2000; weighted, car drivers only; N = 1552

Men drove much more than women did (57% vs. 16%). Younger people drove much more than older people did (59% vs. 32%). These differences exist in all countries. This means also that younger women drove more than older women did (16% vs. 4%).

In both eastern and western Germany, the elderly travelled fewer kilometres than in the other countries; two thirds of these respondents drove less than 10,000 km a year. In the other countries, this percentage was a little higher than 60% and in Finland around 50%. Finland and Italy had a relatively high share of elderly who drive more than 20,000 km (17 and 14%, respectively). The difference between urban and rural areas was small, although the people from the rural area tended to drive rather shorter distances. These differences were not as clear as one would expect based on the longer distances in the countryside. Women drove fewer kilometres than men did. Age also had a negative influence on how many kilometres a person drove.

An interesting question concerns whether elders drive less than they did before. It appears that most, older respondents do drive less than before, though a small percentage actually drives more. The latter group consisted of relatively more women than men. This could be related to the fact that more women become widowed, which may force them to drive themselves. This is valid for the younger age group, where 16% of married women drove themselves, compared to 19% of the widowed and 31% of separated and divorced women. The difference between the two age categories, in the rural as well as in the urban areas, was rather large, except in the Netherlands. Perhaps this can be explained by the relatively urban character of the Dutch rural area compared to the other countries.

Reasons for driving less differ per country. Health was a reason mentioned in every country, but other concerns were more important. Many elderly mentioned financial reasons (Finland, eastern and western Germany), that traffic is getting too hectic (eastern and western Germany, Italy), or the ability to reach and do everything without a car (western Germany and Italy). Another, less important reason was difficulty finding a parking place (eastern and western Germany).

All car drivers were asked if they avoid certain traffic situations completely or if possible (Table 5.8). Driving under poor weather conditions was mentioned by most, except in the Netherlands where driving long distances was avoided slightly more often. Other situations that were frequently mentioned include: driving at dusk or at night, bad roads (especially in the Italian urban area) and driving long distances. Infrequent mention was made of complicated junctions, driving on motorways (except for Italy) and busy roads. Looking at the differences between urban and rural areas, people in the urban areas more often avoided driving under poor weather conditions, while people in the rural areas avoided driving on motorways. In the rural areas of Finland and eastern and western Germany, more people avoided complicated junctions than in the urban areas. In the rural areas of Finland, as well as in eastern and western Germany, people did not like driving on unknown routes or in strange areas. In rural Italy, people avoided driving on busy roads. In the Netherlands, the differences between the rural and urban areas were rather small, except for driving on bad roads, which more people in the urban area avoided.

Table 5.8:   Persons who avoid specific situations as a driver by country and area (%)

Situation	Finland		Eastern Germany		Western Germany		Italy		The Netherlands	
	urban	rural	urban	rural	urban	rural	Urban	rural	urban	rural
Driving at dusk or at night	55	44	35	38	38	39	56	45	30	31
Driving on bad roads	38	37	37	39	50	43	75	62	41	28
Complicated junctions	12	27	15	18	14	22	29	33	16	16
Driving at rush hour	41	49	29	27	39	33	41	33	41	36
Busy roads	20	22	12	23	23	30	30	46	28	24
Driving long distances	32	33	24	32	35	46	50	62	43	46
Driving unknown routes or strange areas	36	43	27	39	30	46	46	44	38	35
Driving on motorways	5	16	6	19	14	37	35	54	8	13
Driving under poor weather conditions	63	64	50	41	55	45	61	56	40	39

Note. MOBILATE Survey 2000; N = 1646, weighted, car drivers only

24% of the car drivers did not avoid any of the situations mentioned in Table 5.8. They might be characterised as self-confident drivers (cf. also Rudinger & Jansen, 2003). The percentage of self-confident drivers varied between countries: there were 13% in Hungary, 15% in Finland, 18% in Italy, 22% in the Netherlands, 31% in western Germany, and 33% in eastern Germany. Women were less self-confident drivers; particularly in the younger age category, women avoided driving under certain conditions considerably more often than men.

The CHAID technique can be used to divide a sample into subgroups with a maximal contrast on the target variable, in this case, whether the respondent was a car driver or not. We analysed subgroups of drivers and non-drivers who differ most in this respect, leaving out the availability of private transport means because of the interrelation between driving and an available car. The physical mobility expressed in the ADL scale is the first indicator, gender a second and the use of public transport and age (four subgroups) are further indicators. The highest percentage of drivers was found in the subgroup of people with no or only slight ADL difficulties (92% and 83%, respectively), both male and no public transport users. A second high group (83% drivers) was found among the young women without ADL difficulty. The lowest percentages were found among the older women with ADL difficulty (3% drivers) or with slight difficulties in performing ADL (13% drivers).

5.1.4   Not driving a car

So far, people who do not drive a car have not been discussed. The total percentage of people who do not drive (any more) and have had a driver's licence was higher in the urban than in the rural areas. Relatively speaking, rural elders and women rarely have possessed a driver's licence (Table 5.9).

Table 5.9:   People who have had a valid driver's licence by country, area, age and gender (%)

	Urban						Rural					
	55 – 74			75+			55 – 74			75+		
	male	female	total	male	female	total	male	female	Total	male	female	total
Finland	69	34	41	56	18	30	45	15	21	20	4	10
Eastern Germany	39	33	34	49	5	23	44	10	20	51	14	28
Western Germany	64	25	37	65	15	35	59	10	24	63	8	28
Italy	50	29	31	57	11	27	9	12	11	18	7	11
The Netherlands	50	35	38	54	17	28	53	21	30	30	21	25

Note. MOBILATE Survey 2000; N = 1869, only respondents who don't drive a car on themselves

Why do elders stop driving? Are there more alternatives, or has driving become too difficult? Easier access to public transportation may be another reason why many elders, especially those in urban areas, no longer have a driving licence.

Reasons for giving up driving varied. One clear difference between the rural and urban areas was that the urban elderly more often reported being able to reach and do everything without a car. This confirms the assumption that better transportation alternatives lead to less driving.

Another frequent reason for not driving any more is health (cf. also Raitanen, Törmäkangas, Mollenkopf & Marcellini, 2003). Younger women less often reported health as a reason, but stressed that they have someone who drives them. Another reason for not driving is that traffic has become too hectic, a feeling more common among women than men. The rural elderly and, especially women of both age categories in the urban areas mentioned having someone who drives them.

Table 5.10 shows whether or not people have someone who will drive them and whether or not they have to pay for it. In Italy most elderly people (96%) reported having someone who will drive them, followed at some distance by Finland (87%), the Netherlands (79%), western Germany (70%) and eastern Germany (64%). It is striking that there were relatively high percentages of people in Finland, especially in the countryside, and eastern Germany who stated that there is no one who will drive them (14% and 12%, respectively). In Finland, paying for a ride was chosen more frequently than in other countries. Almost a quarter of the respondents who do not drive themselves in eastern and western Germany stated that they do not need anyone.

Table 5.10: Availability of other driver paid or not-paid (%, multiple answers possible)

	Finland	Eastern Germany	Western Germany	Italy	The Netherlands
No, there is no one	14	12	7	3	10
No, I do not need it	6	24	23	1	11
Yes, and I pay	23	6	8	2	7
Yes, but I do not pay	64	58	62	94	72

Note. MOBILATE Survey 2000; N = 2245, weighted

Among those who have someone to drive them, 38% receive assistance anytime and 46% only if they really need it. In comparing these figures for people who pay or do not pay, an interesting difference can be observed: 30% were willing to pay only in urgent situations whereas 22% were willing to pay at any time. If one does not have to pay, then this transport was available for 13% in urgent situations and for 41% any time. In short, it seems that people will only pay in rather urgent situations.

5.1.5   The use of a bicycle

The respondents from Finland had the highest rate of bicycle ownership (72%) and those from Italy had the lowest (31%). The main question, however, is whether or not they use their bicycles. In Italy, the bicycle does not belong to the lifestyle of elderly people. Nearly 70% of the owners reported never using a bicycle. In Hungary and Finland, followed by eastern Germany and the Netherlands, between 37% and 48% of the owners used their bicycles daily. In western Germany the use of a bicycle lagged slightly behind (Table 5.11).

Table 5.11: Bicycle use by owners of different age, gender and area (%).

	Urban				Rural			
	55-74		75+		55-74		75+	
	male	female	male	female	male	female	male	female
Daily or almost every day	31	38	32	24	38	37	37	25
1 or 2 times per week	24	21	23	21	21	29	22	22
Less often	33	24	19	17	21	19	12	9
Never	12	18	26	38	20	15	29	44
Total N=	281	221	130	66	386	367	249	177

Note. MOBILATE Survey 2000; N = 1877, only users of a bicycle

The different areas did not show a clear difference in the use of bicycles. Even age was not a factor. Older women used their bicycle less frequently than older men did. Bad weather, darkness, long distances and unknown areas were avoided most by all older (75+) cyclists. Traffic related aspects such as complicated junctions, busy traffic or rush hour, were avoided less (Table 5.12).

Table 5.12: Persons who avoid specific situations as cyclists (%)

Situation	% of bicycle owners	
	55-74	75+
Riding at dusk or at night	57	68
Riding on bad roads	37	49
Complicated junctions	24	32
Riding at rush hour	33	41
Busy roads	34	40
Riding long distances	55	67
Riding unknown routes or in strange area	48	64
Riding under poor weather conditions	60	69

Note. MOBILATE Survey 2000; weighted; N = 1877, only users of a bicycle

5.1.6 Elderly people as pedestrians

Walking is a common mode of transportation for old people. In the following analysis, all people who can walk are compared with a subgroup of people who evaluated their physical mobility as poor or very poor with respect to their behaviour in specific situations.

Table 5.13 Pedestrians avoiding specific situations (%)

Situation	% of pedestrians who can walk	% of poor or very poor physical mobility
Crossing the road at dusk or at dark	48	78
Bad roads	47	78
Walking in rush hour	42	74
Crossing the road without a pedestrian crossing	44	70
Walking along a busy road which does not have sidewalks	56	76
Going to unfamiliar places	52	80
Busy traffic	51	77
Poor weather conditions	62	85
Insufficient light in the street	60	83
Total N =	**3728**	**542**

Note. MOBILATE Survey 2000; weighted; N = 3950

Nearly half of the group of pedestrians who can walk avoided specific situations, if possible. This means that these older people were conscious of specific hindrances in the outdoor environment. Poor weather and insufficient light received high scores, followed by walking along busy roads without sidewalks. Walking in rush hour and crossing roads were avoided less frequently, but still by more than 40% of the respondents (Table 5.13).

Comparing this total group with the subgroup who felt that their physical mobility is rather poor, we see that avoidance behaviour is much higher among those with self-reported poor mobility. More than 70% of frail persons avoided specific situations. Poor weather and insufficient light again received high scores but were followed closely by unfamiliar places, crossing roads at dusk, and bad roads.

In general, avoidance was lower in each subgroup in the rural areas, with the exception of unfamiliar places and poor weather. The oldest age group showed more avoidance behaviour than the youngest age group. Within these groups, women avoided more situations. Older women in the urban areas showed the most avoidance of specific situations. More than 50% tried to avoid poor weather.

Every one of the pedestrians avoided certain situations. Apparently, pedestrians feel less self-confident than car drivers. And in fact, pedestrians are the most vulnerable traffic participants.

5.1.7   The role of public transport

As we have seen, public transportation does not play a leading role in the mobility of the average older individual; walking and car driving are more important. Still, how satisfied are people with public modes of transportation?

Table 5.14: Satisfaction with public transport (means)

	mean	std. deviation
Finland	7.3	2.5
Eastern Germany	6.8	2.5
Western Germany	6.4	2.7
Hungary	7.1	2.4
Italy	5.7	2.8
The Netherlands	6.4	2.0

Note. MOBILATE Survey 2000; weighted, N = 3950
11 point scale: 0 = very unsatisfied, 10 = very satisfied

Italians are most negative about public transport, followed by the Dutch and western German elders. In Finland and Hungary, people were most positive, followed by persons from eastern Germany. Rural elders were less satisfied with public transport, probably due to low availability. Within these rural areas, women were the least satisfied.

Respondents were asked how frequently they used various means of public transportation. The bus was used most often in Hungary (42% regularly) and the Netherlands (37%). The tram was used most often in western Germany. The tram is an essential part of public transport in Mannheim (17% regularly). The train was used most in the Netherlands (19% regularly) and the least in eastern Germany (41% never). The taxi was not part of daily life in Hungary (58% never). In the Netherlands (6%) and Finland (4%), some people used this transport mode regularly.

Why don't the elderly use public transport? Most mentioned that they have no need of public transport because they have a car. Fewer Hungarians made this assertion (46%). They mentioned more often that all they need is in within reach (56%). In Finland, about 20% mentioned that there is no public transport in their housing area. The high costs of public transport were mentioned most often in eastern Germany (13%) and in western Germany (12%). In eastern Germany, the availability and quality of public transport were more often cited as reasons: stops too far away (17%), low frequency (18%), too inconvenient (13%) or inconvenient lines (13%). The inconvenience of public transport was also frequently mentioned in Italy (14%). These findings confirm the statement of Rosenbloom (2003). She tells us to debunk the myth that elderly people first lose the ability to drive, and then use public transport, after that walk and finally use special transport. Long before they lose the ability to drive they are unable to board and ride public transport.

Again, the CHAID analysis enables us to divide the dependent variable into subgroups as regards different independent variables. Here, it was used to divide the users of public transport into subgroups. 57% of the total sample used public transport. In the urban areas, use was 73% versus 41% in the rural areas. The next variable used to split these subgroups was the level of physical activity. The group with the highest level of activity did not show the highest use of public transport; rather, the moderately active group did. The same pattern of findings was found for the rural areas. The percentages were 83% and 54%, respectively. For the most active group, the lack of private modes of transportation, such as a car or a bicycle, were important indicators of public transportation use. The group with the highest public transport use (93%) consisted of people with no car or bicycle, moderate physical activity level and who were living in an urban area. Use of public transportation was the lowest for people with low income, low physical activity and who were living in a rural area.

5.1.8   Relative importance of transport modes

We have seen that walking is the most common mode of transportation, public transport less so. What is the importance of these different modes in the opinions of older people?

Table 5.15: The importance of transport modes by age, gender and area (mean)

	Urban				Rural			
	55-74		75+		55-74		75+	
	male	female	male	female	male	female	male	female
Car	3.7	2.3	2.6	1.4	3.7	2.4	2.7	1.5
Bicycle	2.4	2.2	1.8	1.4	3.1	3.1	2.6	2.0
Moped	1.2	1.1	1.2	1.1	1.4	1.2	1.4	1.2
Car passenger	2.4	3.4	2.8	3.2	2.7	3.8	3.2	3.7
Public transport	3.1	3.9	3.2	3.3	2.4	2.8	2.4	2.4
Special transport	1.5	1.6	1.7	1.9	1.4	1.5	1.6	1.8
Walking	4.4	4.6	4.3	4.2	4.4	4.5	4.3	4.3

Note. MOBILATE Survey 2000; N = 3950
   Rated on a five-point scale: 1 = not important at all to 5 = very important

Walking was the most important mode of transportation for all categories of persons. The car was second in ranking for younger male respondents. For younger women in the urban area, public transport was important, whereas use of the car (as a passenger) and the bicycle both ranked highly in the rural areas. For older respondents, use of the car (as a passenger) was important and so was public transport in the urban areas (see also Mollenkopf, Marcellini, Ruoppila et al., 2002).

5.1.9   Accidents

90% of the respondents did not have an accident over the last few years. In Germany, this percentage was even higher (95%), while in Finland, it was considerably lower (79%). In the rural areas, people appear to have had fewer accidents than in the cities. Age and gender influenced the frequency of accidents. Older women had fewer accidents than younger women, except in Finland. Older men seem to have had more accidents than younger men, except in Hungary and Italy. In Finland, Hungary and the Netherlands, women tend to have had more accidents than men, and in Italy and Germany, men seem to have had more accidents.

The way in which people were involved in an accident differed by country. In Finland, most people were involved in an accident as a pedestrian, or secondly as a cyclist or a car passenger. In Germany, most people involved in accidents were car drivers; the second most frequent accidents were as a car passenger (in eastern Germany) and as a pedestrian (in western Germany). In Hungary most people experienced an accident as a pedestrian, secondly as a cyclist and thirdly as a car driver. In Italy, people were most often involved in an accident as a car driver, then as a pedestrian and thirdly as a moped-/motorcyclist. In the Netherlands, most accidents were experienced by car drivers, followed by pedestrians and finally, cyclists.

In urban areas, men experienced most accidents as a car driver. Older men also had more accidents as pedestrians and cyclists. For women in the urban area, the situation was different. They experienced most of their accidents as pedestrians and secondly as car drivers. In the older age group, most were involved in accidents as pedestrians, followed by public transport users, and then as car drivers. In rural areas the situation for men was almost the same except for the fact that in many accidents, the respondent was a cyclist. In both age groups of women, almost 30% experienced the reported accident while riding a bicycle.

Only 40% of the people who have had an accident indicated that the accident had no repercussions. Most (42%) mentioned consequences for their health; far fewer reported ensuing financial problems or decline in well-being. Nonetheless, 18% experienced financial consequences and 17% felt more insecure than before.

Table 5.16: How people were involved in an accident by area, gender and age (%)

	Urban				Rural			
	male		female		male		female	
	55-74	75+	55-74	75+	55-74	75+	55-74	75+
Pedestrian	11	19	46	63	16	21	31	60
Cyclist	8	12	19	7	12	21	29	31
Car driver	72	58	31	11	62	41	26	6
Moped/motorcyclist	4	6	0	0	4	18	0	3
In public transport	0	4	7	15	0	0	0	0
Passenger of a private vehicle	6	2	7	4	6	0	14	0
Total N =	*53*	*52*	*68*	*46*	*50*	*34*	*35*	*35*

Note. MOBILATE Survey 2000; N = 373

5.1.9.1 Experience with traffic today

The respondents were asked to react to a list of statements on today's traffic situation (adapted from Wittenberg, 1986). 49% stated that cars and motorcycles drive too fast. 46% agreed with the statement that it should be forbidden to cycle on the sidewalk. 39% agreed with the statement that there are not enough cycle lanes, and 38% with the statement that cars drive so fast that one sees them at the last second. The respondents were the least negative about the closing of doors on buses (11%), the abrupt acceleration in buses (15%), readability of timetables (17%) or feelings of helplessness in traffic (17%) (Table 5.17).

Table 5.17: General statements on the traffic today (% of total agreement to respective item; adapted from Wittenberg, 1986)

	All respon-dents	Urban				Rural			
		55-74		75+		55-74		75+	
		male	female	male	female	male	female	male	female
Many cars and motorcycles are going too fast when they approach the pedestrian crossing, and so you never know whether they will brake or not.	49	45	57	49	50	47	49	46	45
Children and adolescents should be forbidden to ride their bicycles on the sidewalk.	46	50	51	51	55	42	38	42	40
There are not enough lanes for bicycles.	39	45	41	41	28	41	44	40	26
Cars and motorcycles drive so fast that you can only see them at the last second.	38	29	39	37	41	36	37	43	43
Many cars and motorcycles drive too near the sidewalks.	37	31	39	39	35	35	37	39	40
Too few people offer their seat in the bus for a person who needs to sit down.	33	41	49	43	36	27	25	22	22
There are not enough seats or shelters at the busstops.	28	26	35	33	32	24	25	27	24
Buses run too infrequently at certain times of the day.	26	20	28	19	18	31	33	29	26
As an elderly person you feel disadvantaged in today's traffic.	25	20	27	27	31	17	23	27	28
The sidewalks are often so narrow that you have to step into the street to make way for other pedestrians.	24	23	30	22	21	24	26	25	22
There are not enough pedestrian crossings and traffic lights with a button for pedestrians to push.	23	24	25	29	23	23	21	22	18
It very often happens that when I am half way across the road, the traffic light has turned red.	21	28	29	31	28	16	16	11	11
Traffic is sometimes so busy that you don't dare to go out on the street.	20	15	23	23	28	14	18	22	23
I have difficulty getting in and out of the bus because of the high steps.	18	12	25	23	32	8	17	13	19
Nowadays I often feel helpless in traffic.	17	12	17	17	23	9	16	18	25
The timetables and route maps are difficult to read and understand.	17	16	24	20	22	10	15	15	13
The buses start too quickly and jerkily such that one is thrown about.	15	14	23	20	27	9	10	9	11
The automatic closing and opening of bus doors is poorly installed, so that you can easily get caught in the door.	11	11	19	16	19	5	7	8	8

Note. MOBILATE Survey 2000; N = 3950

5.2   Journeys in the MOBILATE diary

Information on actual mobility (e.g., the number of journeys or trips made) was reported in a diary, which was journey based. A journey consists of leaving home and returning to the home. Each journey can be divided into trips: a trip is each part of a journey with a specific motive or purpose. A simple change in transport mode does not constitute a new trip; rather only a change in trip purpose does. For example, if the subject travels from home to a shop, then to a bank and on the way back, visits a friend, then the journey consists of four separate trips: shopping, banking, visiting a friend, and returning home.

Respondents reported all of the journeys they made over the course of two days. Information was gathered on the mode of transportation used, the motives for the journey, the departure time from home, and the arrival time back at home. Journeys often cover a long period of time and entail several different activities and different transport modes. In the present analysis, only the journeys can be described with regards to duration. Describing the distribution of activities over the day means that sometimes two or more activities go together. If someone goes out shopping and on the way back home visits a friend, then this journey was counted as a shopping trip and a visiting trip. If each trip was counted separately, some statistics (e.g., the number of persons going out) would be inflated. On the other hand, by focusing our analysis on journeys, we can describe their essential characteristics, including the time of the day that people go out for specific activities.

Below, we present general information about journeys. Note that if a respondent made no trip on a given day, this information was recorded. We therefore make a distinction between people who did not fill in the diary and people who did not make a trip.

5.2.1   General information on journeys

A total of 10,218 forms were filled in by 3,950 persons over the course of two days. But of these, 2,843 forms indicated that no trip was made. This means that 7,375 forms with a journey were filled in, which results in 1.86 journeys pro person during two days. On average, 1,422 persons made no journey on one of these days or on both days. 925 made no journey on both days (23%), 1,300 only on the first day and 1,543 only on the second day. The mobile people (3,025 persons: 77%) made 7,373 journeys during this time, which results in 2.4 journeys over the observation interval.

The differences between the urban and rural areas were rather small, but the number of journeys was lower in rural areas, except for western Germany. Table 5.19 shows that elderly people in rural areas made fewer journeys than those in urban areas, women made fewer journeys than men, and older respondents made fewer journeys than younger ones.

Table 5.18: Mean number of journeys a day by country and areas

Journey mean	Finland**	Eastern Germany	Western Germany	Hungary**	Italy	The Nether- lands**	Total**
Urban	1.4	0.9	0.9	0.9	1.2	0.8	1.4
Rural	1.2	0.9	1.0	0.6	1.1	0.5	1.2
Total N =	*1.3*	*0.9*	*0.9*	*0.7*	*1.1*	*0.6*	*0.9*

Note. MOBILATE Diary ; N = 3950, weighted
** Significant difference between urban and rural areas (p<0.01).

When differentiated by country, the same pattern of relationships was observed. The younger Finnish men in the urban area made the most journeys per day, and older Hungarian women in the countryside made the fewest, along with the older men from the Dutch rural area.

Table 5.19: Mean numbers of journeys a day by country, areas, age and gender

	Urban				Rural			
	55-74		75+		55-74		75+	
	male	female	male	female	male	female	male	female
Finland	1.8	1.4	1.1	0.9	1.5	1.3	1.0	0.7
Eastern Germany	0.9	1.0	0.9	0.8	1.1	0.8	0.7	.0.5
Western Germany	1.0	0.9	0.5	0.6	1.1	1.1	0.9	0.6
Hungary	0.9	1.0	0.9	0.6	0.6	0.7	0.5	0.3
Italy	1.6	1.2	1.2	0.5	1.6	0.9	1.2	0.5
The Netherlands	0.8	0.9	0.6	0.5	0.6	0.6	0.3	0.4

Note. MOBILATE Diary; N = 3950

5.2.1.1   Chaining of trips in journeys

A trip chain, or a journey consisting of three or more trips, is an important unit of analysis. Of the 7,373 journeys, at least 1,390 journeys (19%) had a second motive, which means that people combined more than one activity in the same journey. 19% of the journeys can be considered to be multiple chains. 5% had a third motive and an additional 1% had a fourth motive. Of the 295 chained journeys with 'shopping' as first motive, 8% had 'attending a bank, post, authority, etc.' as a second motive, and again 14% 'shopping' as motive.

5.2.1.2   Motives

In total, 9,291 motives were given for a (part of) the journey. The 6,822 trips back home (as final destination also of walking and cycling tours) have been excluded from this analysis. The motive mentioned most often (31%) was shopping. 15% of all shopping motives were mentioned as a further motive in the same journey. Visiting (12%) was the second and walking or touring (11%) the third most commonly cited motive. Work was reported as motive in 8%, attending a bank etc. in 7%, and health care in 6% of all cases.

Some differences between countries were found. Shopping was the most important motive of single journeys (with one motive) in all countries, ranging from 41% of all cases in Hungary to 21% of all cases in Finland. This motive was followed in Finland and both parts of Germany by 'strolling around'.

Meeting friends was another motive of importance, counting as a primary motive in Hungary, Italy and the Netherlands. Likewise, health care was also important. Some striking findings were the rather high scores for 'visiting religious events or cemetery' in Italy (13%) and Hungary (9%) (a motive in only 2% of cases in Finland). In Finland, frequent motives were banking, and going to the post office (9%). Working was more frequently a primary motive in western Germany (10%) and Finland (9%) and less often in the other countries (roughly 5% to 6%)

5.2.1.3   Choice of mode

People can use more than one mode for the same journey. The slow modes like cycling and walking were often a means of accessing public transport. An overview of the chosen mode of transportation for the first motive gives one an impression of the relative importance of each transportation mode. Of the 7,373 journeys, 48% were, at least partly, made on foot. 26% were made as a car driver and 11% as a car passenger. In 10% of the cases, respondents used a bicycle and in 9%, some type of public transport (of which 2% were special kinds of transport). The total shows that some people used more than one transport mode. Walking was by far the mode of transportation used most often and the car (either as driver or passenger) a strong second mode of transportation.

One way to simplify the results on transportation modes, which often involves many different modes, is to focus on the main transport mode (Bróg, Erl & Glorius, 2000; CBS, 2000). This variable is made by using a specific order of modes, implicitly based on a ranking of modes related to speed and distances. Thus, if a respondent used a train, then this mode is the main mode of transportation for this journey. The next is public transport (BTM: Bus, Tram, Metro), followed by the car, the bicycle and by foot. Table 5.20 lists the frequencies for this variable.

Even using this scheme, the pedestrian journey was the most common, followed by the car. The slow modes were often used as a means of access or egress for public transport, and these trips disappear partly in the analysis of the main mode of transportation. The share of public transport in the analysis is rather low (6%). About 30% of the answer forms were empty, which means that no journeys were made on that particular interview day. In our further analysis, these were left out.

Table 5.20: Distribution of the main transport mode

	Frequency	Percent
No trip	2843	28
Train	5	0
BTM	637	6
Car	2750	27
Bicycle	769	8
Foot	3214	31
Total N =	*10217*	**100**

Note. MOBILATE Diary; weighted

Also within the different age groups, the same differences can be seen (Table 5.21). Women, particularly younger ones, used cars less. Women also went more often by foot and used slightly more public transport. But, age played a role as well: older men used cars less and older women went more often by foot. Both age and gender influence the choice of transportation, and together, the effects of these two demographic variables are even stronger. In each category, bicycle and car use were higher in the rural areas, whereas public transport use was lower.

Table 5.21: Use of the main transport modes by age, gender and area (%)

| | Urban | | | | Rural | | | |
| | 55-74 | | 75+ | | 55 -74 | | 75+ | |
	male	female	male	female	male	female	male	female
Train	0	0	0	0	0	0	0	0
BTM	8	15	13	18	5	3	8	4
Car	48	28	27	17	51	34	33	26
Bicycle	8	9	6	3	13	16	13	9
Foot	37	48	54	62	30	47	46	60
Total N =	*1506*	*1674*	*270*	*471*	*1494*	*1363*	*264*	*336*

Note. MOBILATE Diary; weighted

The motives for the journeys have been reduced to eight categories:

Motive	motive in diary
Work:	work
Visiting:	visiting, baby-sit, care for someone
Shop:	visit to shops, attending services, health care facilities
Recreation:	having coffee, cultural event, association, gardening, short trip
Sport:	sport, fishing
Walk:	walk
Other:	religious, accompany, education
Home:	not active outdoors.

The journeys with work as one of the motives were mostly made using a car as the main mode and least often by foot. Visiting and shopping are activities which were done more on foot. The same tendency was observed for recreational activities, but with this motive, the car and even public transport come slightly more into the picture. Sport facilities were visited more often by car and less often by foot. Sport facilities are often on the outskirts of the cities or villages and it is possible that therefore respondents did not go by foot or bicycle to sport facilities.

5.2.2   Temporal aspects of the mobility behaviour of older people

In many explanations of the mobility behaviour of people the temporal aspects play an important role. Time is a limited commodity, and people must be efficient in their use of it. Time influences mobility in two ways. In the time paths, as described by Hägerstrand (1970), the point in time and the amount of time needed to cover distances determine the spatial range people have and the opportunities they have to carry out different activities (Chapin, 1974; Parkes and Thrift, 1986; Pred, 1984; van Reisen, 1997; Dijst, 1995). Time is thus essential to understanding travel behaviour. Those interested in traffic management are also concerned with the temporal aspects of the mobility of older people because their number is increasing and within this group the proportion of very old people. They have grown up in a time with more spatial mobility and their action radius has increased as well. Better financial conditions for (early) retirement means that today's elderly have more time, more money and more cars, all of which increase mobility (OECD, 2001). Does the actual travel behaviour of the present generation of older people constitute a threat? Today's traffic problems, especially the increasing number of traffic jams, are related to the concentration of persons commuting for work or recreational purposes. Will the mobility of elderly people contribute to traffic bottlenecks, or does their mobility take place outside the peak hours and in conjunction with slower modes of transportation, such as cycling and walking?

First, the distribution of activities over the course of the day is described. The graphs presented below are based on unweighted data. To obtain smooth-lined graphs, we employed a progressive mean calculated as the mean of five periods.

5.2.3   Distribution of mobility over a day

We use the departure and arrival time of the journeys for an overview of the activities during the day. In the following graphs, the time between six and nine has been divided into periods of five minutes.

The graphs depict the percentage of those who were active outdoors over the course of the day. Figure 5.1 shows that the peak of out-of-home activity was around 11:00 o'clock, when nearly 60% of the respondents were away from home. During lunchtime some went home, and a new peak occurred between 15:00 and 16:00 o'clock with nearly 50% of the older people outdoors.

Figure 5.1:   People active outdoors from 6:00 - 21:00 in five European countries in total

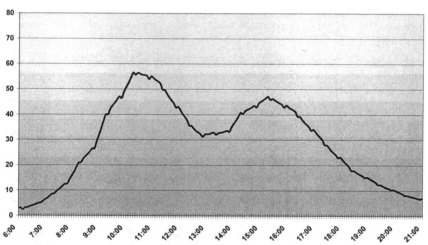

MOBILATE Diary 2000; N = 3950

Figure 5.2:   People active outdoors from 6:00 - 21:00 by country

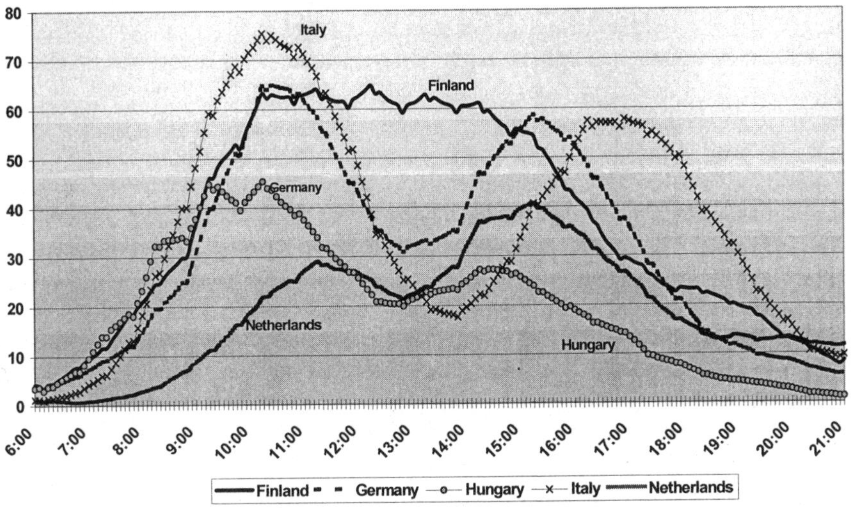

MOBILATE Diary 2000; N = 3950

Figure 5.2 shows the diversity between countries. Italy had the highest peak of out-of-home mobility in the morning. Between 10:00 and 11:00 o'clock, more than 70% of the people were not at home. This peak was a little bit earlier in Italy than in the other countries. These had a clear dip around lunchtime, and in the late afternoon, out-of-home activity started again with a peak between 16:00 and 17:00 o'clock, when about 50% of people were away from home. Finland showed a very different pattern of mobility. Finns started their activities later in the day; between 10:00 and 14:00 o'clock around 60% of people stayed out of home. The other countries all showed two peaks of activity: one in the morning and one in the afternoon. In Hungary this afternoon peak was rather low and in the Netherlands, it was higher than in the morning. The Dutch respondents seem to be slow starters, but in the evening they are relatively often away from home.

In Figures 5.3 to 5.8, the motives for the journeys have been reduced to eight categories, as described in section 5.2.1.3. These graphs illustrate clearly the differences between the countries. All of the countries had a clear distribution of two peaks and a dip during lunchtime. Only Finland showed a completely different pattern and the dip during lunchtime did not take place. The Finnish respondents went out rather frequently. During a large part of the day, between 09:00 and 16:00 o'clock, about 60% of the activities took place outside of their home, and no clear dip was evident. A relatively large part of the Finnish sample still worked, and they started rather early. Visiting other people had no clear peak, but visits were often spent during lunchtime and the early afternoon. Also shopping and attending services and (health) facilities were rather equally distributed over the day.

In the Netherlands, Italy and Hungary, a small proportion of the sample was still working, even at this older age. In Germany this is shared between these countries and Finland. Both parts of Germany differ only slightly in this respect. Shopping, attending services and (health) facilities are typical morning activities. In the Dutch and Finnish samples, such a peak was not very evident. In eastern Germany and Italy, relatively more time was spent on recreational activities. Sport activities were not popular in any country except Finland. Going for a walk, however, was popular in Italy and both parts of Germany. In the Netherlands and Hungary, participation in out-of-home activities was rather low. In Hungary most people went out in the morning while in the Netherlands, more people went out in the afternoon. The two high peaks of activity and the deep dip during lunchtime observed in Italy are typical of this country. Is this a remainder of the siesta? Climate is a part of the explanation of the striking differences between Italy and Finland. The shorter day in Finland could explain why people stay outdoors more often during a shorter part of the day.

An interesting next step in the analysis is the effect of other characteristics of the sample. Variables such as urban and rural, gender and age were introduced. Differences in activity patterns between urban and rural areas ran in the expected direction. Urban elders went out more often. In the rural areas, during the morning peak, about 50% stayed outdoors. In the urban areas, 65% did so. The main differences were observed in shopping, attending services, and recreational activities. These facilities are more available in cities, which might explain different patterns of activity. The hypothesized warmer social climate in rural areas was not evident in the figures for recreational activities or visiting.

Age could be another explanatory variable. During the busy morning peak, 70% of the younger people aged 55 to 74 years were out of their home compared to only 40% of the people aged over 75 years. Most of this difference can be explained by retirement, though it is also due, in some small part, to decreases in activities such as shopping and attending services.

Figure 5.3:   People active outdoors from 6:00 - 21:00 in Finland

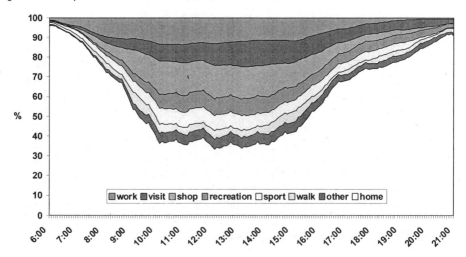

MOBILATE Diary 2000; N = 610

Figure 5.4:   People active outdoors from 6:00 - 21:00 in Hungary

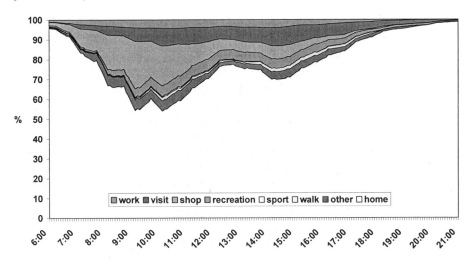

MOBILATE Diary 2000; N = 605

Figure 5.5:   People active outdoors from 6:00 - 21:00 in Eastern Germany

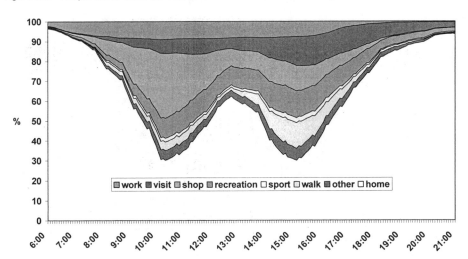

MOBILATE Diary 2000; N = 768

Figure 5.6: People active outdoors from 6:00 - 21:00 in Western Germany

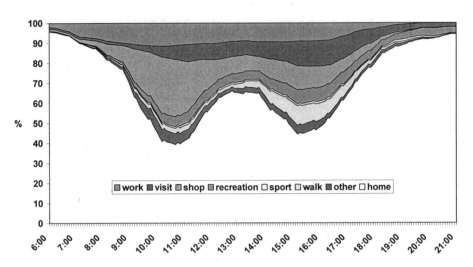

MOBILATE Diary 2000; N = 751

Figure 5.7: People active outdoors from 6:00 - 21:00 in Italy

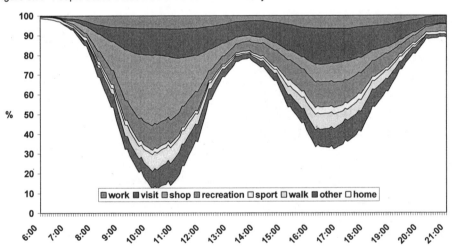

MOBILATE Diary 2000; N = 600

Figure 5.8:   People active outdoors from 6:00 - 21:00 in the Netherlands

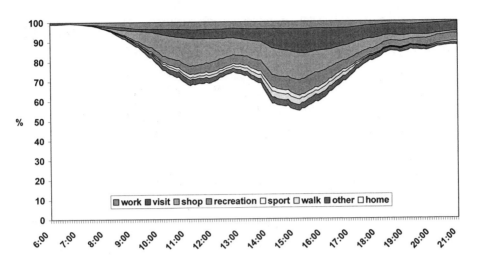

MOBILATE Diary 2000; N = 616

In general, the decrease can be explained more by the reduction of obligatory activities than of voluntary activities. Early in the evening, the younger elderly were more often outdoors than those over 75 years of age. Gender is also part of the explanation. During the busy morning peak, only 20% of the men stayed at home compared to more than 50% of the women.

5.2.4   Comfort of journeys

The mobile elderly do not complain of lack of comfort. Only 7% of the journeys were judged to be uncomfortable, and the differences between the countries were rather small. The Italians were the most negative, followed by respondents in Finland and eastern Germany. Of the 476 uncomfortable journeys, 26% were uncomfortable for a specific reason. For 22%, heavy traffic was the reason for the discomfort and for 16%, personal health. For 6% to 7% of the difficult journeys, 'too many people on streets or in shops', 'parking problems', 'long .way and strenuous trip', and 'rough and narrow sidewalks' were the reasons for discomfort. Very few people chose the other possibilities listed. 'Health problems' got high scores in Finland (42%), while 74% of the respective respondents mentioned a specific reason. Heavy traffic was mentioned in all countries, except for Finland and Italy. 'Parking problems' received a rather high score (21%) in eastern Germany compared to other countries (between 1% and 9%).

Conversely, 93% of the journeys were comfortable due to 'broad and plain sidewalks' (22%), 'light traffic' (21%), 'traffic calmed area' (14%), and 'good parking places' (10%) as well as minor reasons such as 'quiet in shops and streets' (4%) and 'I had company' (4%). In Germany the item 'broad and plain sidewalks' received a high score, perhaps due to the combination of pedestrian path and cycle path frequently encountered there. The 'traffic calmed area' was mentioned most in Hungary and in Italy. 'Light traffic' received a rather high score (22% - 29%) in all countries except for the Netherlands and Hungary. Journeys made in rural areas were slightly more comfortable. Journeys made by older people were more often felt to be less comfortable (Table 5.22).

Table 5.22: Journeys (un)comfortable by area, age and gender (%)

	Urban				Rural			
	55-74		75+		55-74		75+	
	male	female	Male	female	male	female	male	female
Comfortable	91	94	89	88	96	96	94	92
Not comfortable	9	6	11	12	4	4	6	8
Total N =	*1052*	*903*	*606*	*489*	*1041*	*832*	*601*	*406*

Note. MOBILATE Diary 2000

5.3   Trips made by elderly people

The diary was based on the journey as the unit of measurement. The idea was that this approach would be nearer to the way of thinking of elderly people: one leaves the home and comes back after some time. However, in international transport literature, the trip is usually the basic unit of analysis. In order to enable a comparison of these figures with national and international statistics, a basic analysis of the trips undertaken is presented below.

5.3.1   Trips in the diary

The trip analysis required a split up of the journeys. The diary entries were structured in such a way that each form contained all the information on a journey and each line in the form contained information on each individual trip. Trip information included the motive, mode of transportation, origin and destination, the range of the trip and whether the individual was travelling with companion or not. The trip is also part of the journey and thus, general information could be applied to the trips. Only the temporal information is spread out over the whole journey.

For the following analysis, journeys were split up into movements made with a specific motive. Unfortunately, answer forms were often incomplete; in particular, the trip back home was not always filled in, and due to this reason the respective mode of transportation was missing. We have decided to complete these trips. When the trip 'back home' was missing, we added such a trip if the trip before was not a tour home-back home (taking a walk, or a cycle tour, or a short trip without a clear destination). Missing information was added from the foregoing trip, but only in the case of a single chain: home-destination-home.

All respondents filled in the diary and only 16 did not fill in one of these days. This means that nearly the whole sample provided data on two days. 23% made no trip at all during the two days. The mean number of trips varied from the highest number of 2.5 for the younger, urban males to 1.1 for the older, rural women. Women made fewer trips than men, rural people less than urban and older less than rural.

Figure 5.9: People making no trip at one day at least

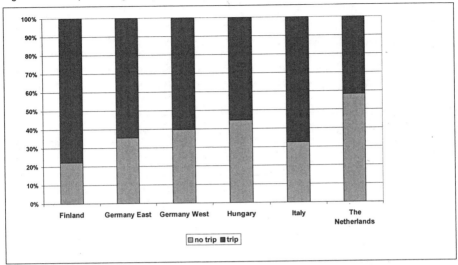

Note. MOBILATE Diary 2000; weighted

Figure 5.9 shows that in Finland, only 22% of persons made no trip on one of the interview days. In the Netherlands, this figure was 58%. Few journeys consisted of chains of trips. The simplest journey consists of two trips: a trip to a destination and a trip back home. Such a journey can be considered to be a single chain with only one motive (or activity) and the return home. Most of the trips concern single chains: from home to a destination and back home. Only about 10% of the journeys consisted of more than two motives (a destination and a way back home), except for Finland where 17% concerned journeys with more motives or multiple chains.

5.3.2 Means of transport for trips

Walking is clearly the most common mode of transportation for trips, as the last column of Table 5.23 shows. This mode was used in 45% of all modes used. Driving a car (28%) and riding in a car (11%) were the second mode of choice, the bicycle (10%) was the third mode and public transport (8%) was the fourth mode. The figures make clear that respondents from the various countries used different modes of transportation. Nonetheless, going on foot was the most common mode in all countries.

Table 5.23: Means of transport used by country (more modes possible) (%)

	Finland	Eastern Germany	Western Germany	Hungary	Italy	The Netherlands	Total
Public transport	6	8	4	15	6	10	8
Car driver	31	22	30	6	42	29	28
Car passenger	14	12	7	4	15	13	11
Bicycle	15	11	8	15	1	15	10
Foot	38	50	53	58	40	30	45
Total N (trips) =	3364	2963	3118	1938	2987	1722	16092

Note. MOBILATE Diary 2000; weighted

Among the countries examined, Hungary had the highest proportion of walkers: 58% of all trips were made, at least in part, on foot. The car was much less of an alternative in this country compared to other countries but it is interesting to note that western Germany and Finland, despite high percentages of car drivers, also had high percentages of pedestrians. In Italy more than half of the trips were undertaken with a car (both as a driver or a passenger). Public transport was used infrequently. In Hungary, it appeared to be an alternative, less so in the Netherlands. The bicycle was used most in Finland, Hungary and the Netherlands, yet hardly at all in Italy.

Table 5.24: Means of transport used by type of areas (more modes possible) (%)

	Urban	Rural
Public transport	12	5
Car driver	25	31
Car passenger	10	12
Bicycle	7	14
Foot	49	40
Total N =	*8577*	*7514*

Note. MOBILATE Diary 2000, weighted

Geography makes a difference. The availability of public transport is better in urban areas than in rural regions; hence, facilities are more accessible. Table 5.24 clearly illustrates these differences. In urban areas, people used public transport or went by foot. In rural areas, longer distances and lack of public transportation necessitated the use of a car or bicycle.

Gender and age are also relevant variables in the explanation of the use of transport means. Men, especially younger ones, drove cars much more often than women. Women were more often car passengers. Women, even older ones, went more by foot apparently due to a lack of a car. Public transport was used more often by older people, and within each age group women used this mode slightly more than men did. Older women rode bicycles the least often. The possibility of using a car seems to be decisive for the choice of mode. When people cannot use this mode because of their age or the lack of a driving licence, they look for alternatives in public transport or in walking.

5.3.3   Motives for the trip

A trip is defined by the motive, making it an ideal unit of analysis (journeys sometimes have multiple motives).

Most of the respondents did not work. Shopping, in the broad sense, was a principal activity especially for Hungarian respondents. Meeting other people was the second most important activity. Strolling or walking were more frequent activities in Finland and eastern Germany, less so in western Germany.

Finland seems to be an 'active' country. Older people more frequently went out for walks, picked berries or went fishing, and did sports; they also went out less frequently for health care. There may be a relationship between more activity and less health care, yet the differences observed were rather small. In Hungary, these activities take a backseat to shopping, which is the main activity in Hungary. Hungarians appeared to walk more out of necessity (lack of cars and public transport). In Hungary and Italy, religious events were more often the motive of a trip. Gardening, which is not only a leisure pursuit but part and parcel of many individuals' daily routine, was more popular in Hungary and eastern Germany. The small differences between urban and rural areas are interesting in this respect. The main difference was found for shopping (34% vs. 28%). In the urban areas, people went shopping more, but in the rural areas, meeting other people was more important (11% vs. 14%). The same pattern was observed for attending religious events or visiting the cemetery (4% vs. 8%)

Table 5.25: Trips made with a specific motive (excluding trips back home (%)

	Finland	Eastern Germany	Western Germany	Hungary	Italy	The Netherlands	Total
Shopping (e.g. supermarket, hairdresser, travel agency)	31	30	30	40	26	34	31
Meeting friends, relatives	10	10	10	14	15	17	12
Strolling, walking tour, cycling	15	16	11	3	9	8	11
Working	9	8	12	6	7	6	8
Attending (e.g. bank, post)	10	6	7	7	4	5	7
Health care (e.g. doctor)	3	7	8	7	5	5	6
Religious service, cemetery	2	3	5	9	11	4	5
Helping someone (in hh)	2	4	4	5	3	2	3
Drinking coffee, lunch	2	3	5	1	5	4	3
Gardening	1	5	2	5	3	1	3
Activities in association	1	1	2	0	3	5	2
Accompanying someone	3	1	2	2	4	2	2
Sport activities (e.g. bowling)	3	3	1	0	2	4	2
Visiting cultural event	2	1	1	0	0	2	1
Short trip, holiday	2	1	0	0	1	2	1
Fishing, picking berries	4	0	0	0	1	0	1
Education (e.g. courses)	0	0	0		1	1	0
Total N (trips) =	*2157*	*1607*	*1738*	*1053*	*1747*	*997*	*9299*

Note. MOBILATE Diary 2000; weighted

Women shopped more than men (36% vs. 28%). Men worked more often (8% vs. 4%), while women more often attended religious events or visited a cemetery. Age was a less discriminating factor regarding the types of activities older people do outdoors. The main difference concerned working, which was more often pursued by younger respondents (9% vs. 2%). Older respondents more often went to meet other people, shop, or walk.

Strolling and walking were not more frequent in rural than in urban areas, and meeting other people was not a typical activity for the smaller rural communities either. Fishing and picking berries were more common in the countryside, especially among the older respondents. Rural elderly, especially the very old, also attended more religious events.

It is also interesting to classify these activities by how strenuous they are. Some activities such as gardening, sport, strolling, and fishing, call for more physical energy. We have defined strenuous activities as being 'active'. Finns and eastern Germans were the most active, while Hungarians were the least. It is surprising that older people pursued more strenuous activities, even when 'work' was taken into account (Table 5.26).

Table 5.26: Trips with an active[1] motive by age, gender and area (without trips back home) (%)

	Urban				Rural			
	55–74		75+		55-74		75+	
	male	female	male	female	male	female	male	female
Not active	81	85	75	79	81	85	80	87
Active	19	15	25	21	19	15	20	13
Total N (trips) =	*1916*	*2169*	*333*	*556*	*1838*	*1742*	*320*	*423*

Note. MOBILATE Diary 2000; weighted
[1] 4 active motives: gardening, sport, strolling, and fishing.

5.4   Spatial aspects of out-of-home behaviour

The activity space of elderly people is quite restricted. 44% of the trips had a destination within a circle of 1 km, and an additional 24% between 1 and 3 km. Only 14% of the trips went further than 10 km from home. In the rural areas, this range was smaller: 46% stayed within a range of 1 km versus 40% in the urban area. In the cities, the activity radius appeared to be slightly larger: 29% of the trips had a destination within a circle of 1 to 3 km whereas in the rural regions, this was 21%. International comparison showed more activity farther from home in the Netherlands and Finland. Maastricht is very close for a number of villages around the city and was often the destination of trips. Maybe, the same is valid for eastern Germany and Italy, where a nearby city has a regional function. In Finland, the city of Jyväskylä is rather far from neighbouring villages, and this can be seen in the larger percentage of Finnish respondents travelling around their own urban area or village.

The distribution over the strata of the sample is more informative. Table 5.27 shows the differences by the main variables used to stratify the sample. Some conclusions:

- Women more often travelled to very close destinations. This can be found for both age groups and localities (rural vs. urban).
- Older people stayed closer to home than younger ones.
- In cities, people travelled more within their own city.
- In the rural areas, people travelled more often to a neighbouring city.
- The range of mobility was larger in rural than urban areas.

Table 5.27: Trips with a destination on a specific distance by region, gender and age (%)

	Urban				Rural			
	55-74		75+		55-74		75+	
	male	female	male	female	male	female	male	female
Near home, neighbourhood (less < 1 km)	31	44	45	55	38	48	51	68
Own urban area or village (between 1 km and 3 km)	30	27	30	29	21	21	21	15
Own city or municipality (3km - 10km)	25	20	18	12	21	15	14	7
Neighbouring city or within region (10-30km)	8	6	5	3	16	12	9	8
Further away (more than 30km)	5	2	3	2	4	4	4	2
Total N =	*1459*	*1312*	*890*	*673*	*1331*	*1136*	*747*	*529*

Note. MOBILATE Diary 2000

5.5 Possible solutions for experienced mobility problems

5.5.1 Improvements in the transport system in general

Some elderly people avoid specific difficult situations. Health condition plays a role in the modal split, trip distances, comfort of trips and trip motives. The use of a car, a bicycle or public transportation is impossible or too strenuous for many elders.

One of the main goals of this project was the enhancement of out-of-home mobility despite these potential constraints. Therefore, we asked the respondents to rate some suggestions for improving the transport system in their personal opinion. According to their responses, it is not the system as such which needs most improvement. On the contrary, the respondents most often stress courtesy (Table 5.28).

Table 5.28: Important improvements in the traffic system (%)

Statement about improvement in traffic system	personally important
More road courtesy	55
Better economic resources for elderly in general	49
More road (traffic) safety	47
Cheaper tickets for public transport	46
More people to help or to accompany frail persons	42
Cheaper driving services for people who have difficulty with walking	40
More park benches in the streets	39
Designing buses according to the needs of elderly	38
More safety in public places, streets, and underpasses by cameras	35
More security in public places, streets and underpasses by personnel	35
More shops and services in easy reach	32
More paths for bicycles	32
Easier accessibility of shops, public buildings (no stairs)	31
Timetables better coordinated	30
Better bus/tram/train connections	29
Clearer and easier information about public transport	28
Longer cycles for crossing at traffic lights	28
More pedestrian crossings (islands)	27
Designing cars according to the needs of elderly	27
Special parking places for people who have difficulty with walking	26
More parking places at bus stops and railway stations	24
Designing trams according to the needs of elderly	18
Designing bicycles according to the needs of elderly	16
Shorter distances between the stops of bus and tram	16
More personal at the bus stops/rail stations	17
Taxi sharing	16
Meeting-points e.g. at big bus stations	11
Women's taxi	4

Note. MOBILATE Survey 2000; N = 3950, weighted data

After this, several items were chosen, which have in common that they concern the economical situation of the elderly people or the costs of travelling. Another more social item concerning the lack of people to help or to accompany the older traveller received high priority. Park benches along the streets were more important than many other suggestions directly related to improving traffic.

The transport systems are rather different between the participating countries, which was reflected in the different choices respondents made. Hungary did not employ all the items, but 'better economic resources for older people' were important to 73% of the older Hungarians and 'cheaper driving services' to 62%. In Italy, 70% found this item to be important, and 80% felt that more helpers were needed for frail people. More road courtesy and safety were rated highly in all countries with percentages between 44% and 70%, except in Hungary, where this item was not assessed. The Dutch demanded more safety and security in public places (58% and 56%). In western Germany, better designing of buses and trams (54% and 46%) were called for. In Italy, respondents felt more benches along the streets would be helpful, which is not surprising, given the steep hills within the city studied. Italians also placed value on having more shops and services nearby (52%), and they felt that buildings should be more accessible (54%).

5.5.2   Flexible demand responsive (public) transport

We have already described the problems elders have when leaving their home. New technology has enabled a new transport service, 'Demand Responsive Transport', which might better fit the needs of older people. Rosenbloom (2003) voices a rather negative opinion about the role special transport can play in the mobility of older people. Her critics are based on paratransit, which is strongly interwoven with public transit with fixed stops and lines. She states that the most significant environmental barrier to the use of specialised transport is the limitation of both services and choices. Even the most disadvantaged traveller rarely uses such systems for many trips because there are serious restrictions and operational problems. She adds that the costs may also create a threshold.

In the Netherlands this type of transport has become commonplace; municipalities are responsible for the accessibility of transport by disabled and handicapped people (and older people make up about 80% of this group). A wheelchair bus typically performs this service, and the trip goes from door to door. The trip must be ordered at least an hour before the desired departure time, and is generally made together with other people, which entails detours to fetch and drop off other passengers. People who are entitled to this type of transport pay a reduced fare. Older people often belong to this target group.

As can be seen in Table 5.29, demand responsive transport not only has advantages, but disadvantages as well, and clients must weigh these against each other. In order to create an efficient and affordable transport service, people were asked to rank five items concerning which concessions they were willing to make (more detailed figures in tables and graphs can be found in Tacken & van Lamoen, 2002).

A wheelchair bus might have stigma attached to it; elders might refuse to use a service for the frail and disabled. However, this was not confirmed by the rankings. Travelling together with other people and travelling in a wheelchair bus both received high scores, which means that these items were the least troublesome. Having to take a detour was the most negative item, except for Hungary, but Hungarian respondents had not actually used the service. The uncertainty of the departure and arrival times were the most negative items in the

Netherlands where people have some experience with this service. Overall, it is difficult to give weight to rankings that come from respondents who have little or no familiarity with the service provided.

Table 5.29:　Averaged rankings of concessions for demand responsive transport (1 = most troublesome to 5 = least troublesome)

	Finland	Eastern Germany	Western Germany	Hungary	Italy	The Netherlands
	Mean	Mean	Mean	Mean	Mean	Mean
You have to order the vehicle at least one hour in advance	2.7	2.7	3.1	3.2	2.8	2.9
The vehicle can be up to 15 minutes early or late	2.4	3.2	3.2	2.8	2.6	2.3
You have to share the vehicle with other passengers	4.0	3.2	3.5	3.8	3.3	3.6
Often a wheelchair bus will be used to carry out the trip	3.2	2.8	3.2	3.7	3.4	4.0
You often have to make a detour in order to pick up or drop off other passengers	2.6	2.2	2.5	3.2	2.9	2.7

Note. MOBILATE Survey 2000; N = 3950, weighted

All in all, our findings confirm the negative image of this mode of transport, as stated by Rosenbloom. Most users complain about the time window for the pickup. They also mention the unreliability about departure and arrival times most often. The most positive elements of the system mentioned by the people are: door-to-door travel, public safety, good service from the driver and travel with other people. People are aware of the subsidised fares, but they do not perceive these as cheap.

5.5.3　The use of new technology

In several ways, new technology intrudes into the lives of older people. In general the new techniques make life easier, but older people are less used to new-fangled ways of doing things. For example, the older generation has not learned to handle menu-controlled user-interfaces (Docampa Rama, 2001). Over the last few decades, much modern equipment has been changed from directly controlled and mechanical to computerized controls, often with multi-layered menus. Clear guidelines and practical training can make things easier. Recent Dutch experiences, one mentioned in the local press (October 2002), viewed the elderly as important users of chip cards (electronic payments). The loader of chip cards was placed in nursing homes in order to compensate for the fact that the branch offices of banks, where people could get their cash money, are disappearing.

In the MOBILATE survey, respondents were asked if they use some of these new technologies and if new devices make life easier. Enormous differences between countries were found. The perception of a new device seems to depend on its availability. The most common device is the automatic teller machine (ATM) for cash money. 63% of the total sample used them, but frequencies varied greatly between countries. In Hungary, only 1% of the older people used ATM versus 89% in eastern Germany. Telebanking was the least used service. In Finland and the Netherlands, about 5% used this service. The Internet was used by 10% of the respondents in the Netherlands and 15% in Finland, but only 1% or less in

Germany and Hungary. Finnish elders were accustomed to using ticket machines and mobile phones, whereas Italians were used to automatic admission systems.

Table 5.30: Users of new technologies by age, gender and area (%)

	Urban				Rural			
	55-74		75+		55-74		75+	
	male	female	male	female	male	female	male	female
Automatic ticket dispenser	35	39	24	24	21	23	16	15
Automatic teller machines, ATM	62	55	34	25	56	51	28	21
Card-operated telephones	28	27	14	9	24	26	7	6
Automatic admission systems	34	36	30	22	25	20	15	7
Electronic cash (PIN)	43	32	17	13	37	30	14	11
Telebanking	5	3	2	3	5	1	1	0
Mobile telephones	38	25	18	10	28	20	10	6
Internet	13	7	3	1	5	3	2	0

Note. MOBILATE Survey 2000; N = 3550, weighted

In all groups, the ATM was the most common form of new technology. The use of the ticket machine was also rather equally distributed over the groups. Younger elders used most of these new technologies more often than older ones. The same can be said for the urban elderly, but ATMs were actually more common in the rural areas (where offices are less available). Automated ticket dispensers were more common in urban areas, because the low density of traffic in rural areas makes these devices less cost effective.

Do people feel that these new technologies enrich life? Respondents who use specific kinds of technological equipment were asked if they enjoy doing so: does this technology make life easier? In eastern Germany, the Netherlands and Finland most users enjoyed the use of the ATMs, but in western Germany and Hungary, users were much less satisfied. Mobile phones seem to be enjoyed greatly. The users' group was not large, but well satisfied. The same can be said for the Internet. In general, it can be said that the users of new technologies were rather positive. In most cases between 70% and 90% of the users enjoyed the new technology, which is a promising development.

5.6   Conclusions

The first conclusion is perhaps a trifle obvious: being able to use a car and having good health are very important for out-of-home mobility. These two factors are strongly related to younger age, male gender, income, and education. Moreover, these characteristics are very strongly interrelated. These factors play decisive roles for out-of-home mobility and for the positive satisfaction of people with their out-of-home mobility possibilities. In rural areas, a car becomes particularly important, because facilities and services are otherwise not accessible.

Regardless of the mode of transportation used, mobility is negatively influenced by bad weather, feelings of insecurity, lack of courtesy demonstrated by fellow travellers, dangerous traffic situations, and financial costs. Technical solutions to these problems include pedestrian crossings, traffic lights, low-floor buses, demand-responsive transport, etc., all of which are basic conditions; but within the range of available alternatives, older traffic participants seem to make their decisions based on present weather conditions and on their own estimation of several social conditions of the traffic system and the larger social context. Older individuals think the current traffic system could be improved by more road courtesy, more road safety and more financial support.

The private modes of transportation, including cars, bicycles or simply going by foot, are preferred. Public transport seems to play a role when no other alternatives are available or when the system is very well organised, with a high frequency of traffic and a dense network of stops, which is often the case in central urban areas.

77% of the sample made at least one journey over the two interview days. Most involved single journeys, i.e., from home to a destination and back home. Shopping was the most common motive for trip making, followed by visiting friends and relatives and going out for a stroll. Going by foot was the most popular mode of transportation, followed by using a car (as a driver or as a passenger). For the oldest age group these pedestrian trips often were the last remaining alternative to get the daily necessities and to maintain a basic level of social contact.

A time analysis of trip-making behaviour over the course of the day showed two peaks: the first in the middle of the morning and a second one in the middle of the afternoon. The elderly people clearly avoid busy traffic hours, which might have been expected, and they stay at home during the late afternoon and night.

23% of the sample made no trip at all during the interview period. The average number of trips for the whole sample was 2.1 trips a day. Going by foot was the most common form of travelling, followed by using the car (as a driver or a passenger). The spatial range of mobility was rather small: 44% of the trips were within a distance of 1 km and an additional 24% were within 3 km.

One important finding related to health was the fact that there are a certain number of aged persons having such great outdoor mobility difficulties and no compensatory means in their use that they have to stay indoors, although most of them are interested in going out for getting necessary services and meeting friends. Especially, among the oldest women there exist persons in need of intensive help for getting out of their homes. This amount varies in relation to age, country, region and gender depending on the compensatory mechanisms in use at different levels. Besides there are much more aged persons who are willing to be more often mobile outdoors than they are able today using the existing compensatory means. Due to autonomy of the aged people being also a very important factor of well-being and quality of life this necessitates different ways to help these people to go out of their homes.

Elders are not very negative about the use of new technology; in fact, people who used some new technologies, were fairly satisfied with them. This appears to be a promising development and may signal a need for new types of transport, such as the demand-responsive system described. Nonetheless, the present system needs improvement: although older people are positive about the idea, they are rather negative about how the present system operates.

References

Brög, W, Erl, E., & Glorius, B. (2000). Germany. In European Conference of Ministers of Transport (ECMT), *Transport and Ageing of the Population.* Report of the 112th round table on transport economics. Paris Cedex, France: OECD Publications.

Centre d'études sur les réseaux, les transports, l'urbanisme et les constructions publiques (CERTU) (2001). *La mobilité des personnes âgées - Analyse des enquêtes ménages déplacements* [The mobility of older people. Analyses of household travel research]. Rapport d'étude. Lyon: CERTU.

CBS (Central Bureau of Statistics) (2000). *De mobiliteit van de Nederlandse bevolking* [The mobility of the Dutch population]. Heerlen: CBS.

Chapin, F. S. (1974). *Human activity in the city, things people do in time and space.* New York: John Wiley and Sons.

Chu, X. (1994). The effects of age on the driving habits of the elderly. Evidence from the 1990 *National Personal Transportation Study.* DOT-T-95-12. Washington D.C.: U.S. Department of Transportation.

Dijst, M. (1995). *Het elliptische leven* [The elliptical life, action space as integral measure for reach and mobility]. Netherlands Geographical Studies (NGS 196). Utrecht: Koninklijk Nederlands Aardrijkskundig Genootschap.

Docampo Rama, M. (2001). *Technology generations handling complex user interfaces.* PhD Thesis, University of Technology Eindhoven. Published by University of Eindhoven.

Fozard, J. L. (2003). Enabling environments for physical aging: a balance of preventive and compensatory interventions. In K. W. Schaie, H.-W. Wahl, H. Mollenkopf, & F. Oswald (eds.), *Aging Independently. Living Arrangements and Mobility* (pp. 31-45). New York: Springer Publishing Company.

Hägerstrand, T. (1970). *What about people in Regional Science?* Paper of the Regional Science Association, Vol XXIV, pp. 7-21.

Leinbach T. & Watkins, J. (1994). *Transportation services, utilization and needs of the elderly in non-urban areas.* DOT-T-95-08. Washington.

Mollenkopf, H., & Flaschenträger, P. (2001). *Erhaltung von Mobiliät im Alter* [Maintaining mobility in old age] (Vo. 197 - Bundesministerium für Familie, Senioren, Frauen und Jugend. Stuttgart). Berlin: Kohlhammer.

Mollenkopf, H., Marcellini, F., Ruoppila, I., Széman, Z., Tacken, M., Kaspar, R., & Wahl, H.-W. (2002). The Role of Driving in Maintaining Mobility in Later Life: A European View. *Gerontechnology 1*, no 4, 231-250.

OECD (2001). *Ageing and Transport, Mobility needs and safety issues.* Paris: OECD.

Parkes, D. N., & Thrift, N. J. (1986). *Time spaces and places, a chrono-geographic perspective.* New York: John Wiley and Sons.

Pred, A. (1984). Place as a historical contingent process: structuration and the time-geography of becoming places. *Annals of the Association of American Geographers,* 74 (1984) 2.

Raitanen, T., Törmäkangas, T., Mollenkopf, H., & Marcellini, F. (2003). Why do older drivers reduce driving? Findings from three European countries. *Transportation Research Part F: Psychology and Behaviour 6*(2), 81-95.

Rudinger, G. & Jansen, E. (2003). Self-initiated compensations among older drivers. In K. W. Schaie, H.-W. Wahl, H. Mollenkopf, & F. Oswald (eds.), *Aging Independently. Living Arrangements and Mobility* (pp. 220-233). New York: Springer Publishing Company.

Rosenbloom, S. (2003). *The mobility needs of older Americans: implications for transportation reauthorisation.* The Brookings Institution Series on Transformation Reform, Centre on urban and metropolitan policy. Washington. www.brookings.edu/urban

Tacken, M., & van Lamoen, E. (2002). *Transport and mobility, differences between European countries in transport behaviour and in realised journeys and trips.* Delft: University of Technology. Info: http://www.bk.tudelft.nl/users/tacken/internet/

Tacken, M. (1998). Mobility of the elderly in time and space in the Netherlands: An analysis of the Dutch National Travel Survey. *Transportation (25)* 4, 379-393.

Van Reisen, A. (1997). *Ruim baan door telewerken* [Telework and its spatial and mobility consequences]. Netherlands Geographical Studies (NGS 22). Utrecht: Koninklijk Nederlands Aardrijkskundig Genootschap.

Wittenberg, R. (1986). Einstellung zum Autobesitz und Unsicherheitsgefühle älterer Menschen im Straßenverkehr [Older People's Attitudes Towards Owning a Car and Feeling Unsafe in Traffic]. *Zeitschrift für Gerontologie*, 19, 400-409.

Enhancing Mobility in Later Life
H. Mollenkopf et al. (Eds.)
IOS Press, 2005

Chapter 6
Health and Leisure Activities

Isto Ruoppila, Mart Tacken and Nina Hirsiaho

6.1   Introduction

The literature on leisure is rich in comments on the difficulty inherent to defining leisure as a term or as an activity. There is no common agreement on the definition of leisure and the field abounds with difficulties generated by the conceptual and measurement problems caused by this lack of clarity. Hamilton-Smith (1991, p. 446) has suggested four constructs with which leisure can be assessed. Of them, leisure as action within time and space is a construct which underlies ideas of recreation. Leisure activities are located in specific time and place contexts, which generally exclude any possibility of confusion with employment and other essential or obligatory activities. The exceptions, in this context, are utility-based leisure activities, such as hunting, fishing, picking berries or gathering mushrooms, and gardening. Hamilton-Smith (1991) argues that this construct provides one of the most useful and appropriate bases for studying leisure activities. She points out that the interaction between time and space often serves to define recreational and leisure activity and set it apart from other kinds of activities. Leisure time and leisure activities are even more difficult to define after a person has retired. Activity patterns show great stability. But when changes in health lead to more difficulties in performing various physical activities of daily living (PADLs) and instrumental activities of daily living (IADLs), or when these tasks require more time and effort, the amount of free time that can be spent on freely chosen leisure activities is reduced.

Health and leisure

It should be emphasized that the same demographic changes which have an effect on the relations between health and outdoor mobility also principally affect the relations between health and leisure. These are the ageing of population and the increase in the number of the very old, especially women. The living arrangements and lifestyles of older women differ from those of older men. Older women generally live alone and are widowed, fewer drive a car (at least in the present cohorts over 60 years of age), and they have smaller pensions. One quite new finding is that the mobility and migration rates of seniors are increasing, especially on a seasonal basis. This kind of mobility may have strong effects on different leisure activities.

Along aging, the number of leisure activities as well as their frequency decrease, first slowly, then after 75/80 years of age, more rapidly. The main reasons for this are diseases, handicaps and various impairments to physical mobility. Generally, outdoor leisure activities decrease to a greater extent, and more rapidly, among women compared to men. In particular, those outdoor leisure activities, which require good health and physical functioning, like travel or rambling, decrease. Within aging, home-based indoor leisure activities as well as media-based leisure activities increase (Iso-Ahola, Jackson & Dunn, 1994). Mollenkopf et al. (1997, p. 302) concluded on the basis of their data: "Quiet, more passive activities within one's home are predominantly important for elderly people who either have no car at their disposal or are limited in their mobility for health reasons".

Lawton (1994) has emphasized the social and environmental factors in leisure activity choice: age, cohort, and history determinants. Schaie (1996) articulated the basic conceptualisation of age changes as consisting of the separate but empirically confounded processes of individual ageing, the socialization experiences of successive cohorts, and the changes that affect people as historical time and events proceed. Lawton (1994), on the basis of the model of selective optimisation with compensation developed by Baltes and Baltes (1989), points out that compensatory leisure activity is an extremely important mechanism in the maintenance of valued activities. Physically less strenuous activities within the same activity type may be adopted. One such change may be from outdoor leisure activities to indoor leisure activities, or beginning to use reminiscence as a substitute for leisure behaviour. In this phase, photographs, picture albums and other different objects depicting subjects' past participatory activities, like travel destinations or products of earlier handicrafts describing the life course of the subjects, may assume important roles.

One important goal in studies concerning leisure after retirement has been to define the level and content of activity. Both are related to successful ageing (Lawton, 1994; Russell, 1990). Generally, participation in leisure activities has been associated with well-being and quality of life (Iso-Ahola, 1994; Mannell, 1993). Social participation and the development of self-knowledge through self-expression are connected to leisure activities. They are held both in theoretical and empirical studies as factors that maintain the health and well-being of elderly persons (Csikszentmihalyi, 1994; Higgins, 1995; Kelly & Ross, 1989).

Higgins (1995) has analysed the problem of how to achieve health through leisure. Leisure has been interpreted as a concept emphasizing self-actualisation and freedom. Health promotion can be defined as "the process of enabling people to increase control over, and to improve, their health" (WHO, 1984, p. 4). The concept of leisure contains some elements similar to those in the concepts of health, functioning ability and health promotion (when health is viewed in terms of physical, psychological and social well-being). The mechanisms of leisure activities, which promote health and well-being, are manifested at different levels, i.e., from the individual through organizational levels to community and societal levels (Higgins, 1995). Both leisure and health promotion seek to enhance quality of life. Health is regarded as more than the mere absence of disease and includes physical, mental, and spiritual well-being (WHO, 1984) and the ability to self-fulfill needs and adapt to the environment. Recreation is a public good, much like public health care services. In addition to the direct benefits of leisure and recreation services, users can expect indirect benefits from leisure in the form of enhanced social interaction and sense of community. It has been suggested that the field of leisure and recreation can be a strategic partner for health and other social services; it can be a potent force in shaping the health of the population (Ball, 1996).

Psychological well-being and leisure

Via leisure activities one can express oneself and one's state of mind. The meaning of leisure activities for psychological well-being has been studied by using different but related outcomes like mental health (e.g. Csikszentmihalyi, 1994; Iso-Ahola, 1994; Mannell, 1993;

Riddick & Daniel, 1984), happiness (e.g. Brown, Frankel, & Fennell, 1991), life satisfaction (Doyle & Forehand, 1984; Kelly, Steinkemp, & Kelly, 1987; Ragheb & Griffith, 1982; Riddick, 1985; Russell, 1987), quality of life (Russell, 1990), self-actualisation (Csikszentmihalyi & Kleiber, 1991) and mood (Csikszentmihalyi, 1990; Hull, 1991; Lawton, 1994). Leisure activities have also been used in treating depression (Patrick, 1994). The findings generally show that different leisure activities enhance people's well-being (Lampinen et al., 2004). This may have been operationalized as mental health, happiness, life satisfaction or as different indicators of mood. People who have many leisure activities and participate in them frequently rate their well-being higher than those who have only a few leisure activities and participate in them only rarely. Although most leisure activities are clearly related to well-being, in some studies, religious and sport leisure activities have not been related to it (Lawton, 1994). Brown, Frankel and Fennell (1991) showed that of the different types of leisure activities, only social and outdoor activities contribute to the well-being of men, while social, household, sedentary and physical activities are all significantly related to the well-being of women. However, social activities are more important to women than to men in terms of well-being.

Iso-Ahola (1994) has summarized the mechanisms by which different leisure activities are assumed to affect health. He emphasizes that an active leisure lifestyle is important for mental health, which is marked by an enhanced sense of freedom and control over one's behaviours. An active leisure lifestyle is conducive to many different health benefits like positive mood. These, in turn, lead to improvement in physical health, e.g., via the secretor immune system. The health benefits of an active leisure lifestyle include flow and self-actualisation experiences (Csikszentmihalyi, 1990, 1997), increased happiness and life satisfaction, improved self-esteem and reduced loneliness. Leisure affects health also by providing buffering mechanisms when there are crises in life. The disease rate stays relatively low regardless of stress for those who maintain an active lifestyle but increases among those who lead a passive and sedentary leisure life. Leisure participation facilitates coping with life stress by fostering companionships, friendships and informal and formal social support networks, and by enhancing a sense of control and mastery of the life course. In particular, leisure-related social contacts are highly effective in buffering stress, whereas obligatory contacts do not (Bolger & Eckenrode, 1991; Rook, 1987). Self-determination also serves as a buffer: perceived freedom in leisure buffers stress so that the disease rate of subjects high in perceived freedom or control of leisure remains low with increasing life stress. Conversely, the disease rate rises dramatically with increasing stress among those low in perceived freedom or control of leisure (Coleman & Iso-Ahola, 1993; Deci & Ryan, 1987; Iso-Ahola & Mannell, 1985).

It is assumed that informal, self-initiated activities rather than formal, organized activities may provide more meaning and satisfaction to the individual, which in turn translate into higher life satisfaction and well-being (McPherson, 1991). Similarly, expressive and instrumental activities may provide more or less satisfaction, depending on the preferences of the older individual. There is no general answer as to which leisure activities will best enhance life satisfaction or well-being in the later years; heterogeneity prevails (McPherson, 1991).

Modernity, or modern society, directs the ageing process and the role-expectations received by elderly persons according to prevailing cultural and ethical notions (Tokarski, 1993). Being free from the roles and role-expectations related to work may interfere with other expectations relating to elderly people's leisure activities (Mahoney, 1994; Pedlar, Sherry, & Gilbert, 1996). Csikszentmihalyi (1994) has emphasized the inability of people in modern society to use their leisure time for themselves. Instead, persons experience frustration and anxiety because of empty time and because of their own inability to make it meaningful and developing.

Life course and leisure

People acquire their interests in youth or in early adulthood, and these interests form the basis of their later leisure activities. Until retirement and before the third age, these activities appear to be stable if the living environment makes them possible. Early in the acquisition of interests, clear culturally related gender differences can be seen. The age differences are small, but cohort differences can be considerable. Additionally, education and occupation strongly determine, not only during working age but also afterwards, what the leisure time of an elderly person will be like and what kind of activities it will include.

Other factors which influence the time spent on leisure activities as well as their content stem from the earlier life-course of an individual. In particular, basic and vocational education, as well as one's profession, have their own roles in the selection of leisure activities. Past patterns of leisure activities affect the way older adults use their time. When people retire, most continue to do the same activities they did before, but at a different pace (Kelly, 1993). The activity patterns of middle age tend to persist into the later years. Gradually, as people become frail, the number of activities decreases, they practice them less frequently than earlier and they modify them so as to be symbolically and meaningfully related to earlier leisure pursuits. The principle of selective optimisation with compensation can be seen in this.

Elderly people adapt their leisure activities. They may be modified on the basis of a person's life situation and the activity potential of one's living environment. In leisure activities, the same basic theme, however, often remains permanent throughout life. This theme may hold the same psychological, sociological and developmental meaning, even though the individual sees him- or herself differently in the different phases of his or her life (Kelly, 1982; Lawton, 1993).

Iso-Ahola et al. (1994) have studied aggregate and intra-personal patterns of leisure behaviour: the starting, ceasing and replacing of leisure activities as a function of successive developmental periods of the life course. Their findings, based on American data, showed that the number of people starting new activities first declined but levelled off in the two oldest age groups, 44 to 63 years of age and 64 years and older. The number of people replacing activities was similar to the number starting new activities. The number of people ceasing leisure activities declined during the life course, while the reverse was true for continuers of participation in the same activities. The authors conclude that although the overall quantity of leisure activities may decrease with age, the data did not indicate that starting different types of activities declines over the life stages: the number of people starting physically demanding outdoor activities decreased with advancing age, but there was a significant increase in the number of people starting home-based activities in later life.

The Finnish Evergreen follow-up study shows that half of the elderly people investigated, aged 65 to 84 years at the first assessment and assessed eight years later, had a leisure activity which they had maintained throughout their life course. Among men the most frequent leisure activities were physical and artistic activities and among women handicrafts

(Pikkarainen & Heikkinen, 1999a; Suutama, Ruoppila, & Laukkanen, 1999). It is assumed that handicrafts are more closely related to the well-being of elderly people than physical activities; it is also possible to pursue handicraft activities into old age, whereas there are restrictions on physical activities (Smale & Dupuis, 1993).

On the basis of the Finnish Evergreen project, leisure activities among two cohorts of male and female Jyväskylä residents aged 65 to 69 years in 1988 (born in 1919 - 1923) and in 1996 (born in 1927 - 1931) were also compared (Heikkinen, Lampinen, & Suutama, 1999; Pikkarainen & Heikkinen 1999b). The leisure activities of both cohorts were quite similar. The predominating leisure activities of both women and men were reading newspapers and magazines, watching TV and domestic travel. The female cohort listened to the radio somewhat less in 1996, but studied more than in 1988. Men's leisure activities were similar in both male cohorts. Of the 1988 cohort, 10% were studying in 1988, compared to 17% in 1996. Men studied more often in 1988, but women studied more in 1996. There were no entirely passive 65 to 69-year-old subjects at either assessment point. About half of both the male and female cohorts had a lifelong leisure activity. Handicrafts were the most popular lifelong leisure activity among women, and sports among men. The main reason for non-participation in one's earlier hobbies was poor health or poor physical functioning. Men's leisure activities, like voluntary working for organizations and engaging in sports, decreased more often and women's activities increased more often during retirement. The main reason for involvement in new leisure activities after retirement was that subjects aged 65 to 69 had more time for leisure.

It should be emphasized that in leisure activities, continuity is the rule. Although ageing and, especially chronic diseases, force the conservation of resources, even the impairments of old age occur in a context where the person remains in control to direct the process of selective optimisation with compensation. Within very broad limits, learning new leisure activities is possible, and is the spice of life (Lawton, 1994).

Financial resources and leisure

Health acts as a threshold factor for leisure activities, similarly to the financial resources, which have a supporting effect. Different leisure activities are differently associated with the financial cost their practice requires. Usually, indoor activities like having visitors, reading, listening to the radio, watching TV or playing games are not high-cost activities. Among the outdoor leisure activities, e.g. walking, rambling, picking berries and gathering mushrooms, visiting the library, attending religious events or doing voluntary or charity work are the inexpensive ones to practice. But there are also those which cost more, such as playing golf, taking courses, pursuing artistic activities, visiting the opera, etc. In some countries, a range of leisure activities are supported by public funding, as in the Universities of the Third Age, which exist for the further education of retired people. Other cultural activities, like the theatre, opera and concerts, may offer discounts for the elderly, therefore meaning greatly varying costs for the elderly individuals living in different countries and regions.

Barriers and hindrances to leisure

Henderson et al. (1988) studied the leisure barriers for women. Their findings showed ten leisure barrier factors. These were time, money, facilities, family concerns, unawareness, lack of interest, decision-making, body image, skills and social inappropriateness. The researchers assumed that women might have more antecedent barriers operant in their lives than men. The antecedent barriers identified in their study were social inappropriateness, body image, and lack of interest. The latter two seemed to be moderately strong barriers. Other factors were identified as intervening barriers.

Mannell (1994) also analysed the types and frequencies of leisure constraints in the context of daily life on the basis of American data consisting of 3,412 self-reports utilising the experimental sampling method and alternative activity probe technique (n = 92 retired older adults). Constraint profiles were formed using this data. The constraint profiles of three of the four groups, active schedule, active enough, and withdrawal, were each dominated by two types of constraints. The fourth, the unconstrained group, reported all six types of constraints with average or below average frequency.

The active schedule group was characterised by being already too busy with leisure activities as well as with many other activity interests. This group obtained the highest scores in the satisfaction measures. The active enough group reported that they were active in leisure activities. However, these subjects had fewer competing interests and clearly lacked interest in increasing their participation. However, this group did not differ from the active schedule group in satisfaction. The withdrawal group, while reporting being busy with daily obligations as frequently as the subjects in the other groups, was inhibited from increasing their leisure activity levels by a lack of energy or wellness and a desire to avoid social contact. About 50% of the retired people in this study were in the unconstrained group. This group was more willing to increase their participation than the other groups.

Although it may seem odd, one of the most important barriers to leisure among older people can be time-related. It may be that some older men and women are not very good at organizing their daily obligations and activities, or they need more time for them because of their lowered health-status, and consequently at arranging time for leisure activities (McGuire, 1984).

The hindrances to leisure activities differ between men and women (Iso-Ahola et al., 1994). Women more easily abandon earlier leisure activities and are also more cautious in beginning new ones because of the so-called women hindrances, which include lack of a companion, care duties, and social obstacles (Henderson, Stalnaker, & Taylor, 1988). Because of women's more frequent loneliness, leisure activities may have the effects of enhancing the self-worth and self-knowledge of elderly women.

Outdoor mobility and leisure

Leisure activities and sport are an important part of the out-of-home activities of older people. For most of them, work no longer serves to structure their time, and they fill their days with several types of activities, which we will term leisure activities, without external pressures. However, the daily activity pattern can be structured by leisure activities and fixed times and arrangements can also become compulsory.

Little information is currently available on specific transport patterns. Most research attention has focused on the modal split and numbers of trips. Mostly the motives of trip-making have been reduced to a few categories, of which leisure is one. In 1997, 47% of the trips made by people aged 75 and older were made for shopping and 36% for leisure (Brög, Erl & Glorius, 2000). Leinbach and Watkins (1994) produced a more detailed analysis of the reasons for trip-making in their study of the transport behaviour of elderly persons in non-urban areas in Kentucky. They made a distinction between 'life maintenance' (shopping, medical and financial) and 'higher-order' (social, religion, dining out and other) trips. They analysed the effect of age, gender and residential location. For gender they concluded that no differences between men and women existed in their data. For location they found that in rural areas, medical trips and essential shopping were more important than in 'periurban' areas and that social trips were less important. With age, the importance of 'life maintenance' increases, especially medical trips.

The Dutch Social and Cultural Planning Office paid attention to leisure activities in its overview study of the elderly. They concluded that the diversity of leisure activities has recently increased, even among the older age groups (SCP, 1997). Analysing this diversity by regression analysis, they found that age, education, transport facilities and income have the most influence. The number of out-of-home activities depends on age, health experiences and income. The positive influence of these factors was stronger in the higher age groups.

Mollenkopf and Flaschenträger (2001) also analysed leisure activities using data rather similar to that in the MOBILATE study. They found out that young people and car drivers were more active, spending more time on walking, cycling, going on tours and playing sports. Men went out more for the purposes of gardening, taking walks and going on cycle tours, whereas women spent more time on visits, going to the theatre, reading etc. Religious events and activities for retired people were more favoured in the oldest group.

Carp (1988) compared leisure in a compact city and a sprawled city and found great differences. In the compact city, 55% went out for entertainment and recreation once a week, whereas only 3% did the same in the sprawled city. The accessibility of public transport and neighbourhood facilities were crucial. After removing work trips Rosenbloom (1988) concluded that older people make more trips than younger people. Shopping, family and personal business trips accounted for more than 50% of all trips. Medical trips were the longest. The Dutch National Travel Survey (CBS, 2000) divides leisure activities into five rough categories: visiting, shopping, tour/walking and recreation and sport. The numbers of trips made for all these purposes decreased with age, as did the total distances travelled for them.

We assume that leisure time activities are more culturally context-bound than health, at least within the western industrialized societies. Health may differently affect participation in leisure activities after the age of 55 years, and participation in leisure activities (to a lesser extent) may differently affect health during the ageing process. The interaction between health and leisure is influenced by culture (country and region), gender, via differing gender-role associated activities, and age/cohort. The general research objective of this chapter is to determine the relation between health and leisure activities during the ageing process and how it varies in different European countries, in urban and rural environments, and in men and women.

6.2   Health and leisure activities in the MOBILATE study

6.2.1   Research questions and hypotheses

The research questions addressed in this chapter are as follows:

1. How satisfied are people aged 55 years and older with their leisure activities, and how active are they in participating in different leisure activities? Moreover, how do these vary between countries, regions, genders and age-groups?

2. How does health relate to the leisure activities pursued by the subjects?

    It is expected that those having better health status will be more satisfied with their leisure activities, will be more likely to have a higher number of different indoor and outdoor leisure activities as well as make more holiday trips lasting at least for one week than those with impaired health status.

3. Does health have different effects on the basis of age, gender, and region in the different participating countries as regards satisfaction with one's own leisure activities, the number of leisure activities and the number of holiday trips made during the previous year?

We assume that younger subjects will be more satisfied with their different leisure activities than older ones, men will be more satisfied than women and urban subjects more satisfied than rural ones. As regards indoor leisure activities, we expect that older subjects, women and people living in rural areas will have more of these than younger subjects, men and urban subjects. We also expect that older subjects, women and people living in rural regions will have fewer different outdoor leisure activities than younger subjects, men and urban subjects. Finally, we assume that younger subjects, men and people living in urban regions will more often make trips lasting at least one week than older subjects, women and people living in rural regions, because generally it is easier for men and for people living in urban areas to make such trips as they might have not only better health, but also more possibilities to do them. There might be different interactions between health, region and gender due to the varying possibilities for outdoor leisure activities because of different (cultural) gender roles, and differences in supply, distances and the costs of participating in these leisure activities. Generally, the above-mentioned hypotheses are based on differences in health and outdoor mobility between the groups to be compared.

6.2.2   Methods

We have information on the leisure activities of elderly people from two main sources. In the questionnaire, subjects reported their personal experiences and judgements regarding leisure activities, and in the diary, they described their actual travel and leisure behaviour. Both sources of information will be analysed here.

In the first part, which focuses on leisure activities as such, a distinction is made between indoor and outdoor activities. Here a variety of outdoor activities has been used. The remaining activities (which were not selected as outdoor ones), are grouped together as indoor activities. This selection is presented in Table 6.4.

In studying the possible effect of health on leisure time activities (the second part), two separate factors were found by factor analysis, namely indoor and outdoor activities. In the figures, the answer categories are calculated as the sum of the 'yes' answers. ('I take part in' 1 = yes and 0 = no)

It should be emphasised that Factor II, 'Outdoor activity', differs slightly from the indicator 'Options of outdoor activities' used in the outdoor mobility index in the further regression analyses (see Chapter 12 and 13). Games, do-it-yourself activities, as well as the artistic activities in the list below are not included in that indicator, because these activities can be pursued both indoor and outdoor. In explaining the number of outdoor activities by social background, health and transport mode-variables (Tables 8.7-8.10), picking berries and making holiday trips lasting at least one week were included like in the indicator of outdoor activities.

Factor I 'Indoor activity' contains the following variables:
- Receiving visits in my home
- Just being cosy at home, looking out of the window
- Reading, solving riddles, collecting stamps and coins
- Watching TV, listening to the radio
- Talking on the phone

The theoretical range of this indoor activity factor varies between 0 and 5.

Factor II 'Outdoor activity', consists of:
- Meeting friends or acquaintances outside of my home
- Going to a café, restaurant or bar
- Games, e.g., bingo, canasta, boccia
- Making small trips or journeys, lasting at least half a day
- Gardening
- "Do-it-yourself", being busy with handicrafts, car, house etc.
- Dancing, bowling
- Hiking, riding a bicycle
- Going out for a walk, stroll through the town
- Actively pursuing sports
- Watching sporting events (not on TV)
- Visiting theatre, opera, concerts, movies
- Visiting a library
- Taking courses (arts and crafts, etc.) and further education
- Religious events, attending church
- Activities in clubs or associations
- Activities for retired people
- Fishing
- Voluntary or charity work
- Artistic activities such as painting or drawing.

The theoretical range of this outdoor activity factor varies between 0 and 20.

The satisfaction obtained from participating in the leisure time activities (0-10, 0 = very unsatisfied and 10 = very satisfied) and the number of holiday trips lasting at least one week made since the beginning of the year 2000 (0 = no trip; 1 = one big trip; 2 = several trips, recoded as number of the trips made) were also analysed.

The least reliable scale used in the present analyses is the indoor leisure activities scale, which varied between 0.55 and 0.62 (Cronbach's alpha). These quite low coefficients mean that caution is advised when interpreting findings based on this scale. The outdoor leisure activities sum-scale had satisfactory reliability: 0.69 - 0.77.

6.3   Leisure activities: description and explanation

6.3.1   Satisfaction with leisure and sport activities

A first general overview shows satisfaction with leisure activities (Table 6.1).

Table 6.1:   Satisfaction with leisure activities by age, gender and residential location (mean)

	Urban				Rural			
	55 - 74		75+		55-74		75+	
	male	female	male	female	−male	female	−male	female
Finland	8.6	8.5	7.8	7.9	8.1	7.8	7.8	7.1
Eastern Germany	7.5	7.3	6.4	5.7	6.3	6.3	6.0	4.9
Western Germany	7.7	7.7	5.5	6.1	7.5	7.6	7.4	7.1
Hungary	8.1	8.0	7.0	6.7	6.3	5.7	6.1	5.7
Italy	8.2	8.0	7.7	6.9	7.2	6.7	7.1	6.2
The Netherlands	7.7	7.3	7.6	7.3	7.5	7.6	7.7	7.1

Note. MOBILATE Survey 2000; N = 3950;
11 point satisfaction scale: 0 = very unsatisfied, 10 = very satisfied

Generally, the Finnish subjects were the most satisfied, the East Germans the least satisfied. In Hungary a clear difference was evident between the urban and the rural respondents. Among the latter, satisfaction was rather low. Younger people were, in general, more satisfied than their older counterparts. People living in urban areas were also more satisfied. This can also be seen in the comparison of the total subgroups, not controlled by country, area, age or gender. In urban areas, satisfaction was, at 7.6, significantly higher (t-test: p<.01) than in the rural areas, where it was 6.9. Age also played a crucial role: the younger age groups were rather similar at 7.5 (55-64) and 7.4 (65-74), but the older age groups were less satisfied with means of 6.9 (75-84) and 5.8 (85^+) (t-test: p<.01). Gender also produced a slight difference between groups, with means of 7.4 (men) and 7.1 (women) (t-test: p<.05).

The transport facilities available seem to affect satisfaction with leisure as well. People with no car or bicycle had a satisfaction score of 6.4; those with one of these modes had a score of 7.2 and with both modes 7.8. Furthermore, a clear relation to activities of daily living (ADL) revealed. People with no problem at all had a score of 8.0 and those with light problems 7.7, but people with serious problems had a score of 6.1.

Table 6.2:   Satisfaction with leisure activities by self-evaluation of physical mobility (means)

Self-evaluation of physical mobility	very poor	poor	fair	good	very good
Satisfaction with leisure activities (m)	3.7	6.0	7.4	7.7	8.1

Note. MOBILATE Survey 2000; N = 3950 weighted;
11 point satisfaction scale: 0 = very unsatisfied, 10 = very satisfied

An even stronger relation can be found for self-reported physical mobility (Table 6.2). Evaluating one's physical mobility as very poor associated with low satisfaction with leisure activities, whereas very good mobility with high satisfaction (F-test: p<.001).

One might suppose that in an urban environment (compared to a rural one), the leisure opportunities available lead to more satisfaction. The significant difference (t-test, p <.01) between 7.6 and 6.9 confirms this assumption. Satisfaction, however, is a measure which is always related to personal experiences and how a person weighs them, rather than to realised behaviour. In the next section, we focus on participation in activities.

6.3.2 Participation in leisure activities

Table 6.3 gives an overview of the participation in different leisure activities. The items have been ordered by their frequency of the total column across countries. This shows clearly that activities at home lead the series. Watching TV, receiving visitors, be cosy at home, reading, and talking on the phone are rather common activities. More than 52% of the respondents do these activities at some time.

Table 6.3: People participating in specific leisure activities (%)

Leisure activity	FIN	G-(E)	G-(W)	HUN	IT	NL	Urban	Rural	Total
Watching TV, radio	85	94	85	95	85	85	90	87	89
Receiving visits at home	72	76	80	67	46	88	76	69	72
Meeting friends (not at home)	72	60	70	59	52	89	71	63	67
Just being cosy at home	51	65	60	78	48	75	66	60	63
Reading, solving riddles	61	53	48	63	46	67	63	49	56
Talking on the telephone	51	60	64	47	29	58	61	43	52
Going out for a walk	57	60	64	28	54	44	63	41	52
Gardening	41	62	43	63	48	49	41	61	51
"Do-it-yourself"	56	31	37	36	42	45	40	41	41
Making small trips	55	44	50	23	18	46	45	35	40
Religious events	39	11	45	38	43	57	33	43	38
Café, restaurant	17	31	51	7	29	54	38	27	32
Hiking, riding a bicycle	38	36	38	10	6	53	31	31	31
Theatre, opera, etc.	41	14	24	8	11	36	29	15	22
Games (e.g. Bingo, Card)	15	16	20	20	23	37	23	20	21
Picking berries, mushrooms[1]	61	19	7	6	8	/	16	18	17
Activities in clubs	22	8	16	4	7	37	15	16	15
Library	36	4	9	6	3	23	16	9	13
Activities for retired	22	10	18	10	6	8	11	14	12
Voluntary or charity	17	6	9	5	12	23	13	11	12
Watching sport	12	6	11	11	7	19	12	10	11
Dancing, bowling	19	8	13	5	9	11	12	9	11
Actively pursuing sport	6	9	11	2	6	26	12	8	10
Others	30	5	5	0	3	6	11	5	8
Fishing	31	4	2	4	3	3	7	8	7
Taking courses	16	4	6	1	3	11	8	5	7
Swimming, gymnastics[2]	23	/	/	2	4	/	6	3	4
Artistic activities	7	2	5	1	4	7	5	3	4
Playing PC games	5	2	2	1	4	7	5	2	3
Surfing the internet	4	2	2	0	2	8	4	2	3
Hunting[3]	9	1	1	/	3	/	1	3	2
Total N =	608	766	750	602	598	610	1960	1972	3935

Note. MOBILATE Survey 2000; N = 3950; weighted
[1] not asked in the Netherlands; [2] not asked in Germany and the Netherlands; [3] not asked in Hungary and the Netherlands

The first out-of-home activity concerns meeting friends elsewhere (67%), followed by going for a walk (52%), gardening (51%), do-it-yourself (41%), and making small trips (40%). Religious events also score rather high with a percentage of 38%, but on this item, large differences appear between countries: Italy, western Germany and the Netherlands have high scores (43-57%) and eastern Germany a very low score with only 11%. Likewise, hiking and cycling were quite frequent activities in other countries, except Hungary and Italy. Visiting a café or restaurant is only a little bit lower, with rather low scores in Finland, Italy and Hungary.

Cultural events obtained low scores in eastern Germany, Hungary and Italy. Activities in clubs and going to a library obtained high scores in Finland and in the Netherlands, as did voluntary work, which can be done through clubs and associations. Picking berries and fishing were activities typical of many Finnish elders. Besides these activities, many Finns took part in swimming and dancing; apparently they enjoy rather sportive activities. Actively pursuing sports obtained a high score in the Netherlands. The Dutch research area showed a high degree of participation in clubs, and sport can be one of their activities.

Table 6.3 also presents the difference between urban and rural areas. In many activities, a difference can be found. The most striking is 'going out for a walk', which was most often done in urban areas; not surprisingly, 'gardening' was most often done in rural areas. In the cities, people went out more to the theatre etc., they also read and solved riddles more as well as called on the phone more frequently than the rural inhabitants. Reading went together with a higher frequency of visits to a library.

A next step was the question: how important do the respondents rate the activities in which they participate? To answer this, we related the numbers of respondents who confirmed an item as important, with the numbers of respondents who participated in each activity (Table 6.4).

Table 6.4 shows an interesting discrepancy with Table 6.3. Table 6.4 is again ordered by the frequencies across countries. The first (most important) activity mentioned is 'swimming, gymnastics, etc.', although this concerns only a few people. Nonetheless, this group views such activity as being very important. Activities with a few participants mostly means a more explicit choice is being made. Active sports, meeting friends elsewhere, voluntary work, going out for a walk and picking berries and mushrooms are important for those who are active in these respects. Being cosy at home is the most important activity at home. What is surprising is the low position of religious events: only in Hungary are these important to those they concern.

Table 6.4:   Importance of leisure activities for people who participate in these activities (%)

	Finland	Eastern Germany	Western Germany	Hungary	Italy	The Netherlands	Total
Swimming, gymnastics[2]	83	/	/	91	90	/	84
Meeting friends (not at home)	75	65	70	78	73	93	79
Actively pursuing sport	74	100	75	0	82	0	78
Voluntary or charity	59	75	58	88	80	89	74
Going out for a walk	63	63	58	88	84	79	72
** Just being cosy at home	62	38	71	83	78	93	72
Picking berries, mushrooms[1]	48	42	58	97	82	/	71
** Receiving visits at home	51	61	72	93	75	77	71
** Playing PC games	63	48	69	84	70	90	71
Taking courses	55	53	50	80	75	80	67
Theatre, opera, etc.	60	38	49	88	77	85	66
Making small trips	52	46	62	80	69	84	65
Dancing, bowling	61	48	43	79	74	84	64
Hunting[3]	55	30	40	/	67	/	63
** Watching TV	55	44	45	84	69	80	63
Café, restaurant	46	43	43	78	78	75	62
** Artistic activities	52	45	52	79	91	88	62
Hiking, riding bicycle	58	56	55	81	83	53	61
** Talking on the telephone	50	41	52	82	73	84	59
** Games (e.g. Bingo, card)	51	36	41	65	64	72	57
** Reading, solving riddles	48	41	51	57	65	80	57
Activities in clubs	54	44	52	74	66	67	57
Fishing	50	43	43	72	58	71	54
Library	49	42	37	86	70	85	54
Activities for retired	60	33	39	83	67	0	54
** Surfing the internet	50	26	41	91	55	75	53
Gardening	39	34	44	72	62	77	52
** "Do-it-yourself"	29	22	43	64	57	58	45
Watching sport	22	14	50	100	57	56	44
Religious events	12	18	44	100	48	45	35

Note. MOBILATE Survey 2000; N = 3950; weighted
each figure presents the percentage of people who mention this activity as important related to the participating people
[1] not asked in the Netherlands
[2] not asked in Germany and the Netherlands
[3] not asked in Hungary and the Netherlands
** included in indoor activities, all other items in outdoor activities.

6.3.3   Variety in indoor and outdoor activities

For the indicators of mobility, we selected also the variety of out-of-home activities. For this purpose a distinction was made between indoor and outdoor leisure activities.

Table 6.5:   Mean numbers of indoor or outdoor activities participated in

	Finland	Eastern Germany	Western Germany	Hungary	Italy	The Netherlands
Indoor activities (10)	5.9	5.9	6.0	5.9	6.7	5.2
Outdoor activities (18)	6.5	4.4	5.3	3.0	3.5	6.2

Note. MOBILATE Survey 2000; N = 3950; weighted

Table 6.5 gives an overview of the variety of indoor and outdoor activities participated in (the distinction between these categories can be seen in Table 6.4). With regards to the 10 indoor and 18 outdoor activities, people participated relatively more often in indoor activities, except for Finland and the Netherlands. This fits in well with the earlier findings on high rates of at-home activity. The differences between countries were not what one would expect on the basis of climate. This again shows that the number of activities does not mean the same as the amount of time spent outdoors. The numbers of indoor and outdoor activities cannot be compared, only the variety in these activities.

9% of the respondents participated in no outdoor activity and the most active 10% mention 9 to 18 activities outdoors. Everyone participated in at least one indoor activity and the most active 10% participated in 8 to 10 indoor activities.

Table 6.6:   Mean numbers of indoor activities (10 activities), in which people participate by age, gender and location

	Urban				Rural			
	55 - 74		75+		55 - 74		75+	
	male	female	male	female	male	female	male	female
Finland	5.7	5.2	6.3	5.7	6.8	5.9	6.7	6.2
Eastern Germany	5.6	5.6	5.4	5.8	6.2	6.3	6.9	6.8
Western Germany	6.2	5.5	6.5	6.2	5.8	5.8	6.7	6.1
Hungary	5.3	5.2	5.7	6.2	6.5	6.3	6.3	6.9
Italy	5.7	6.3	6.4	6.7	7.1	7.2	7.5	7.4
The Netherlands	5.3	5.2	5.6	5.5	5.2	5.0	5.9	5.4

MOBILATE Survey 2000; N = 3950

Table 6.6 shows that in the rural areas, people generally engaged in more different activities indoors, except in the Netherlands. Women, in general, engaged in a lower variety of indoor activities, especially in western Germany. Given the traditional role of women in this generation as housewives, this finding is surprising.

In most countries people in the oldest age group participated in fewer outdoor activities. In the youngest group these differences are not always in the same direction. In Italy women are less active in out-of-home activities (Table 6.7).

As regards the association between age and outdoor activities, there was a slight tendency for the variety in outdoor activities to fall with age. This was not valid for Finland, where the older men were more active outdoors. One possible explanation for this is the fact that the men in the younger age-group were still working and did not have as much time for these activities as the older men. Another trend was that men pursued more activities outdoors than women. This holds true, in particular, for Italian men and for older men in rural areas which fits in well with their traditional roles, according to which men more often take care of external activities.

Table 6.7: Mean numbers of outdoor activities (18 activities), in which people participate by age, gender and residential location

| | Urban | | | | Rural | | | |
| | 55 - 74 | | 75+ | | 55 - 74 | | 75+ | |
	male	female	male	female	male	female	male	female
Finland	7.6	8.6	5.4	4.7	6.0	6.7	4.1	3.3
Eastern Germany	5.1	5.0	3.6	2.6	4.7	4.5	3.3	2.6
Western Germany	5.9	5.9	3.0	3.6	6.0	5.9	4.3	3.4
Hungary	3.8	3.9	2.8	2.2	2.3	2.9	2.4	1.7
Italy	5.7	4.0	3.7	2.1	4.0	2.4	2.6	1.3
The Netherlands	6.4	6.3	4.6	4.4	6.7	7.1	5.0	4.4

Note. MOBILATE Survey 2000; N = 3950

As Mollenkopf and Flaschenträger (2001) propose, one might expect that self-rated health and the availability of a car, bicycle or the use of public transport play a role in this question. Table 6.8 demonstrates clearly the relation between two health variables. People with rather poor health status engaged in more indoor activities and fewer outdoor activities. Healthy people showed less variety in indoor activities and much more in outdoor activities.

Table 6.8: Mean numbers of indoor and outdoor activities by combinations of ADL problems (PADL + IADL) and self assessed physical mobility

Elderly persons by mobility	mean # indoor activities (10 activities)	mean # outdoor activities (18 activities)
Serious ADL problems, very poor physical mobility	7.0	1.0
Light ADL problems, fair physical mobility	5.8	4.9
No ADL problems, very good physical mobility	5.4	7.2

Note. MOBILATE Survey 2000; N = 3950

A similar relation revealed between available modes of transport and the location of activities (Table 6.9). If older and younger people had no transport facilities available, they did more indoor activities. They were much more active outdoors if they used a variety of transport alternatives. The differences between indoor activities were small; most of these activities were rather commonplace. The situation was different for participation in outdoor activities where much greater differences could be seen. The analysis shows that health, age, location, available modes of transport and gender played an important role.

Table 6.9: Mean numbers of indoor and outdoor activities by age, availability of a car or bicycle and use of public transport (PT).

Elderly persons by mobility	mean # indoor activities	mean # outdoor activities
55 – 64, no car, no bicycle, no PT-user	6.4	2.1
55 – 64, car, bicycle, PT-user	5.6	7.1
65+, no car, no bicycle, no PT-user	6.7	1.6
65+, car, bicycle, PT-user	5.8	5.5

Note. MOBILATE Survey 2000; N = 3950; not-weighted

To find the relative meaning of the explanatory variables, we carried out a stepwise regression analysis. For health we chose a variable which describes the level of physical activity on a scale from 'hardly any physical activity' to 'physical exercise regularly and several times a week'. The variables of the ADL scale, self-estimated physical mobility and physical activity level all correlate highly with one another, and therefore, we chose the one which explains the most variance. For the availability of private modes of transport (most used), we chose both car and/or bicycle. Both offer a discretionary opportunity to go out beyond walking distance (which is already included in level of physical activity). After the first step, only the significant variables were included in the analysis.

Table 6.10: Model summary of the stepwise regression analysis with outdoor activities as dependent variable

Model	R	R Square	Adjusted R Square	Std. Error of the Estimate
Physical activity (1=hardly any; 4=several times a week)	.506	.256	.256	2.739
+ income (1=low; 3=high)	.555	.308	.307	2.643
+ attachment to living area (1=not; 10=very attached)	.588	.346	.345	2.569
+ mean number of trips made	.612	.374	.374	2.512
+ age (55 – 98)	.624	.390	.389	2.482
+ car in hh (0=no car; 1=car available)	.631	.398	.397	2.465
+ use of public transport (1=no; 2=yes)	.638	.408	.406	2.446
+ years of education (0 to 30 yrs)	.641	.411	.410	2.439

Note. MOBILATE Survey 2000; N = 3950

The regression explains in total 41% of the original variance (R-square) in the range of outdoor activities. Physical activity level explained the most variance, followed by income, feelings of attachment to the living area, mean number of trips made, age, available car in the household, use of public transport and the years of education. Gender and location were not significant and therefore left out of this analysis. Health makes it possible to be active and the accessibility of the broader environment is conditioned by income. The residential environment is used more when people feel attached to it. The availability of a car and the use of public transport offer both more opportunities to go out. Education can give a broader interest in what happens in a more extended context.

We have seen which variables explain most of the differences in outdoor activity. We were, furthermore, interested in subgroups of people who show a specific outdoor activity pattern. The HOMALS-analysis (Figure 6.1) or a multiple correspondence analysis shows how the respondent's characteristics can be placed in a two-dimensional space. The most homogeneous items will come close to each other. By doing this, it is possible to find the most homogeneous subgroups in the sample.

One's level of outdoor activity mainly explained the first dimension, though physical activity and age were strongly related to this dimension also. In the upper right corner we find the eldest age group, with no physical activity and no outdoor activity. Closest to these categories come no trips made, no public transport used and no car or bicycle available. In the other extreme of the upper left corner, we see that a high level of physical activity was associated with the youngest age group and a high level of outdoor activity, with the availability of a car and a bicycle, high education, high income and highest number of trips made.

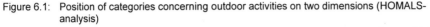

Figure 6.1:   Position of categories concerning outdoor activities on two dimensions (HOMALS-analysis)

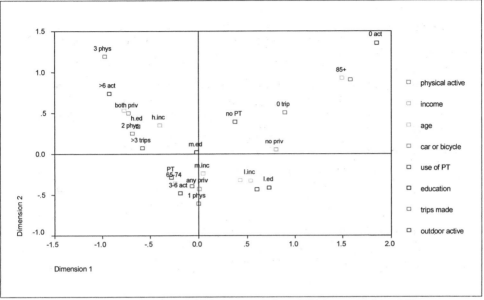

Note. Physical active: 1=low - 3=high; income: 1=low - 3=high; age: 55-74 and 75+; car or bicycle: 1=no use of car and bicycle – 3=use both; use of PT: 1=no - 2=yes; education: 1=low – 3=high; trips: 0=no trip - 3=>3 trips; outdoor active: 0 activity - >6 activities)

6.3.4   Comparison of the variety in outdoor activities in survey and in diary

Up to now, the overview of indoor and outdoor activities was based on questions in the questionnaire about the participation in a list of leisure activities in and out of the home. In the trip diary, respondents mentioned among others, the trips they made for leisure activities. We thus have also information on realised outdoor mobility, and the leisure activities mentioned there offer an opportunity to link both approaches to the variety in outdoor activities.

In the diary we have counted the number of different activities performed outdoors. The numbers can not be compared with those on the list of leisure activities in the questionnaire because they are different, but we can compare the variety in outdoor activities; the great variety in the survey matches the great variety in the diary, and enables us to see if people actually participate in these activities which they say they participate in.

The correlation between the variety of activities in the survey and in the diary is, at 0.30, not very high. Comparing both variables directly in a cross table shows that 5% made no trips at all and participated in no activity, and that an additional 20% participated in different activities, but no trip with any stated motive was made. On the other hand 90% of people who made 4 or more trips for different reasons also reported participating in 3 or more outdoor activities. The group in between cannot be so clearly divided into subgroups.

In the survey people can easily claim to do the activity in question, whereas the diary reflects more directly the actual activity pattern. However, not all activities take place on each day of the reporting period of the diary. Religious events, for example, take place on Sunday and club activities on a specific day, weekly or monthly. Still, one might expect a higher participation rate (in the diary) for people who report participation (in the survey). Table 6.11 shows this relation for some of the variables which are comparable between the survey and the diary.

Table 6.11: Relation between reported participation and realised activities (%)

Activity	% of total participating (based on the questionnaires)	N	% of realised activities (based on the diary entries)	N
Meeting friends	64	2510	25	635
Visiting café or restaurant	30	1162	13	151
Gardening	48	1878	8	151
Clubs, voluntary work	20	803	13	103
Visiting the theatre	19	747	5	38
Taking courses	5	208	4	9

Note. MOBILATE Survey 2000; N = 3950

The second column in Table 6.11 represents the people who reported that they participate in these activities and the fourth column gives the percentages of the people who made at least one trip with this motive. The difference between the columns tells us about the relation between the two types of information. 25% of the people who reported meeting friends also did this during one or both days of the diary. For visiting a café or restaurant, visiting a club, or doing voluntary work, these percentages were high (13%), especially when compared with the 8% for gardening. For this last figure the season is relevant: autumn is not the busiest time in the garden. These figures were all together high when we realise that most of these activities do not belong to the daily activity routine.

6.3.5 Changing leisure behaviour

Respondents in Hungary and Italy mentioned more often than others that they have reduced their out-of-home activities. These two countries have the fewest respondents who mentioned no changes. Some engaged in more activities, but this group was quite small in Western Germany and in Hungary. Retirement could lead to an increase in discretionary activities (Table 6.12).

Table 6.12: More or fewer out-of-home activities than a few years ago (%).

	FIN	GER-(E)	GER-(W)	HUN	IT	NL
No change	42	54	51	29	34	53
Fewer activities	39	29	38	63	51	34
More activities	19	12	4	5	15	13
No changes, but more intensive		4	7	2		1
Total N =	609	768	750	599	600	553

Note. MOBILATE Survey 2000; weighted

Table 6.13: More or fewer out-of-home activities than a few years ago by age, gender and location (%)

	Urban				Rural			
	55 - 74		75+		55 - 74		75+	
	male	female	male	female	male	female	male	female
No changes	53	46	35	39	47	48	36	29
Fewer activities	28	35	58	58	38	38	57	67
More activities	16	18	5	3	12	10	3	3
No changes, but more intensive	4	2	2	0	3	4	3	1
Total N =	531	523	430	449	539	543	431	432

Note. MOBILATE Survey 2000

Young, urban elderly people engaged in slightly more activities, particularly gardening, strolling in the city, hiking or riding a bicycle and swimming, and women also mentioned being busy with handicraft and taking courses. The younger age groups reported having more time and being retired, both of which mean having more free time. Having a better state of health and the need to be together with other people were additionally mentioned.

Slightly more than one out of five respondents (914) would like to be more active outdoors. Meeting friends, making small trips, gardening and going to the theatre were mentioned most often, but these numbers were low. Nearly half of the respondents (48%) mentioned health as the main reason for the discrepancy between preferred and realised behaviour, whereas 18% mentioned lack of time, 13% lack of an opportunity nearby, and 11% high costs.

6.3.6 Travel and satisfaction with this activity

Holiday trips lasting at least one week are not part of older people's daily life. About 60% of the younger elders and almost 85% of the elders aged 75 years or older reported having made no such trip during the last twelve months before the interview (autumn 2000)(Table 6.14). Roughly 20% had made one and 10% more than one of such trips. The German elders travelled most while the Hungarians travelled least.

More urban than rural elders, slightly more men than women (not shown in the Table) and – not surprisingly – more younger than older respondents made a trip of at least one week in the course of about one year. These patterns were found in all countries, and the differences were highly significant between urban and rural areas and age groups. Correspondingly, elder urbanites and the young old showed higher satisfaction with travelling than older people living in the countryside and persons aged 75 years and older. More important were, however, the differences in satisfaction between persons who did not travel (age 55-74: M=6.8; age 75+: M=6.0) and persons who made one or several big journeys (between M=8.0 and 8.8). Again, this pattern holds for all participating countries.

All in all, these findings indicate that today's elders are not permanently travelling about but that obviously this activity is of great value to them, because those who occasionally are able to travel for at least one week are significantly more satisfied in this regard than people who for any reason do not or cannot pursue such kind of activity.

Table 6.14: Number of performed journeys lasting at least one week during the last 12 months and satisfaction with travel possibilities.

	Finland		The Netherlands		Eastern Germany		Western Germany		Hungary		Italy		All countries	
	55-74	75+	55-74	75+	55-74	75+	55-74	75+	55-74	75+	55-74	75+	55-74	75+
Journeys undertaken (%)														
no journey	54.9	78.8	58.9	79.7	47.0	80.7	50.2	80.0	84.7	92.9	76.0	88.3	60.7	83.4
one journey	25.9	11.9	28.2	11.1	36.4	15.2	37.1	14.4	8.2	4.8	14.9	9.2	26.2	11.3
two or more journeys	19.1	9.3	12.9	9.2	16.6	4.1	12.7	5.7	7.1	2.3	9.1	2.5	13.1	5.3
Travel satisfaction (M)														
no journey	7.2	7.3	7.1	6.9	6.6	4.8	6.3	3.8	7.1	6.4	6.4	5.6	6.8	6.0
one journey	8.3	7.7	7.9	8.2	8.5	8.0	8.7	8.4	7.8	8.6	7.4	7.2	8.3	8.0
two or more journeys	8.4	8.4	8.4	8.1	9.3	9.0	9.4	9.1	7.7	8.5	8.9	8.8	8.8	8.6

Note. MOBILATE Survey 2000
Satisfaction scale from 0 = very unsatisfied to 10 = very satisfied.

6.4   The relationship between health and leisure time activities

6.4.1   Health and satisfaction with possibility to participate in leisure activities

Like with respect to mobility (see Chapter 4), the health-related factors of heavy and light ADL, satisfaction with state of health, visual acuity and the Digit Symbol Substitution Test were added together to form a more condensed health-sum variable (Cronbach's alpha 0.80, varying between 0.76 and 0.82) in order to analyse the relations between health and leisure time activities: satisfaction with the possibility to participate in them, both indoor and outdoor, and the number of holiday trips made lasting at least one week. When analysing the relationships between health and leisure time activities, it has to be remembered that the effect of age on health was originally very strong.

The significant 3-way country*region*health-sum interaction with regards to satisfaction with the possibility of participating in the various leisure activities showed that in each country and region, the subjects with better health were more satisfied, as expected 8.15). The effect of health on satisfaction with leisure activities was, however, different between countries and location (Figure 6.2). In the urban and rural locations of eastern Germany, especially, and in the urban location of western Germany, health indicated strong effects on satisfaction.

Figure 6.2:   The effect of health on satisfaction with participation in leisure activities in different countries and localities

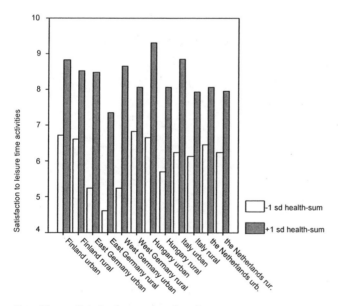

Note. The predicted values are based on the women

In the rural localities of western Germany and Italy, and in both the urban and rural localities of the Netherlands and Finland, health status, on the other hand, had the smallest effects on satisfaction with the leisure activities. This leads us to believe that in these locations, the supply of possible leisure time activities to different groups of people might be better, or it may be that people in these regions are more adapted to the leisure time activities available to them.

The values +1 sd health-sum and -1 sd health-sum refer to the means of subjects belonging to those who were one standard-deviation above the average (+1sd) and one standard-deviation below the average (-1sd). There were altogether 541 subjects with better health status and 678 subjects with poorer health status.

6.4.2   Health and indoor leisure activities

Indoor activities consisted of: receiving visits, being cosy at home, reading and solving riddles or collecting stamps and coins, watching TV and listening to the radio, and talking on the telephone. Because the reliabilities (Cronbach's alphas) of the sum scores of these indoor activities were only moderate, varying between 0.55 -0.56 for subsamples and being 0.58 for the total sample, caution is necessary when drawing conclusions on the basis of the statistical data analyses.

Three significant interactions emerged between indoor leisure activities and the health-sum variable, country, location and gender. These were country*location, country*gender and country*health-sum variable. The urban-rural differences were different in the participating countries (Figure 6.3).

Figure 6.3: Number of indoor leisure activities by country, residential location and gender

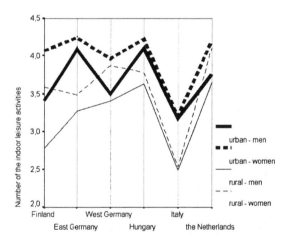

In eastern Germany and Italy, but also in Finland and Hungary, the urban subjects showed clearly higher means for indoor activities compared to the rural subjects; in western Germany and the Netherlands this was also the case but to a lesser extent. A possible explanation for engaging more in indoor activities in urban localities might be found in the fact that in rural areas, more daily domestic chores have to be done also outdoors while this is not necessarily so in urban settings. Another explanation may be that in urban areas there are fewer attractive opportunities to be out and about. The effect of gender on the frequency of indoor activity also differed in the participating countries. Women in Finland, in particular, had higher means for indoor activity compared to men. This pattern was also evident in western Germany and the Netherlands, and to a lesser extent in eastern Germany and Hungary. In Italy, however, this was not the case (Figure 6.3) .

Similarly, the effect of health on the mean level of indoor activity differed in the participating countries. In Figure 6.4 it can be noted generally that the better their health, the more likely people were to take part in indoor leisure activities.

Figure 6.4: Number of indoor leisure activities by countries and health status

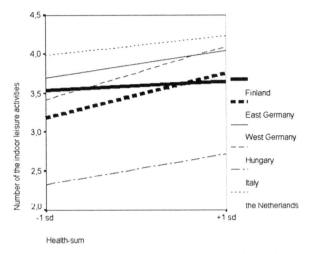

Health-sum

Note. The predicted values are based on those for the rural women

Health had the most obvious relation to the number of indoor leisure activities in Hungary and eastern Germany, whereas in Finland, no clear relationship between health and the number of indoor activities was found. Irrespective of their health status, the subjects from the Netherlands practised more indoor leisure activities, and the Italian subjects less than in the other participating countries. The above-mentioned interactions can be explained only after analysing the relationship between health and outdoor leisure activities, as time, even among retired people, imposes limits on the number of possible activities.

6.4.3   Health and outdoor leisure activities

Outdoor leisure activities consisted of the 20 activities mentioned in Section 6.2.2, above. The sum-variable formed from the above mentioned items had satisfactory reliability. Two significant interactions country*location*health-sum and country*gender will be interpreted. In each country and location, the subjects with better health showed higher mean levels of outdoor leisure activities, as was expected. The interaction country*location*health shows that the effect of health on the number of outdoor leisure activities was, however, different between countries and locations (Figure 6.5). Both in urban and rural Finland, the Netherlands and western Germany, those in better health had a greater variety of outdoor leisure activities than those in poorer health. In the rural locations of Hungary, Italy and eastern Germany, the effect of health was not as strong as in the urban locations of these countries.

Figure 6.5:   Number of outdoor leisure activities by country, location and health

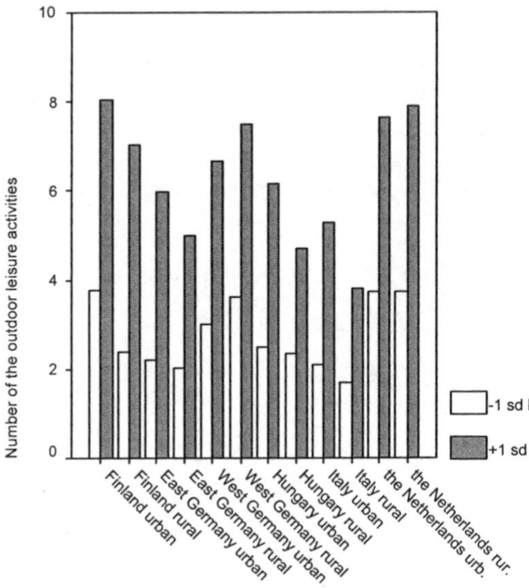

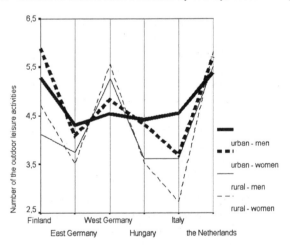

Note. The predicted values are based on those for the women

Figure 6.6:   Number of outdoor leisure activities by country, location and gender

The country*gender interaction showed that the effect of gender on the number of the outdoor activities also differed in the participating countries (Figure 6.6). The women in Finland, especially, and in western Germany had higher means for outdoor activities than the men, whereas in Italy and to a lesser extent in eastern Germany and Hungary, this pattern was totally reversed. In the Netherlands, there were only minor differences between men and women in the number of outdoor leisure activities. These differences might be the result of different role-expectations in the countries studied.

6.4.4   Health and holiday trips lasting at least one week during the last year

Trips lasting at least for one week and made for leisure and recreation are one leisure activity which requires quite good health; coping successfully with difficulties, such as one encounters on a long flight, requires personal resources, and the ability to adapt physically, psychologically and socially to other life circumstances during this period. For those reasons, health might be an especially important factor, besides economic resources, to be able to make trips of this kind.

The analysis shows that gender had no effects on the number of trips lasting at least one week. There was, however, a significant country*location*health-sum variable interaction (Figure 6.7). In each country and region, the subjects with better health made more trips lasting at least one week. Generally, health had a greater effect on the number of trips made by urban dwellers, especially in eastern Germany, Hungary and Italy. In Finland, there were, however, no differences between the urban and rural dwellers, whereas in the Netherlands the rural dwellers were more affected by their health as regards the number of trips made. It was noted that among the healthier subjects, 24% made two or more trips, 35% one trip and 41% no trips. Among the subjects in poorer health, these numbers were, respectively by 1%, 5% and 94%. There was thus a considerable difference between health-status groups in this respect.

Figure 6.7:   Number of holiday trips by country, location and health status

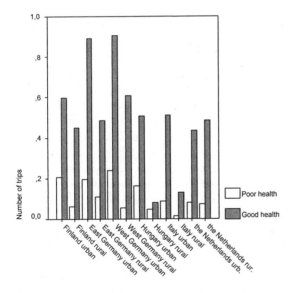

Note. The predicted values are based on those for the women

6.5   Discussion

The aim of the chapter on leisure and health was to clarify the relation between health and leisure activities during the ageing process and how it varies in the different participating European countries, in urban and rural environments and in men and women.

When studying leisure time and leisure activities, especially among older people, one must be aware of the fact that there is no commonly accepted definition of leisure. An approximation to such a definition could be the subjects' own definitions, i.e., the activities a person willingly participates in could be defined as leisure activities. However, this would require an idiographic approach (as opposed to nomothetic approach), which would prohibit statistical comparisons between individuals. In the MOBILATE project, we selected a nomothetic approach to assess leisure activities. This meant providing the subjects with a rather long list of different groups of leisure activities, and they were asked to select those they participated in. This selection of options can not cover all the possible leisure activities elderly people may pursue in different countries and environments. For this reason, the selected list included the most common alternatives, as well as a few activities which are frequent in only one or the other of the participating countries. The list we employed may thus favour different countries, locations and gender differently, necessitating great caution when comparing the leisure activities of the different strata of the MOBILATE study. In particular, some indoor activities may have been absent from the list, and clearly some of the outdoor leisure activities are popular only in one or a few of the participating countries. Also, it has to be pointed out that our leisure activity data do not describe the frequency or intensity of the different leisure activities elderly people engage in, but whether they pursue it and whether it is important to them.

At the individual level, regression analyses show health to be the most important factor affecting participation in both indoor and outdoor leisure activities. In addition, education and economic resources like income level and owning a car, as well as attachment to one's living area and age, explain the number of different outdoor leisure activities pursued. At the mode of transport level, car and bicycle ownership, as well as the frequent use of public transport and in general the number of trips made, also explain, although to a lesser extent, the number of outdoor leisure activities engaged in.

It is easy to understand why health is so important for participation in different leisure activities. Health is a necessary but not a sufficient condition for participation in any kind of leisure activity. On the other hand, the resources which an individual has gained through education are very important ones in providing the knowledge base and skills specifically needed for successful participation in many leisure activities. Economic resources e.g., having one's own car and bicycle, also facilitate participation. Furthermore most leisure activities require sometimes considerable financial means to participate in them. If a person has the necessary financial resources, he or she can greatly broaden the variety of his or her leisure activities. Similarly, the greater the number of modes of transport available to a person, the better possibilities he or she has of accessing desired leisure activities. Moreover, it is important to see how attachment to place is also connected to participation in leisure activities. This relation goes perhaps in both directions: enjoying leisure activities increases attachment to place and vice versa. This hypothesis, however, can only be examined by using longitudinal data. It is also important to know that, in addition to the above-mentioned predictive factors, age still explains a part of the variance in participation in leisure activities. Precisely how age influences participation, however, is a question for further studies.

Leisure activities are culturally or contextually bound activities: how they are favoured varies with time and place. They are socio-culturally bound according to age, gender, social class, location and country. They also vary seasonally: different outdoor leisure activities are popular in the summer, and some in other seasons. Because our data were gathered in autumn, this allows a great variety of leisure activities to be found in the diary data except those requiring warm summer or winter circumstances.

An important finding was the rather low correspondence between the leisure activities a respondent reported doing (in the questionnaire) and those she or he actually described doing (over a two-day period in the diary). This discrepancy deserves further study. However, a period of two days is a very short one; many outdoor leisure activities like concerts, theatre, club meetings, religious activities and sport events, are often offered only on a weekly or less frequent basis.

The analysis of the selection between leisure activities and health was based on sum-variables formed by combining the different leisure activities our subjects reported engaging in. Thus, the analysis needs to be continued by constructing more homogeneous classes of leisure activities (see Mollenkopf et al. 1997, for an example) or even by studying the factors related to different individual leisure activities. We expect that considerable variation in the factors connected to the different individual leisure groups or leisure activities will be found. Similarly, the factors connected to different leisure activities can also be expected to vary from country to country and from location to location depending on ease of access, distances and the costs needed to participate in them. This will also require further analyses of the available data. One important research question is the importance of different psychological factors like cognitive processing and coping-processes in people's participation in different leisure activities.

Further analyses are needed on the variables constituting the health-sum indicator, as well on the impact of other possible factors like one's social network.

6.6   Conclusions

Elderly people have no work to structure their daily activity pattern after retirement. Leisure activities, however, play an important role in their lives. People appear to be rather satisfied with their leisure activities. Those in the urban locations were more satisfied than those in the rural environments, where the oldest age group, in particular, was less satisfied.

At-home activities head the list of leisure activities. The first outdoor activity, ranked as third, concerns meeting friends elsewhere, and the next one, going out for a walk, is ranked seventh. Meeting friends was also perceived to be the most important activity after dancing and bowling, which was perceived to be very important by those who participate in them. Active sports and voluntary work were also judged to be important. People who attend religious events find them to be less important. The most variety in indoor activities was found in the rural locations, and women performed more indoor activities, whereas men were more active outdoors.

Health was strongly related to participation in indoor and outdoor activities. Moreover, the more means of transport available, the more people went out. In a more comprehensive analysis, level of physical activity explained most of the variance, followed by income, attachment to living area, age, car in household, use of public transport and years of education. These differences were also seen in the subgroups, distinguished by the HOMALS technique.

The correlation between the variety of participation mentioned in the survey and the variety in the realised motives for a trip was rather low (0.30).

For some people, the number of activities increased, mostly as a result of retirement; 20% would like to be more active. Meeting friends, small trips, gardening and going to the theatre were mentioned most, but were often prevented by state of health.

At least one week lasting holiday travel was not part of older people's daily life: 30% made at least one such trip during the previous year. However, people were very satisfied with the amount of travelling they do.

Subjects with better health showed higher satisfaction with the possibility of participating in different leisure activities, as expected. However, the strength of the association between health and satisfaction varied between countries and localities. The weakest association was found in Finland and the Netherlands. The strongest associations were in the urban and rural areas of eastern Germany and in the urban location of western Germany. A possible explanation may concern the quality of access to leisure activities or the costs of participation. Different countries and locations may have different role-expectations concerning the participation of elderly subjects in leisure activities. One hypothesis is that people in Finland and the Netherlands compared to the German subjects are more happily adapted to their possibilities for participating in leisure activities. We intend to test some of these hypotheses at a later date.

The better their health, the more likely people were to take part in indoor leisure activities. Health showed the strongest relation to the frequency of indoor leisure activities in Hungary and eastern Germany, whereas in Finland, no such relationship was found. This could mean that continuity exists with earlier indoor leisure activities. Those previously active were still active later and vice versa. Irrespective of health, the subjects from the Netherlands practiced indoor leisure activities more and the Italian subjects less than those in the other participating countries.

The urban subjects took part more often in indoor leisure activities than the subjects from the rural areas. However, there were differences between countries in the frequency of indoor activities. These differences may be caused by the quite low reliability of the indoor leisure activity indicator. Generally, the gender differences show that except for Italy, women had more indoor leisure activities than men, as had also been assumed. In Italy, urban dwellers showed higher means for indoor activities, since people in rural areas prefer to spend their leisure outside the house, and their activities are more manual than mental. The reason could also be that the leisure indoor activities assessed did not reflect the everyday life of Italian women, whose activities such as cooking, cleaning, caring for grandchildren, sewing, knitting, etc. take most of their time.

Health status was related to the number of outdoor leisure activities in each country and location. The subjects with better health showed higher mean levels for outdoor leisure activities, as was expected. The strength of this relation, however, differed between countries and locations. Both in the urban and rural areas of Finland, the Netherlands, and western Germany, health showed a rather similar and strong association with the number of outdoor leisure activities. In the rural areas of Hungary, Italy, and eastern Germany, this relation was not as strong as in the urban areas of these countries. Further analyses are needed which take into account possible differences in the outdoor leisure activity profiles of these countries and locations. A possible explanation may lie in personal and cultural habits; people in rural locations are probably more accustomed to going out even when they have some health problems.

The country*gender interaction showed that women in Finland, and to a lesser extent, women in western Germany, had higher means for outdoor leisure activities compared to men. In Italy and to a lesser extent also in eastern Germany and Hungary, this relation was reversed. Culturally differing gender-role expectations may explain this. It may be considered more 'suitable' for women in Italy, eastern Germany and Hungary to engage in fewer outdoor leisure activities than men. In countries like Finland and western Germany, where women have more outdoor activities than men, clear gender-related differences in acceptable outdoor activities for women and for men may no longer exist.

Holiday trips lasting at least one week were more often undertaken by the healthier subjects. The country*region*health-sum interaction additionally indicated that the effect of health on the number of such trips was stronger in the urban than rural areas, except in Finland. Also, considerable differences between countries were found: the German urban subjects travelled most, the Hungarian and Italian rural subjects least. The urban subjects in good and poor health made generally more such trips than their rural counterparts.

References

Ball, J. (1996). Preventative medicine: The recreation edge. *Parks and Recreation Canada*, *54*, 11-13.

Baltes, P. B., & Baltes, M. M. (1989). Optimierung durch Selektion und Kompensation: Ein psychologisches Modell erfolgreichen Alterns [Optimization with selection and compensation. A psychological model of successful aging]. *Zeitschrift für Pädagogik*, *35*, 85-105.

Bolger, N., & Eckenrode, J. (1991). Social relationships, personality, and anxiety during a major stressful event. *Journal of Personality and Social Psychology*, *61*, 440-449.

Brown, B. A., Frankel, B. G., & Fennell, M. (1991). Happiness through leisure: The impact of type of leisure activity, age, gender and leisure satisfaction on psychological well-being. *Journal of Applied Recreation Research*, *16*, 368-392.

Brög, W, Erl, E., & Glorius B. (2000). Germany. In ECMT (Ed.), *Transport and Ageing of the Population.* Report of Round Table 112. Paris: OECD Publications Service.

Carp, F. (1988). Significance of mobility for the well-being of the elderly. In Transportation Research Board/ National Research Council (TRB), *Transportation in an aging society. Improving mobility and safety for older people.* Washington: TRB.

CBS (Central bureau of Statistics) (2000), De mobiliteit van de Nederlandse bevolking 1999 [The mobility of the Dutch population 1999]. Heerlen/Voorburg: CBS.

Coleman, D., & Iso-Ahola, S. (1993). Leisure and health: The role of social support and self-determination. *Journal of Leisure Research*, *25*, 111-128.

Csikszentmihalyi, M. (1990). *Flow: The psychology of optimal experience.* New York: Harper & Row.

Csikszentmihalyi, M. (1994). The consequences of leisure for mental health. In D. M. Compton & S. E. Iso-Ahola (Eds.), *Leisure & Mental Health* (pp. 34-41), Vol.1. Park City, UT. U.S.A.: Family Development Resources, Inc.

Csikszentmihalyi, M. (1997). *Finding flow*. New York: Basic Books.

Csikszentmihalyi, M., & Kleiber, D. A. (1991). Leisure and self-actualization. In B. L. Driver, P. J. Brown & G. L. Peterson (Eds.), *Benefits of Leisure* (pp. 91-102). State College, Pennsylvania: Venture Publishing.

Deci, E. L., & Ryan, R. M. (1987). The support of autonomy and the control of behaviour. *Journal of Personality and Social Psychology, 53,* 1024-1037.

Doyle, D., & Forehand, M. J. (1984). Life satisfaction and old age: A reexamination. *Research on Aging, 6,* 432-448.

Driver, B. L. (1990). Focusing research on the benefits of leisure: Special issue introduction. *Journal of Leisure Research, 22,* 93-98.

Hamilton-Smith, E. (1991). The construction of leisure. In B.L. Driver, P.J. Brown & G.L. Peterson (Eds.), *Benefits of leisure* (pp. 445-450). State College, Pennsylvania: Venture Publishing, Inc.

Heikkinen, E., Lampinen, P., & Suutama, T. (1999) (Eds.). Cohort differences in the functional capacity, health and leisure activities of 65-69 year-old persons. Observations from the cohort comparisons of the Evergreen project in 1988 and 1996. Helsinki: The Social Insurance Institution, Finland, Studies in Social Security and Health, 47.

Henderson, K. A., Stalnaker, D., & Taylor, G. (1988). The relationships between barriers to recreation and gender-role personality traits for women. *Journal of Leisure Research, 1,* 69-80.

Higgins, J. W. (1995). Leisure and recreation: Achieving health for all. *Journal of Applied Recreation Research, 20,* 17-36.

Hull, R. B. (1991). Mood as a product of leisure: Causes and consequences. In B. L. Driver, P. J. Brown, & G. L. Peterson (Eds.), *Benefits of leisure* (pp. 249-262). State College, Pennsylvania: Venture Publishing, Inc.

Iso-Ahola, S. E. (1994). Leisure lifestyle and health. In D. M. Compton (Ed.), *Leisure & Mental Health,* Vol. 1 (pp. 43-60). Park City, UT, U.S.A.: Family Development Resources Inc.

Iso-Ahola, S. E., Jackson, E. & Dunn, E. (1994). Starting, ceasing, and replacing leisure activities over the life-span. *Journal of Leisure Research, 3,* 227-249.

Iso-Ahola, S. E., & Mannell, R. C. (1985). Social and psychological constraints on leisure. In W. Wade (Ed.), *Constraints on Leisure* (pp. 111-151). Springfield, IL: Charles C. Thomas.

Kelly, J. R. (1982). Freedom and leisure learning. In J. R. Kelly (Ed.), *Leisure* (pp. 157-179). Englewood Cliffs, NJ: Prentice-Hall.

Kelly, J. R. (Ed.) (1993). *Activity and aging. Staying involved in later life*. Newsbury Park: Sage Publications.

Kelly, J. R., & Ross, J. (1989). Later-life leisure: Beginning a new agenda. *Leisure Sciences, 11,* 47-59.

Kelly, J. R., Steinkemp, M. W., & Kelly, J. R. (1987). Later-life satisfaction: Does leisure contribute? *Leisure Sciences, 9*, 189-199.

Lampinen, P., Heikkinen, R-L., Kauppinen, M., Heikkinen, E. (2004). Activity as a predictor of mental well-being among older adults. Manuscript.

Lawton, M. P. (1993). Meanings of activity. In J. R. Kelly (Ed.), *Activity and aging. Staying involved in later life* (pp. 25-41). Newsbury Park: Sage Publications.

Lawton, M. P. (1994). Aging and activity: A theoretical perspective. In D. M. Compton (Ed.), *Leisure & Mental Health*, Vol. 1 (pp. 61-78). Park City, UT, U.S.A.: Family Development Resources, Inc.

Leinbach, T., & Watkins, J. (1994). *Transportation services, utilization and needs of the elderly in non-urban areas. Patterns in two Kentucky Communities* (DOT-T-95-08). Washington: U.S. Department of Transportation.

Mahoney, A. R. (1994). Change in the older-person role: an application of Turner's process role and model of role change. *Journal of Aging Studies, 8*, 133-148.

Mannell, R. C. (1993). High-investment activity and life satisfaction among older adults. Committed, serious leisure, and flow activities. In J. R. Kelly (Ed.), *Activity and aging. Staying involved in later life* (pp. 125-145). Newbury Park: Sage Publications.

Mannell, R. C. (1994). Constraints, leisure participation and well-being among older adults. In D. M. Compton, & S. E. Iso-Ahola (Eds.), *Leisure & Mental Health*, Vol. 1 (pp. 79-97). Park City, UT, U.S.A.: Family Development Resources, Inc.

McGuire, F. A. (1984). A factor analytic study of leisure constraints in advanced adulthood. *Leisure Sciences, 6*, 313-326.

McPherson, B. D. (1991). Aging and leisure benefits: A life cycle perspective. In B. L. Driver, P. J. Brown, & G. L. Peterson (Eds.), *Benefits of leisure* (pp. 423-430). State College, Pennsylvania: Venture Publishing, Inc.

Mollenkopf, H., Marcellini, F., Ruoppila, I., Flaschenträger, P., Gagliardi, C., & Spazzafumo, L. (1997). Outdoor Mobility and Social Relationships of Elderly People. *Archives of Gerontology and Geriatrics, 24*, pp. 295-310.

Mollenkopf, H., & Flaschenträger, P. (2001). *Erhaltung von Mobiliät im Alter* [Maintaining mobility in old age] (Vo. 197 - Bundesministerium für Familie, Senioren, Frauen und Jugend. Stuttgart). Berlin: Kohlhammer.

Patrick, G. D. (1994). A role for leisure in treatment of depression. In D. M. Compton, & S. E. Iso-Ahola (Eds), *Leisure & Mental Health*, Vol. 1 (pp. 175-190). Park City, UT, U.S.A.: Family Development Resources, Inc.

Pedlar, A., Sherry, D. & Gilbert, A. (1996). Resumption of role status through leisure in later life. *Leisure Sciences, 18*, 259-276.

Pikkarainen, A., & Heikkinen, R.-L. (1999a). Changes in leisure activities among elderly Finnish persons in an eight-year follow-up study. In T. Suutama, I. Ruoppila, & P. Laukkanen (Eds.), *Changes in functional abilities among elderly people. Findings from an eight-year follow-up study by the Evergreen project*. Helsinki: The Social Insurance Institution, Finland, Studies in Social Security and Health, 42, 199-216.

Pikkarainen, A., & Heikkinen, R.-L. (1999b). Leisure activities among 65-69-year-old people in 1988 and 1996 in Jyväskylä. In E. Heikkinen, P. Lampinen, & T. Suutama (Eds.), *Cohort differences in the functional capacity, health and leisure activities of 65-69 year-old persons. Observations from the cohort comparisons of the Evergreen project in 1988 and 1996.* Helsinki: The Social Insurance Institution, Finland, Studies in Social Security and Health, 47, 81-96.

Ragheb, M., & Griffith, C. A. (1982). The contribution of leisure participation and leisure satisfaction to life satisfaction of older persons. *Journal of Leisure Research, 14,* 295-305.

Riddick, C. C. (1985). Life satisfaction determinants of older males and females. *Leisure Sciences, 7,* 47-63.

Riddick, C. C., & Daniel, S. N. (1984). The relative contribution of leisure activities and other factors to the mental health of older women. *Journal of Leisure Research, 16,* 136-148.

Rook, K. S. (1987). Social support versus companionship: Effects on life stress, loneliness, and evaluations by others. *Journal of Personality and Social Psychology, 52,* 1132-1147

Russell, R. V. (1987). The importance of recreation satisfaction and activity participation to the life satisfaction of age-segregated retirees. *Journal of Leisure, 19,* 273-283.

Russell, R. V. (1990). Recreation and quality of life in old age: a causal analysis. *Journal of Applied Gerontology, 9,* 77-90.

Schaie, K. W. (1996). *Intellectual development in adulthood: The Seattle Longitudinal Study.* New York: Cambridge University Press.

Social and Cultural Planning Office (SCP) (1997). *Rapportage ouderen 1996* [Report of elderly people 1996]. Report nr. 135. The Hague: SCP.

Smale, B. J. A., & Dupuis, S. L. (1993). The relationship between leisure activity participation and psychological well-being across the lifespan. *Journal of Applied Recreation Research, 18,* 281-300.

Suutama, T., Ruoppila, I., & Laukkanen, P. (1999) (Eds.). *Changes in functional abilities among elderly people. Findings from an eight-year follow-up study by the Evergreen project.* Helsinki: The Social Insurance Institution, Finland, Studies in social security and health, 42.

Tokarski, W. (1993). Later life activity from European perspectives. In J. R. Kelly (Ed.) *Activity and aging. Staying involved in later life* (pp. 60-67). Newsbury Park: Sage Publications.

WHO (World Health Organization) (1984). *Health for all.* Geneva, Switzerland: World Health Organization Publications.

Enhancing Mobility in Later Life
H. Mollenkopf et al. (Eds.)
IOS Press, 2005

Chapter 7
Psychological Aspects of Outdoor Mobility in Later Life

Frank Oswald, Hans-Werner Wahl and Roman Kaspar

7.1   Introduction

Within the interdisciplinary scope of variables of MOBILATE, psychological constructs have found considerable attention with the scientific aim to add to the description and explanation of individual differences in outdoor mobility patterns. Psychological aspects are addressed in order *to describe similarities and differences of mobility-related psychological factors between urban and non-urban regions* and *to better understand the impact of psychological factors on mobility and on subjective well-being*. In this chapter, emphasis is put on the basic description of project data, bivariate steps of data analysis, as well as some on multivariate analyses with a wide range of psychology variables linked to the different aggregate outdoor mobility indicators as introduced in an earlier chapter of this book (i.e., transport modes, outdoor activities, everyday trips), and mobility satisfaction. The effect of psychological aspects in conjunction with other mobility-related variables (such as socio-structural and health data) on these indicators as well as on quality of life in more general terms, that is, the full interdisciplinary analytical model of MOBILATE, is described in Chapter 12. However, the psychology input into this final integrative model is prepared in this chapter.

Because psychological constructs are major individual resources and outcomes of outdoor mobility, basic cognitive abilities, control beliefs, coping strategies, the experience of place attachment, and emotional well-being were assessed in the MOBILATE study. Regarding the quality of the psychological assessment conducted in MOBILATE, it should be noted from the beginning on that the majority of instruments and measures used are internationally well-known and well established.

Psychological aspects can be related to an older person's outdoor mobility in a variety of ways. To navigate through the complexity of these processes, we suggest a three-fold role of psychological factors for mobility - predictive, mediating, and outcome - each of which is framed within a hypothesis. Although we expect these hypotheses to hold generally, MOBILATE also offers one the opportunity to check for differences across regions and countries. It should be noted that this will be done in this chapter in a rather exploratory manner, i.e., no concrete hypotheses are suggested at this stage of data analysis in any cross-cultural direction.

Hypothesis 1: Psychological resources are important predictors of outdoor mobility in later life. With this hypothesis, we assume that psychological resources of the ageing individual fundamentally and directly influence outdoor mobility in old age. Cognitive abilities (perceptual motor processing speed in particular) are especially emphasised in this regard.

Rationale behind Hypothesis 1:

Outdoor mobility in all its variety is a complex human behaviour which is highly likely to be influenced by basic intellectual abilities. For instance outdoor mobility orientation and way-finding, the interpretation of mobility-related information, as well as decision-making, all of which strongly depend on cognitive functioning. Perceptual motor processing or *visumotoric coordination* has repeatedly been found to be a major indicator of basic cognitive functioning, frequently described in the literature as fluid intelligence or the mechanics of intelligence (e.g., Baltes, 1993). This cognitive ability is also an important ability underlying outdoor mobility related cognitive functioning as just described. Speed of perceptual motor processing is closely related to ageing (Lindenberger & Reischies, 1999). Decreases in functioning of almost one percent per year have been found in healthy adults between 25 and 75 years of age, supporting a tentatively linear decrease of speed-dependent cognitive functioning in old age. Such empirical evidence deserves qualification, however, since pronounced inter-individual variability can be observed even in very old individuals (Madden, 2001; Lindenberger & Reischies, 1999; Salthouse, 1985). It seems as if some elders compensate better than others for their loss of cognitive functioning, which may lead to quite different outdoor mobility patterns in the same chronological age stratum.

Hypothesis 2: Psychological resources play a major mediating role within the complexities of predicting outdoor mobility in later life. With this hypothesis, it is assumed that some psychological processes can indirectly impact on mobility outcomes in old age. Control beliefs, coping styles, indoor place attachment, importance of being out, and indoor/outdoor motivation were especially emphasised in this regard. In contrast to cognitive abilities, these processes probably will not directly impact on outdoor mobility, but may well exert indirect influence via personal dispositions regulating self-world relations in the aging individual (control beliefs, coping styles) or via environment-related processes that achieve special importance in old age (indoor place attachment, importance of being out, indoor/outdoor motivation).

Rationale behind Hypothesis 2:

Control beliefs. Personal control beliefs have been found to reflect a major driving force in explaining the course and outcome of ageing (Heckhausen & Schulz, 1995; Levenson, 1973; Smith, Marsiske, & Maier, 1996). If individuals perceive events as highly contingent upon their own behaviour, an *internal locus of control* is assumed. If they perceive events not being related on their own actions, but on *powerful others*, or *luck, chance or fate*, one may consider them as having an *external locus of control*. Empirical evidence supports the notion that external control increases in old age, whereas internal control tends to stay stable in adult life (Clark-Plaskie & Lachman, 1999; Lachman, 1991). Control beliefs may influence outdoor mobility in a variety of ways. For example, the experience of being in control over one's life circumstances may strongly motivate an ageing individual to invest much time and effort in maintaining a maximum level of outdoor mobility, even when confronted with health decrements. Similarly, high internal control beliefs may overwrite adverse environmental aspects such as mobility-relevant barriers in the outdoor environment frequently encountered in rural regions.

Coping style. To examine coping strategies from a dispositional perspective, we relied on a concept of age-related coping which draws from the distinction between *assimilative* versus *accommodative* tendencies of maintaining the self and well-being in the later years (Brandtstädter & Renner, 1990). From an environmental and mobility perspective, these two complementary strategies can be expected to be of critical importance (see also Slangen-de Kort, 1999). Whereas assimilation involves active modification of the environment in accordance with life goals ('Changing the world'), accommodation involves adjustment of personal goals to external resources and remaining functional capacity ('Changing the self'). This is similar to the differentiation between 'proactivity' and 'docility' suggested by Lawton in terms of how older people deal with environmental options and barriers (Lawton, 1989, 1990, 1998). On a more general level, measures of coping strategies are aimed to address the individual's behaviour to adapt or proactively shape the environment in order to regain, maintain or enhance healthy ageing. To take the words of Lawton: "This hypothesis suggests that the greater the competence of the person, the more likely the person's needs and preferences will be successfully exercised to search the environment for resources to satisfy the needs (…). In fact, the essence of a proactively created environment is its dynamic, temporally changing quality and its inability to be separated from the user. Examples of such transactional environmental resources are (…) the perceived (…) environment, the local amenities that are used, the state of maintenance of a home, (…) and so on" (Lawton, 1989, p. 18f). Outdoor mobility probably is an important behavioural expression of these personal tendencies.

Indoor place attachment, importance of being out, and indoor/outdoor motivation. The basic assumption here is that attitude- and affect-related links to physical-spatial locations as condensed in one's "place attachment" (Altman & Low, 1992; Oswald & Wahl, 2005; Rowles, Oswald, & Hunter, 2004; Rubinstein & Parmelee, 1992), as well as the motivation to use the outdoor environment as a major opportunity structure, both are important for the explanation of interindividual differences in outdoor mobility (Oswald, Wahl, Mollenkopf, & Schilling, 2003). Indoor place attachment and importance of being out addresses cognitive and emotional bonding to the own home, while indoor/outdoor motivation is predominantly seen as a personal behavioural tendency that varies according to biographical experiences and preferences that have developed across the life span (Oswald & Wahl, 2003). Due to the lack of widely acknowledged measures of these constructs, we implemented global self-ratings of personal, emotional, and cognitive place attachment (differentiated according to indoor and outdoor contexts) based on empirical experience with these measures in our earlier studies on outdoor mobility (e.g., Mollenkopf, Oswald, & Wahl, 1999) and urban neighbourhood attachment (Oswald, Hieber, Wahl, & Mollenkopf, 2005). These measures examine whether people who are well attached to their immediate indoor (indoor place attachment) and/or outdoor (importance of being out) environment are better able to cope with bad objective living conditions or with functional disabilities and whether they are thus more satisfied. Since the literature suggests that attachment to the indoor and outdoor environment among rural and urban elders and among elders with and without severe mobility impairments might differ, two ratings that separately address the indoor and the outdoor environment were implemented. In addition, the motivation-oriented attitude towards the indoor versus outdoor home environment was assessed, the so-called global rating on the indoor/outdoor type. This self- rating served to address the participant's ideal position between the extremes of staying at home versus being on the go as much as possible.

Hypothesis 3: Psychological adaptation is a major outcome of outdoor mobility in later life. With this hypothesis, we assume that existing patterns of outdoor mobility in later life have an impact on psychological outcomes. In particular, the general hypothesis is that the aging individual who uses his or her outdoor mobility capacity as much as possible (depending on a variety of influencing factors) is related to better emotional quality of life. Thus, emotional well-being is emphasised as a major variable in this regard.

Rationale behind Hypothesis 3:

Staying mobile in old age must not only be seen as a result of several objective and subjective preconditions, but is itself a precondition for subjective well-being and life satisfaction. To further strengthen the idea of well-being as an outcome of outdoor mobility on the measurement level, we extended the one-item self rating of psychological well-being used in earlier research (which is heavily weighted towards the cognitive aspects of well-being) with an affect-oriented scale of emotional well-being. In particular, a now classic measure to assess positive and negative affect was introduced for this purpose, namely the Positive and Negative Affect Scale (PANAS; Watson, Clark, & Tellegen, 1988; see also Baltes, Freund, & Horgas, 1999; Kercher, 1992). The literature suggests that positive affect decreases with age, while negative affect does not (Staudinger, Freund, Linden, & Maas, 1999). In conjunction with outdoor mobility, the expectation would be that higher scores in the basic modes of outdoor mobility (transport modes, outdoor activities, everyday trips, and mobility satisfaction) is related to more positive and fewer negative feelings.

In line with the basic descriptive nature of this chapter, we have no intention of comprehensively testing the three hypotheses presented above. Instead, this chapter only provides the first steps in this direction, which are followed in a more integrated and the needed interdisciplinary manner in Chapters 11, 12 and 13 of this book.

Finally, it should be noted that the results reported in this chapter are based on weighted data by applying the Statistical Analysis System (SAS). Correlation analyses were carried out as Pearson correlations. Also, a comment of caution is in place in terms of the statistical significance of reported findings. Although the level of accepted significance was set, in accordance with other MOBILATE analyses, to $p < .01**$ and $p < .001***$, respectively, significant effects occur with regularity in large samples. To be concrete, the absolute threshold for reaching the $p < .01$ level is about $r = .04$ in the aggregated sample (including all countries) and $r = .09$ regarding country-specific analyses. Hence, the absolute size of the correlations reported here (instead of the mere statistical significance of the correlations reported) should always be taken into consideration in data interpretations. Regarding the effect sizes of correlation coefficients, one may follow the now classical proposal by Cohen (1988), arguing that correlations between r = 0.1 and 0.3 are considered as a "small effect", between r = 0.3 and 0.5 as a "medium effect", and above r = 0.5 as a "large effect".

7.2 In-depth description of psychological measures, psychometric analyses, and basic intercorrelations

In this section the psychometric properties of the measures used in MOBILATE are described in more detail. This step is important in order to determine whether the measures have worked well in all countries and research sites (and which must be excluded due to unsatisfactory reliability).

7.2.1 Description of measures and their psychometric properties

An overview of all measures and a short characterization of each of these measures can be found in Table 7.1.

Table 7.1: Overview on Psychological Measurements

Digit-Symbol-Substitution
(Oswald & Fleischmann 1995; Wechsler, 1958)
• Basic cognitive abilities in terms of *visumotoric coordination*, perceptual motor processing speed and working memory indicating fluid intelligence
• One test-sheet, non verbal test revealing a single score, i.e., number of correct substitutions in 90 seconds
Locus-Of-Control Beliefs Scale
(Smith, Marsiske, & Maier, 1996)
• Psychological *self-regulative mechanisms*, i.e., control beliefs for internal and external control (powerful others and chance)
• 14-item questionnaire, items rated on a 5-point scale
Tenacious Goal Pursuit and Flexible Goal Adjustment
(Brandtstädter & Renner, 1990)
• Assimilative and accomodative *strategies of coping*, i.e., Tenacious Goal Pursuit (TGP) and Flexible Goal Adjustment (FGA)
• 30-item questionnaire, each item rated on a 5-point scale, aggregated into two subscales scores
Place Attachment and Indoor/Outdoor-Type
(Mollenkopf, Oswald, & Wahl, 1999)
• Cognitive and affective *environmental bonding* (i.e. indoor place attachment and importance of being out) and perceived *environment-related motivation* in terms of indoor/outdoor-type of person
• Three global self-evaluation ratings, i.e., three single-item ratings on an 11-point rating scale
Positive and Negative Affect Schedule (PANAS)
(Watson, Clark & Tellegen, 1988)
• *Emotional well-being*, i.e. positive and negative affect
• 20-item list revealing frequencies of experienced emotions during last year, aggregated into a positive and negative affect total score

Digit-Symbol-Substitution. Basic cognitive abilities in terms of perceptual motor processing or *visumotoric coordination* and working memory indicating fluid intelligence were assessed with the subtest provided in the Nuremberg Age Inventory / Nürnberger-Alters-Inventar (NAI) (Oswald & Fleischmann, 1995). Participants were asked to complete a row of letters with each letter belonging to a certain symbol. According to the instructions, the task is to complete the row of letters using the digit-symbol combination shown above on the sheet as quickly as possible. The test is considered as a tentatively *culture fair* one. Hence, the assumption is that different cultural backgrounds should not substantially impact on test performance, that is, to test for the basic information processing capacity of the human mind. The number of correctly implemented letters within a timespan of 90 seconds was recorded. Test-retest reliability was established based on older age norm-groups (r_{tt}: .89-.97; Oswald & Fleischmann, 1995). It should also be noted that the digit-symbol substitution test addresses the range of normal cognitive functioning in ageing individuals and is thus not meant to be an indicator of mental health.

Locus-Of-Control Beliefs Scale. The instrument administered to the MOBILATE sample was the control beliefs questionnaire used in the Berlin Aging Study (Baltes, Freund, & Horgas 1999; Smith, Marsiske, & Maier 1996), in which the dimensions of 'Internal Control' (6 items), 'External Control: Powerful Others' (4 items), and 'External Control: Chance' (4 items) were assessed. Whereas 'Internal Control' means that events are perceived as highly contingent upon one's own behaviour, 'External Control: powerful other' means that other persons are seen as being responsible for one's life or that the expectation is such that things happen by mere luck, by chance, or by fate ('External Control: Chance'). Participants were instructed to judge to what extent they personally agree or disagree with each statement on a five-point scale from 1 = 'not at all' to 5 = 'very much'. The scale on Internal Control includes statements such as "It's up to me to arrange for all the good things in my life". The scale 'External Control: Powerful other' includes statements such as "I depend on others to ensure that there are no problems in my life". The scale 'External Control: Chance' includes statements such as "The good things in my life are for the most part a matter of luck". It should be noted that the BASE questionnaire originally differentiated between internal control over positive versus negative events, but factor analysis of the MOBILATE sample confirmed a three-factor solution (internal control, external control: powerful others, external control: chance), explaining about 47% of the variance (Maximum-Likelihood criteria, orthogonal varimax transformation). We thus decided to retain these three dimensions in all MOBILATE data analyses of control beliefs.

Internal consistencies of the scales in all sites were calculated for 'Internal Control': Cronbach's α = .44 to .81, for 'External Control: Powerful other': Cronbach's α = .67 to .89, and for 'External Control: Chance': Cronbach's α = .37 to .72 (see Table 7.2, which also gives the according scores for all other measures). Due to low internal consistencies (Cronbach's α. < .50) in at least one subscale of the Locus-of-control Beliefs scale in Hungary and the Netherlands (see numbers in italics in Table 9.2), we decided not to use these measures in the data analyses concerned with these countries. Reasons for these low internal consistencies across countries might be due to translation difficulties as well as the relatively small number of items in each scale.

Table 7.2:   Report on the internal consistencies of psychological scales in different research sites of
MOBILATE Survey

Cronbach's α [a]	Finland	Eastern Germany	Western Germany	Hungary	Italy	The Netherlands
Locus-Of-Control Beliefs Scale						
Internal Control (6 items)	.62	.79	.81	.70	.66	*.44*
External Control: Chance (4 items)	.52	.55	.70	*.34*	*.51*	*.48*
External Control: Powerful Others (4 items)	.68	.90	.86	.83	.79	.69
Positive and Negative Affect Schedule (PANAS)						
Positive Affect (10 items)	.88	.89	.92	.74	.84	.77
Negative Affect (10 items)	.85	.81	.87	.78	.74	.77
Tenacious Goal Pursuit and Flexible Goal Adjustment						
Flexible Goal Adjustment (FGA) (15 items)	.65	.64	.71	-	-	-
Tenacious Goal Pursuit (TGP) (15 items)	.75	.79	.80	-	-	-

Note. MOBILATE Survey, 2000
Calculation based on standardized Cronbach's α. Low internal consistency ($< .50$) in
subscales is marked with italic numbers.

Tenacious Goal Pursuit and Flexible Goal Adjustment. Assimilative and accommodative
strategies of coping (Brandtstädter & Renner, 1990), also labelled as 'Tenacious Goal Pursuit'
(TGP) (15 items) and 'Flexible Goal Adjustment' (FGA) (15 items) by Brandtstädter and
Renner (1990) were assessed only in Finland and Germany due to the psychology expertise
available at both of these research sites. Participants were instructed to indicate to what extent
they personally agree with each statement on a five-point scale from 1 = 'strongly disagree' to
5 = 'strongly agree'. The 'Tenacious Goal Pursuit' scale includes statements like "The harder
a goal is to achieve, the more appeal it has to me". The 'Flexible Goal Adjustment' scale
includes statements like "When everything seems to be going wrong, I can usually find a
bright side to a situation". As can be seen in Table 7.2, all internal consistencies regarding
'Tenacious Goal Pursuit' (Cronbach's α = .77 to .80) and 'Flexible Goal Adjustment'
(Cronbach's α = .69 to .74) were quite satisfactory both in Germany and Finland.

Indoor place attachment, importance of being out, and Indoor/outdoor type. The home
environment is not only a part of the physical space around us, defined through equipment
and everyday behaviour. Home can also be a place to call home, a place one is attached to, in
terms of pleasure, feelings of security, familiarity, and privacy, or a place that reminds one of
memories of persons and events (e.g., Rowles, Oswald, & Hunter, 2004). The same is true for
the immediate outdoor environment. The neighbourhood is also not only a part of the physical
space around us, defined through buildings, streets, and outdoor behaviour. Neighbourhood
can also be a place to call home, a place one is attached to, in terms of pleasure, feelings of
security, familiarity, and privacy, or a place that reminds one of persons and events. To assess
such cognitive and affective environmental bonding, participants were instructed to indicate
to what extent they personally feel attached to their indoor home environment and how
important being out is to them on an 11-point Likert-type scale from 0 = 'absolutely not
attached'/'absolutely not important' to 10 = 'a great deal of place attachment' or 'very
important'. In addition, participants were asked to judge what kind of person they are in terms
of indoor/outdoor relation. For this purpose, they were instructed to judge if they perceive

themselves as being a person who more often likes to stay at home, or as a person who likes to be on the go on an 11-point Likert-type scale ranging from 0 = "I would like to be at home all the time, if possible" to 10 = "I would like to be on the go all the time, if possible". In terms of the psychometric properties of these new measures used in MOBILATE, we know from earlier work that they have sufficient variability, that their age correlation is - as expected - only in a low to medium range, and that they show consistent relations with factors related to outdoor mobility (e.g., Oswald, Wahl, Mollenkopf & Schilling, 2003; Wahl, Heyl, & Schilling, 2002).

Positive and Negative Affect Schedule (PANAS). Personality development in adulthood and adaptation in later life is often discussed in association with the regulation of emotional states. Many studies have shown that a positive affect balance is associated with higher life satisfaction and other indicators of psychological well-being (e.g., Staudinger, Freund, Linden, & Maas, 1999). Among the best known and reliable constructs of psychological well-being in gerontology are life satisfaction and emotional well-being. A now classic measure to assess positive and negative affect also is the 20-item Positive and Negative Affect Schedule (PANAS) (Watson, Clark, & Telegen, 1988; Staudinger, Freund, Linden, & Maas, 1999; Kunzmann, Little, & Smith, 2002). The PANAS affords separate scores for negative (10 items) and positive affect (10 items), each of which represents a separate dimension. A score for emotional balance (i.e., the difference between the frequencies of positive and negative affect) can be calculated as well, but this option was not used in the MOBILATE analyses (in line with the majority of the literature; see Kunzmann, Little, & Smith, 2002, for the latest analyses of BASE data). Positive and negative affect were assessed comparable to the format used in the Berlin Aging Study (Baltes, Freund, & Horgas, 1999; Staudinger, Freund, Linden, & Maas, 1999; Kunzmann, Little, & Smith, 2002). Participants were instructed to judge to what extent they experienced each emotion during the last year on a five-point scale from 1 = 'not at all' to 5 = 'very often'. The positive affect scale includes statements such as 'interested', 'excited', or 'inspired'. The negative affect scale includes statements such as 'upset', 'guilty', or 'afraid'. The internal consistencies of the scales for positive affect ranged between Cronbach's α = .76 to .81, for negative affect between Cronbach's α = .74 to .86, and were thus quite acceptable (see Table 7.2).

7.2.2   Intercorrelations of psychological constructs, age, and gender

To approach the validity of the different psychological instruments and constructs in MOBILATE, only *overall* correlations between the different measures, age and gender are provided in Table 7.3. For the sake of clarity, differences between research sites are neglected, because this step of the analysis merely serves a psychometric purpose.

Note once again that intercorrelations on this global level quite often attain statistical significance simply due to the large sample size. The correlations between the psychological variables were generally very low taking into consideration the great heterogeneity of the sample as regards, age, location and country. On the whole, however, the results wereas expected as far as similar constructs and relations are portrayed in the existing ageing literature. It is known, for example, that chronological age is associated with a decrease in processing speed, internal control, positive affect, and tenacious goal pursuit and an increase in external control beliefs; all of these relations were observed in the current data set. Gender-related relations indicate that women tend to be higher in flexible goal adjustment (.10***) and lower in tenacious goal pursuit (-.13***) compared to men. Some further correlations between the different psychological measurements included a negative correlation between internal and external control beliefs (-.05***; -.29***), a zero-correlation between positive and negative affect (.01), a positive but low correlation between indoor and outdoor place attachment (.16***), and a zero-correlation between flexible goal adjustment and tenacious goal pursuit (-.04); again, most of these relations correspond well with what other researchers have found. Other relations have not yet been reported in the ageing literature due to the fact that such measures were introduced by the MOBILATE group for the first time. However, these correlations, such as the ones between outdoor place attachment and external control: powerful others (-.22***) and positive affect (.23***) were in the expected direction.

Table 7.3: Intercorrelations between psychological constructs, age, and gender

All research sites (N = 3950)	Age	Gender (m = 0)	Processing speed	Internal control	External control: chance	External control: p. others	PANAS: positive affect	PANAS: negative affect	Indoor place attachment	Importance of being out	Indoor / outdoor type	Goal adjustment: FGA
Processing speed	-.41 ***	-.03										
Internal control [a]	-.10 ***	-.08 ***	.18 ***									
External control: chance [b]	.19 ***	.05 **	-.20 ***	-.05 **								
External control: p. others	.33 ***	.06 ***	-.27 ***	-.29 ***	.34 ***							
PANAS: positive affect	-.32 ***	-.01	.35 ***	.26 ***	-.16 ***	-.31 ***						
PANAS: negative affect	-.06 ***	.12 ***	.01	-.16 ***	.09 ***	.18 ***	.01					
Indoor place attachment	<.01	.03	-.04	.09 ***	-.04 **	-.08 **	.02	-.09 ***				
Importance of being out	-.17 ***	-.06 ***	.19 ***	.17 ***	-.06 ***	-.22 ***	.23 ***	-.16 ***	.16 ***			
Indoor / outdoor type	-.17 ***	-.13 ***	.16 ***	.15 ***	-.07 ***	-.18 ***	.27 ***	-.05 **	-.11 ***	.33 ***		
Goal adjustment: FGA [c]	.01	.10 ***	<.01	.13 ***	.04	-.09 ***	.06 **	-.27 ***	.22 ***	.18 ***	.01	
Goal adjustment: TGP [c]	-.26 ***	-.13 ***	.27 ***	.14 ***	-.27 ***	-.31 ***	.43 ***	-.03	-.03	.17 ***	.21 ***	-.04

Note. MOBILATE Survey, 2000
Correlations p < .01**; p < .001***; [a] Not applicable in The Netherlands; [b] Not applicable in Hungary and The Netherlands; [c] Not applicable in Hungary, Italy, and The Netherlands

7.3 Psychological constructs and outdoor mobility: bivariate relations across geographical locations

In the following, differences and similarities in psychological measurements between research sites are presented by country and geographic location (urban vs. rural). Additionally, relations with age, gender, and mobility outcomes are presented in terms of correlations. In accordance with the three main hypotheses underlying this research, results are presented first on psychological constructs as predictors of mobility (3.1), second as mediators of mobility (3.2), and third as outcomes of mobility (3.3).

7.3.1   Psychological constructs as predictors of outdoor mobility

Visumotoric coordination is viewed as a direct and major predictor of mobility. Results are presented in Table 7.4 and in Figure 7.1. Interpreting psychological measures such as visumotoric coordination across different European countries should be done with great caution. In general, higher scores in The Netherlands, Germany and Finland versus lower scores in Hungary and Italy should not be misinterpreted as 'better' functioning per se, but may be regarded in terms of cultural variations. Note that processing speed is - in principal - *not* expected to be substantially related to educational levels in the same way as a knowledge-based cognitive test would be. Nonetheless, the results are probably related to education and illiteracy, to practice and motor performance (such as whether or not one has had to write a great deal over the lifespan), which might explain part of the observed differences. Another portion of variance could come from health differences (e.g., regarding cardio-vascular diseases), which are related to central information processing (Schaie, 1996).

As far as geographic location is concerned, significant differences in visumotoric coordination between urban and rural elders occur, with the exception of the Netherlands and eastern Germany. Urban elders tend to have higher mean scores, which again might be explained best by the reasons discussed above. Regarding the eastern German and Dutch settings, one should note that in the Netherlands, differences between urban and rural settings were minimal.

Table 7.4:   Results on the relation of visumotoric coordination and outdoor mobility in the different sites

Variable *M (SD)* [a]	Finland		Eastern Germany		Western Germany		Hungary		Italy		The Netherlands	
	28.5 (14.0) (range: 1-62)		34.1 (15.5) (range: 1-67)		31.1 (14.6) (range: 1-67)		23.9 (13.3) (range: 1-67)		21.4 (13.0) (range: 1-65)		37.8 (13.9) (range: 1-67)	
	Urban	Rural	Urban	Rural	Urban	Rural	Urban	Rural	Urban	Rural	Urban	Rural
Cognitive abilities: Visumotoric coordination (1-67) (*N* = 3392)	32.9 *** (14.2)	23.8 *** (12.1)	33.2 (15.6)	34.9 (15.4)	33.8 *** (15.8)	28.6 *** (13.0)	28.3 *** (13.3)	19.7 *** (11.8)	26.0 *** (13.9)	16.6 *** (10.1)	38.2 (14.0)	37.4 (13.9)
Age	-.68 ***		-.34 ***		-.36 ***		-.41 ***		-.52 ***		-.33 ***	
Gender (male = 0)	.05		<.01		-.08		.01		-.15		-.06	
Mobility satisfaction (0-10)[b]	.23 ***		.13 ***		.22 ***		.20 ***		.39 ***		.19 ***	
Transport modes (0-13) [c]	.48 ***		.18 ***		.36 ***		.40 ***		.61 ***		.27 ***	
Outdoor activities (0-1) [d]	.44 ***		.40 ***		.38 ***		.41 ***		.48 ***		.29 ***	
Everyday trips [e]	.40 ***		.19 ***		.13 **		.30 ***		.47 ***		.13 **	

Note. MOBILATE Survey, 2000
[a] Weighted data. Urban-Rural differences are calculated by GLM-procedure with $p < .01$**; $p < .001$*** (also for correlations).
[b] Self-evaluation rating on an 11-point rating scale, higher scores indicating higher satisfaction.
[c] Number of used options per person (0-13).
[d] Relative number of reported options per person (0-1).
[e] Number of realised trips per day and per person.

Age effects are substantial and all in the expected direction, that is, visumotoric coordination is clearly and consistently negatively related with age in all countries. It is nevertheless important to note differences between countries which also appear in Figure 7.1, which depicts age-visumotoric relations in a scatterplot manner. One interesting observation against the pronounced variability found in all samples, is that the regression lines start at quite different levels; they are highest in the Netherlands, followed by Finland and Germany, while Hungary and Italy are somewhat lower. Another interesting observation is that there seems to be a substantial portion of older adults in the younger age group (aged 55-74 years) with rather high visumotoric coordination scores in Germany and the Netherlands. This pattern was less apparent in Hungary and Italy, even less so in Finland. This seems to produce part of the clearly higher negative age-visumotoric coordination correlation in Finland, which is also true with respect to Hungary and Italy.

Figure 7.1: Scatterplots of the relations between chronological age and visumotoric coordination across countries

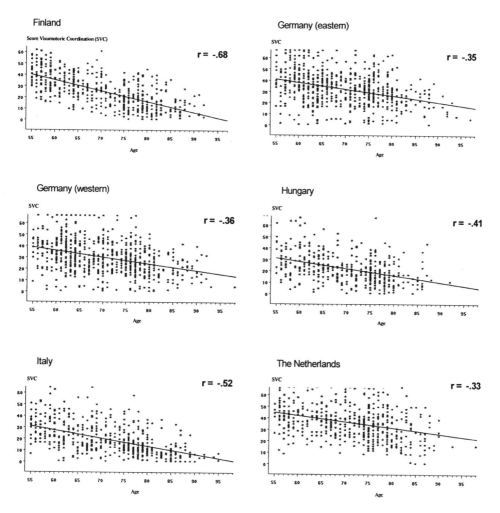

In sum, scatterplots support the view that Germany and the Netherlands are similar in the sense that they start on a comparable level and reveal a comparable age-related loss around r = -.35, which tends to be lower than reported in other studies. In addition, Hungary and Italy are similar in that they start at a lower level, but reveal quite substantial age loss, perhaps higher than in Germany and the Netherlands. Finally, Finland is unique in terms of starting on a by and large comparable level with Germany and the Netherlands, but with a much stronger rate of decline across age. The underlying reasons for these different trends in the 'hard' domain of a basic cognitive capacity are difficult to identify in definite manner. One explanation might be that the Finnish sample is more heterogeneous regarding health-related aspects in the younger group. However, a satisfactory explanation for these results remains to be found.

In terms of additional results, no significant relation of processing speed with gender was observed. As far as mobility-related outcomes are concerned, visumotoric coordination was consistently and positively related with all indicators of mobility in all countries, although the strength of this relation varied considerably between sites. Consequently, Hypothesis 1, which assumed a positive link between visumotoric coordination and outdoor mobility, was well supported by these findings.

7.3.1.1   Psychological constructs as mediators of outdoor mobility

In this part of the present chapter, control beliefs (internal versus external locus of control), coping styles (i.e., assimilative and accommodative tendencies of behaviour) and indoor place attachment (cognitive and emotional bonding to the indoor environment), the importance of being out, as well as environment-related motivation (indoor/outdoor-type of person) are examined, that is, those constructs that theoretically have been conceptualised as mediators of mobility. Results are presented in Tables 7.5 - 7.7.

Concerning control beliefs (see Table 7.5), mean scores were rather comparable across different countries (as mentioned above, results from some subscales are not considered in the Netherlands and Hungary). Consistent with the general literature on control beliefs, belief in the control of powerful others tended to be lower compared to internal control and external control: chance across all countries.

The age effects observed in the MOBILATE samples were generally in accordance with the literature in the field (e.g., Lachman, 1991). Higher chronological age was associated with lower perceived internal and higher external control, which is especially true for the age-related increase in the perceived powerful others control dimension. But once again, cultural variation seems to be an issue in the age-control relation. In particular, internal control in Finland was positively related with age, but the magnitude of this correlation was rather low.

As far as gender effects are concerned, men perceived slightly higher internal control in Finland and Italy, whereas in Italy and eastern Germany, women perceived higher external control (powerful others). One explanation for this finding might be that the control-related results from Italy reflect a somewhat more traditional view of responsibilities within the current cohort of elders characterized by clearly divided roles for men and women, leaving the women with few responsibilities.

Table 7.5:   Comparisons of internal control, external control: chance, and external control: powerful others in different sites

Variable M (SD) [a]	Finland		Eastern Germany		Western Germany		Hungary		Italy		The Netherlands	
	Urban	Rural	Urban	Rural	Urban	Rural	Urban	Rural	Urban	Rural	Urban	Rural
Locus-of-control Beliefs: Internal control (1-5) (N = 3798)	3.3 (0.6) (range: 1.3-5)		3.7 (0.7) (range: 1.3-5)		3.5 (0.8) (range: 1-5)		3.1 (0.7) (range: 1-5)		3.2 (0.6) (range: 1.3-4.8)		- f)	
	3.2** (0.6)	3.4** (0.5)	3.7 (0.6)	3.7 (0.7)	3.4** (0.8)	3.6** (0.8)	3.1 (0.7)	3.0 (0.7)	3.3*** (0.6)	3.1*** (0.6)	- f)	
Age	.14 ***		-.20 ***		-.12 **		-.22 ***		-.10		- f)	
Gender (male = 0)	-.13 ***		-.05		-.02		-.05		-.20 ***		- f)	
Mobility satisfaction (0-10)[b]	.03		.26 ***		.25 ***		.29 ***		.14 ***		- f)	
Transport modes (0-13) [c]	-.11 **		.15 ***		.16 ***		.28 ***		.25 ***		- f)	
Outdoor activities (0-1) [d]	-.09		.28 ***		.25 ***		.30 ***		.31 ***		- f)	
Everyday trips [e]	-.06		.18 ***		.20 ***		.16 ***		.21 ***		- f)	
Locus-of-control Beliefs: External control: Chance (1-5) (N = 3814)	3.2 (0.7) (range: 1.3-5)		2.8 (0.7) (range: 1-4.8)		2.9 (0.8) (range: 1-5)		- f		3.2 (0.6) (range: 1-4.8)		- f)	
	3.1*** (0.7)	3.3*** (0.6)	2.8 (0.7)	2.8 (0.6)	2.8*** (0.8)	3.0*** (0.8)	- f		3.1*** (0.7)	3.4*** (0.5)	- f)	
Age	.28 ***		.27 ***		.08		- f		.24 ***		- f)	
Gender (male = 0)	.07		.09		.02		- f		.06		- f)	
Mobility satisfaction (0-10)[b]	-.14 ***		-.28 ***		-.13 ***		- f		-.18 ***		- f)	
Transport modes (0-13) [c]	-.21 ***		-.35 ***		-.17 ***		- f		-.29 ***		- f)	
Outdoor activities (0-1) [d]	-.20 ***		-.32 ***		-.17 ***		- f		-.19 ***		- f)	
Everyday trips [e]	-.16 ***		-.16 ***		-.09		- f		-.22 ***		- f)	
Locus-of-control Beliefs: External control: Powerful others (1-5) (N = 3834)	2.4 (0.6) (range: 1-4.8)		2.3 (1.0) (range: 1-5)		2.2 (1.0) (range: 1-5)		2.3 (1.0) (range: 1-5)		2.6 (0.8) (range: 1-5)		2.5 (0.6) (range: 1-5)	
	2.3** (0.6)	2.5** (0.6)	2.3 (1.0)	2.3 (1.1)	2.2 (1.0)	2.2 (1.0)	2.1** (1.0)	2.4** (1.0)	2.4*** (0.8)	2.8*** (0.8)	2.5 (0.7)	2.5 (0.6)
Age	.25 ***		.49 ***		.28 ***		.26 ***		.37 ***		.28 ***	
Gender (male = 0)	.01		.09 **		.04		.07		.13 **		.01	
Mobility satisfaction (0-10)[b]	-.11 **		-.47 ***		-.31 ***		-.25 ***		-.35 ***		-.19 ***	
Transport modes (0-13) [c]	-.22 ***		-.52 ***		-.31 ***		-.30 ***		-.40 ***		-.27 ***	
Outdoor activities (0-1) [d]	-.19 ***		-.45 ***		-.39 ***		-.31 ***		-.35 ***		-.30 ***	
Everyday trips [e]	-.15 ***		-.30 ***		-.24 ***		-.19 ***		-.34 ***		-.15 ***	

Note. MOBILATE Survey, 2000

[a] Weighted data. Urban-Rural differences are calculated by GLM-procedure with $p < .01$**; $p < .001$*** (also for correlations).

[b] Self-evaluation rating on an 11-point rating scale, higher scores indicating higher satisfaction.

[c] Number of used options per person (0-13).

[d] Number of reported options per person (0-17).

[e] Relative number of reported options per person (0-1).

[f] Not reported because of low stability (< .50) in this subscale.

As far as mobility-related outcomes are concerned, internal control beliefs were positively related to all mobility-related outcomes in all countries, with the exception of Finland (why this is the case can not be explained at this point in time; the magnitude of the correlation was $r = -.11$, which was quite low). Inversely, external control beliefs were, for the most part, negatively related to mobility outcomes at all research sites. Again, this was especially and most consistently true for the powerful others control dimension.

Next, results on 'Flexible goal adjustment' (FGA) and 'Tenacious goal adjustment' (TGP) are presented, bearing in mind, that the first serves to indicate assimilative, i.e., proactive coping strategies, whereas the latter serves to indicate accommodative, i.e., reactive coping strategies, both of which critical in order to modify or adjust to the socio-physical environmental in old age (see Table 7.6). Both scales were assessed only in the Finish and German research sites.

Table 7.6:   Comparisons of 'Flexible Goal Adjustment' and 'Tenacious Goal Pursuit' in different sites

Variable M (SD) [a]	Finland		Eastern Germany		Western Germany	
Coping Styles: Flexible Goal adjustment (FGA) (1-5) (N = 1833)	3.5 (0.4) (range: 2.4-4.7)		3.4 (0.4) (range: 2.3-4.7)		3.5 (0.5) (range: 2.3-4.7)	
	Urban	Rural	Urban	Rural	Urban	Rural
	3.5 (0,4)	3.6 (0,4)	3.4 (0,4)	3.3 (0,4)	3.4 (0,5)	3.5 (0,4)
Age	.01		-.11 **		.07	
Gender (male = 0)	.14 **		.04		.11 **	
Mobility satisfaction (0-10) [b]	.11 **		.21 ***		.16 ***	
Transport modes (0-13) [c]	-.03		.21 ***		.03	
Outdoor activities (0-1) [d]	.02		.21 ***		.04	
Everyday trips [e]	-.04		.09		.06	
Coping Styles: Tenacious Goal Pursuit (TGP) (1-5) (N = 1836)	3.1 (0.5) (range: 1.4-4.9)		3.0 (0.5) (range: 1.4-5.0)		3.0 (0.6) (range: 1.1-4.6)	
	Urban	Rural	Urban	Rural	Urban	Rural
	3.1 (0,5)	3.0 (0,5)	3.1** (0,5)	3.0** (0,5)	3.1*** (0,6)	2.9*** (0,6)
Age	-.35 ***		-.27 ***		-.21 ***	
Gender (male = 0)	-.06		-.15 ***		-.15 ***	
Mobility satisfaction (0-10) [b]	.11		.30 ***		.14 ***	
Transport modes (0-13) [c]	.20 ***		.33 ***		.23 ***	
Outdoor activities (0-1) [d]	.24 ***		.37 ***		.33 ***	
Everyday trips [e]	.21 ***		.16 ***		.19 ***	

Note. MOBILATE Survey, 2000
[a] Weighted data. Urban-Rural differences are calculated by GLM-procedure with $p < .01$**; $p < .001$*** (also for correlations).
[b] Self-evaluation rating on an 11-point rating scale, higher scores indicating higher satisfaction.
[c] Number of used options per person (0-13).
[d] Relative number of reported options per person (0-1).
[e] Number of realised trips per day and per person.

In general, mean scores were comparable in the different countries with a tendency that TGP was somewhat lower compared to FGA. As far as differences due to geographic location are concerned, urban-rural effects reached statistical significance only in Germany. However, absolute differences in the means were quite comparable and should not be interpreted any further.

Age effects occurred in all countries in the expected manner, showing that with increasing age, assimilative (i.e., proactive) coping strategies were lower (Brandstädter & Renner, 1990). Interestingly, in eastern Germany, this was also the case for accomodative (i.e., reactive) coping strategies (FGA). As far as gender effects are concerned, basically women tended to be more accommodative (i.e., reactive) whereas men tended to be more assimilative (i.e., proactive). This might possibly have something to do with life-long learned social roles for men and women in this cohort of elders. However, note that these latter results did not always reach statistical significance.

With regard to mobility-related outcomes, assimilative strategies (TGP) were positively and substantially related with all outcomes in all countries, whereas accommodative strategies (FGA) were not, except for eastern Germany. Both coping styles, however, were positively related to mobility satisfaction, underscoring that both proactive and reactive ways of coping play a role in the subjective evaluation of older people's outdoor mobility.

Finally, indicators for emotional and cognitive environmental bonding (indoor place attachment and importance of being out), as well as environmental motivation (indoor-outdoor type of person) are considered, assessing another set of potential moderators for mobility (Table 7.7). In general, indoor place attachment tended to be higher than the importance of being out, except in the Netherlands. Finnish elders were extremely high in both scales. Importance of being out differed to a greater extent between the countries compared to indoor attachment ratings. Importance of being out was especially low in Hungary and Italy, and again particularly low in the Hungarian and Italian rural areas. As far as motivational aspects are concerned, older adults in Finland were mostly indoor-oriented, whereas elders in the Netherlands were highly outdoor-oriented. Concerning this motivational rating, there was also a large difference between indoor-oriented western and outdoor-oriented eastern German elders.

In terms of geographic location the results were generally quite mixed. Moreover, urban-rural effects reached statistical significance only in some sites. We thus refrain from any attempt to interpret these differences in a substantial manner. Nevertheless, it does not seem to be the case that outdoor place attachment in general is lower in urban settings and higher in rural ones, or vice versa. Age effects occurred at all sites except the Netherlands. Whereas there were no effects of age on indoor place attachment, importance of being out was significantly lower among the older age groups in most sites. In addition, age was positively related to motivational indoor-orientation at most sites (except the Netherlands and Italy). As far as gender effects are concerned, women tended to be more indoor-oriented, whereas men tended to be more outdoor-oriented at most sites (except for the Netherlands and western Germany). Especially in Italy, men were more attached and oriented towards the outdoor environment compared to women, possibly due to culture-specific life-long socialisation toward home-related environments in this cohort of elder women.

With respect to outdoor mobility-related results, importance of being out and the outdoor-oriented type of motivation were both positively and consistently correlated with all indicators of mobility in all countries, whereas this was not the case regarding indoor place attachment. But note here that SDs were quite low in the case of indoor place attachment, pointing to a ceiling effect with the measurement of this variable which would also undermine correlations.

Table 7.7:   Comparisons of 'Indoor place Attachment'; 'Importance of being out' as well as of 'Indoor/Outdoor Type' in different sites

Variable M (SD) [a]	Finland		Eastern Germany		Western Germany		Hungary		Italy		The Netherlands	
	Urban	Rural	Urban	Rural	Urban	Rural	Urban	Rural	Urban	Rural	Urban	Rural
Indoor Place Attachment (0-10) (N = 3939)	9.7 (0.7) (range: 4-10)		8.9 (1.3) (range: 0-10)		9.1 (1.5) (range: 0-10)		9.3 (1.2) (range: 1-10)		9.0 (1.5) (range: 0-10)		7.9 (1.8) (range: 0-10)	
	9.7 (0.6)	9.7 (0.7)	8.8*** (1.4)	9.1*** (1.2)	9.0 (1.7)	9.2 (1.3)	9.5** (1.0)	9.2** (1.4)	9.5*** (1.3)	8.6*** (1.6)	7.9 (2.0)	8.0 (1.6)
Age	.06		<.01		.06		-.08		-.02		-.02	
Gender (male = 0)	.21 ***		.05		.01		.05		.07		< -.01	
Mobility satisfaction (0-10)[b]	.08		.16 ***		.22 ***		.17 ***		.10		.20 ***	
Transport modes (0-13) [c]	.02		.04		-.03		.10		.11 **		.11 **	
Outdoor activities (0-1) [d]	.07		.13 ***		.05		.20 ***		.09		.15 ***	
Everyday trips [e]	<.01		.08		.08		.15 ***		-.04		.05	
Importance of being out (0-10) (N = 3936)	8.9 (1.4) (range: 0-10)		7.7 (2.4) (range: 0-10)		7.1 (2.7) (range: 0-10)		6.7 (2.6) (range: 0-10)		7.0 (2.6) (range: 0-10)		8.0 (1.5) (range: 1-10)	
	8.9 (1.2)	8.8 (1.6)	7.4** (2.4)	7.9** (2.3)	6.9** (2.7)	7.4** (2.6)	7.3*** (2.5)	6.1*** (2.6)	7.4*** (2.4)	6.7*** (2.7)	7.8 (1.8)	8.1 (1.8)
Age	-.15 ***		-.21 ***		-.21 ***		-.16 ***		-.22 ***		-.10	
Gender (male = 0)	-.05		-.08		-.07		<.01		-.18 ***		<.01	
Mobility satisfaction (0-10)[b]	.28 ***		.46 ***		.43 ***		.31 ***		.41 ***		.18 ***	
Transport modes (0-13) [c]	.20 ***		.33 ***		.27 ***		.24 ***		.27 ***		.10	
Outdoor activities (0-1) [d]	.29 ***		.38 ***		.40 ***		.30 ***		.27 ***		.25 ***	
Everyday trips [e]	.17 ***		.05		.23 ***		.23 ***		.29 ***		.10 **	
Indoor-Outdoor Type (0-10) (N = 3929)	3.5 (2.3) (range: 0-10)		5.1 (2.4) (range: 0-10)		4.4 (2.2) (range: 0-10)		4.3 (2.7) (range: 0-10)		4.7 (3.1) (range: 0-10)		5.3 (2.3) (range: 1-10)	
	3.8** (2.3)	3.3** (2.2)	5.0 (2.1)	5.1 (2.6)	4.7** (2.1)	4.2** (2.4)	4.7*** (2.8)	3.8*** (2.6)	4.9 (3.0)	4.4 (3.2)	5.3 (2.5)	5.4 (2.1)
Age	-.20 ***		-.16 ***		-.23 ***		-.23 ***		-.08		-.10	
Gender (male = 0)	-.10 **		-.15 ***		-.07		-.13 **		-.31 ***		-.05	
Mobility satisfaction (0-10)[b]	.13 ***		.27 ***		.21 ***		.19 ***		.26 ***		.08	
Transport modes (0-13) [c]	.26 ***		.20 ***		.30 ***		.25 ***		.31 ***		.15 ***	
Outdoor activities (0-1) [d]	.34 ***		.24 ***		.30 ***		.33 ***		.21 ***		.15 ***	
Everyday trips [e]	.23 ***		.16 ***		.23 ***		.21 ***		.28 ***		.12 **	

Note. MOBILATE Survey, 2000

[a] Weighted data. Urban-Rural differences are calculated by GLM-procedure with $p < .01$**; $p < .001$*** (also for correlations).

[b] Self-evaluation *rating* on an 11-point rating scale, higher scores indicating higher satisfaction.

[c] Number of used options per person (0-13).

[d] Relative number of reported options per person (0-1); [e] Number of realised trips per day and per person.

In sum, results on control beliefs, coping styles and place attachment support the usefulness of Hypothesis 2, but also call for qualification with respect to some variables which we have considered to be mediators of outdoor mobility in later life. Control-beliefs in general were related in a consistent way with mobility outcomes; this was clearly evident with external control: powerful others. Constructs taken from other theoretical frameworks, however, produced mixed results. For example, tenacious goal pursuit was found to be far more consistently related to 'objective' outdoor mobility outcomes than the flexible goal adjustment. Importance of being out and the motivational indoor-outdoor type were found to relate in a quite consistent manner with the different outdoor mobility indicators, yet this was not true with respect to indoor place attachment.

7.3.1.2   Psychological constructs as outcomes of mobility

In this part of the chapter emotional well-being (i.e., positive and negative affect) is examined as a theoretical outcome of mobility. Results are presented in Table 7.8.

In general, some interesting differences among countries were observed, although most of these were relatively small. In particular, urban Italian elders tended to be highest in positive, rural Hungarian elders in negative affect, whereas rural Finnish elders (together with western German elders) tended to be lowest in both. Thus, as far as differences due to geographic location are concerned, urban-rural effects were somewhat mixed with a slight tendency that both positive and negative affect tend to be higher in urban compared to rural settings.

With respect to the relation between affect and age, positive affect was negatively correlated with age at all research sites, that is, positive affect decreased with age as was also observed in other studies (Baltes, Freund, & Horgas, 1999; Staudinger, Freund, Linden, & Maas, 1999). Considerable inconsistency, however, was observed with regards to the findings on negative affect: whereas in Finland, *younger* elders were substantially higher in negative affect, there was little or no substantial effect for this domain in the other countries. Although we have no explanation to offer for this finding, one might remember here that the Finns, especially the younger subjects, tended to have lower scores on cognitive functioning compared to respondents from Germany and the Netherlands.

Gender effects were consistent with most of the international literature: Women scored higher on negative affect, whether or not this reflects a 'true' result or is simply a methodological artefact (e.g., women are less inhibited about reporting negative feelings). In contrast, no relation between gender and positive affect was observed.

As far as mobility-related results are concerned, positive affect was consistently and positively correlated with all outcomes in all countries, whereas the relations between negative affect and the outcomes were quite mixed. By and large, this supports the usefulness of Hypothesis 3 which postulated a meaningful relation between outdoor mobility and major psychological outcomes such as positive affect. However, the assumption does not apply as well to negative affect.

Table 7.8:   Comparisons of Positive and Negative Affect in different sites

Variable M (SD) a)	Finland		Eastern Germany		Western Germany		Hungary		Italy		The Netherlands	
	Urban	Rural	Urban	Rural	Urban	Rural	Urban	Rural	Urban	Rural	Urban	Rural
Emotional Well-being: Positive affect (1-5) (N = 3761)	3.0 (0.7) (range: 1-4.9)		3.3 (0.7) (range: 1-4.7)		3.1 (0.8) (range: 1-4.9)		3.2 (0.7) (range: 1-4.7)		3.3 (0.7) (range: 1-4.9)		3.4 (0.5) (range: 1.3-4.7)	
	3.1*** (0.7)	2.9*** (0.7)	3.4*** (0.6)	3.2*** (0.7)	3.3*** (0.7)	3.0*** (0.9)	3.3 (0.7)	3.2 (0.6)	3.5*** (0.7)	3.2*** (0.7)	3.4 (0.6)	3.4 (0,5)
Age	-.48 ***		-.34 ***		-.27 ***		-.22 ***		-.40 ***		-.19 ***	
Gender (male = 0)	-.02		-.06		-.02		.08		-.10		.08	
Mobility satisfaction (0-10)b)	.33 ***		.28 ***		.22 ***		.31 ***		.52 ***		.20 ***	
Transport modes (0-13) c)	.45 ***		.37 ***		.34 ***		.31 ***		.41 ***		.27 ***	
Outdoor activities (0-1) d)	.52 ***		.49 ***		.54 ***		.42 ***		.50 ***		.34 ***	
Everyday trips e)	.34 ***		.25 ***		.35 ***		.28 ***		.35 ***		.16 ***	
Emotional Well-being: Negative affect (1-5) (N = 3802)	2.0 (0.6) (range: 1-4.1)		2.1 (0.5) (range: 1-3.5)		2.1 (0.6) (range: 1-4)		2.2 (0.7) (range: 1-4.2)		2.3 (0.6) (range: 1-4.1)		2.2 (0.6) (range: 1-4.1)	
	2.1** (0.6)	2.0** (0.6)	2.1 (0.5)	2.1 (0.5)	2.3*** (0.6)	2.0*** (0.6)	2.1*** (0.6)	2.4*** (0.7)	2.3 (0.6)	2.2 (0.6)	2.3*** (0.6)	2.1*** (0.5)
Age	-.29 ***		.11 **		-.02		-.09		-.04		-.02	
Gender (male = 0)	.07		.14 ***		.05		.12 **		.22 ***		.16 ***	
Mobility satisfaction (0-10)b)	-.04		-.25 ***		-.31 ***		-.22 ***		-.22 ***		-.19 ***	
Transport modes (0-13) c)	.23 ***		-.18 ***		-.05		-.09		-.06		-.10	
Outdoor activities (0-1) d)	.23 ***		-.23 ***		-.14 ***		-.20 ***		-.05		-.09	
Everyday trips e)	.13 **		-.17 ***		-.01		-.17 ***		-.06		-.08	

Note. MOBILATE Survey, 2000

a) Weighted data. Urban-Rural differences are calculated by GLM-procedure with $p < .01**; p < .001***$ (also for correlations).

b) Self-evaluation rating on an 11-point rating scale, higher scores indicating higher satisfaction.

c) Number of used options per person (0-13).

d) Relative number of reported options per person (0-1).

e) Number of realised trips per day and per person.

7.4   Psychological constructs and outdoor mobility: multivariate relations across countries

In this more complex step of analysis, we included those psychological resources which have revealed quite consistent bivariate relations with mobility outcomes and demonstrated sufficient reliability in all countries (see section 7.2). As a result of this selection process, only visumotoric coordination, external control: powerful others, importance of being out, and indoor-outdoor type could be retained as independent variables. In order to consider potential interrelations between all four mobility outcomes, we used multivariate analysis of variance

(MANOVA) as our data analysis strategy. The findings are depicted in Table 7.9 in a somewhat aggregated manner to ensure clarity.

The main result is that all four psychological variables revealed a very consistent relation with outdoor mobility in all countries. The only exception was the role of 'external control: powerful others' in the case of Finland. In this context, one should note that the bivariate relations between this variable and all outdoor mobility indicators were the weakest in the Finnish sample to begin with (see again Table 7.5). However, aside from this hard-to-explain difference, it is clear that these results provide additional support for the hypothesis of a major link between a set of well-selected psychological variables and a multifacetted concept of outdoor mobility (as is done in MANOVA analysis) in all of the countries participating in MOBILATE.

Table 7.9: Results of MANOVA analysis separately conducted for four psychological constructs with four outdoor mobility indicators treated as dependent variable [a]

Variable	Finland	Eastern Germany	Western Germany	Hungary	Italy	The Netherlands
Visumotoric Coordination	+	+	+	+	+	+
External Control: Powerful Others		+	+	+	+	+
Importance of being out	+	+	+	+	+	+
Indoor-Outdoor-Type	+	+	+	+	+	+

Note. MOBILATE Survey, 2000

    [a] Results are based on the results of the SAS procedure GLM. "+" means that the data analysis revealed a significant effect at least at the .01 level consistently in four major test statistics suggested in the SAS for MANOVA (Wilk's Lamba, Pillai's Trace, Hotelling-Lawley Trace, Roy's Greatest Root).

The results were less clear when coping styles (flexible goal adjustment and tenacious goal pursuit) were also included in the analyses (these could only be carried out in Finland and Germany). None of these coping modes remained a significant ($p < .01$) predictor of outdoor mobility in Finland. Tenacity did not predict mobility in eastern and western Germany either. In fact, flexible goal adjustment was the only construct to play a significant role, and only in the western Germany region. However, both tenacity and flexibility were significant predictors of mobility when data from eastern and western Germany were integrated into one set.

7.5   Summary and conclusions

In this section, descriptive results from the MOBILATE study have been presented, illustrating the role of psychological variables in outdoor mobility in later life. It is important to note in this context that psychological processes have typically been neglected in outdoor mobility analysis or were considered only in a marginal sense in earlier research. In MOBILATE, psychology processes are, to our knowledge for the first time, explicitly addressed based on state-of-the-art geropsychology constructs and procedures designed specifically to measure them.

Consequently, a first major step of this report concentrated on the psychometric properties of the measures used in MOBILATE with - on the whole - quite satisfactory findings across countries and regions in terms of internal consistency and construct validity.

Nevertheless, some of the psychometric properties of these tests were unsatisfactory, leading us to drop certain variables from specific analyses.

In terms of content, the rationale to address psychological resources as relevant for outdoor mobility was channelled into three hypotheses. In short, psychological constructs were hypothesised to have a three-fold effect on outdoor mobility. First, basic functioning at the cognitive level (operationalised as visumotoric coordination/processing speed) was expected to directly influence the performance of outdoor-related behaviours. Second, a range of personality- and person-environment-related constructs (i.e., control beliefs, coping styles, indoor place attachment, importance of being out) was expected to serve as a mediating force regarding outdoor mobility. Third, it was assumed that outdoor mobility may also serve as an antecedent variable for major psychological outcomes such as emotional adjustment (e.g., positive affect).

All of these hypothesis could be basically supported, but some qualification is necessary in terms of evaluating their importance with respect to outdoor mobility outcomes, even at the simple bivariate level of analysis. Whereas processing speed or control-beliefs were related quite consistently with mobility outcomes at all research sites, the coping style 'tenacious goal pursuit' was more strongly related to outdoor mobility than the coping style 'flexible goal adjustment'. Differential relations can be assumed furthermore between indoor place attachment vs. importance of being out and mobility outcomes (which were stronger related to importance of being out) and between mobility outcomes and positive versus negative affect (positive affect revealed itself to be more consistently related to mobility). In a more complex step of data analysis, high consistency was found with respect to those variables considerable in *all* countries (visumotoric coordination, external control: powerful others, importance of being out, indoor-outdoor type) and an aggregate view of all four outdoor mobility indicators across countries. That is, letting aside some country-specific differences, participants who were good in visumotoric coordination, who considered themselves not be too dependent on other persons (external control beliefs), and who liked to be out and about as much as possible (outdoor motivation), generally had higher scores in outdoor mobility outcomes.

Finally, the substance of this chapter should be qualified once again in that the data analyses presented were not intended to address more complex relationships inherent in our hypotheses. Only multivariate analyses such as structural equation modelling can test the assumption of direct, indirect and outcome-related effects of psychological resources in the context of outdoor mobility. The results of such comprehensive analyses will be reported in Chapter 13 of this book.

References

Altman, I., & Low, S. M. (Eds.) (1992). *Human Behavior and Environment, Vol. 12: Place Attachment.* New York: Plenum.

Baltes, M. M., Freund, A. M., & Horgas, A. L. (1999). Men and Women in the Berlin Aging Study. In P. B. Baltes & K. U. Mayer (Eds.), *The Berlin Aging Study,* (pp. 259-281). Cambridge: Cambridge University Press.

Baltes, P. B. (1993). The aging mind: Potential and limits. *The Gerontologist,* 33, 580-594.

Brandtstädter, J., & Renner, G. (1990). Tenacious Goal Pursuit and Flexible Goal Adjustment: Explication and age-related analysis of assimilative and accommodative strategies of coping. *Psychology and Aging*, 5, 58-67.

Clark-Plaskie, M., & Lachman, M. E. (1999). The sense of control in midlife. In S. L. Willis, & J. D. Reid (Eds.), *Life in the middle: Psychological and social development in middle age* (pp. 181-208). San Diego, CA: Academic Press.

Cohen, J. (1988). Statistical power analysis for the behavioral sciences. Hillsdale, New Jersey: Erlbaum.

Heckhausen, J., & Schulz, R. (1995). A theory of control and its implication for the life-span. *Psychological Review*, 102, 284-304.

Kercher, K. (1992). Assessing Subjective Well-Being in the Old-Old. *Research on Aging*, 14 (2), 131-168.

Kunzmann, U., Little, T., & Smith, J. (2002). Perceiving control: a double edged sword in old age, *Journal of Gerontology*, 57B, 484-491.

Lachman, M. E. (1991). Perceived control over memory aging: developmental and intervention perspectives. *Journal of Social Issues*, 47, 159-175.

Lawton, M. P. (1989). Environmental proactivity in older people. In V. L. Bengtson, & K. W. Schaie (Eds.), *The Course of Later Life* (pp. 15-23). New York: Springer.

Lawton, M. P. (1990). Residential Environment and Self-Directedness Among Older People. *American Psychologist*, 45 (5), 638-640.

Lawton, M. P. (1998). Environment and aging: Theory revisited. In R. J. Scheidt, & P. G. Windley (Eds.), *Environment and Aging Theory. A Focus on Housing*, (pp. 1-31). Westport (CT): Greenwood Press.

Levenson, H. (1973). Multidimensional locus of control in psychiatric patients. *Journal of Consulting and Clinical Psychology*, 41, 397-404.

Lindenberger, U., & Reichies, F. M. (1999). Limits and potentials of intellectual functioning in old age. In P. B. Baltes, & K. U. Mayer (Eds.), *The Berlin Aging Study. Aging from 70 to 100* (pp. 329-359). Cambridge, U.K.: Cambridge University Press.

Madden, D. J. (2001). Speed and timing of behavioural processes. In J. E. Birren, & K. W. Schaie (Eds.), *Handbook of the psychology of aging* (5 ed., pp. 28-312). San Diego: Academic Press.

Mollenkopf, H., Oswald, F., & Wahl, H.-W. (1999). *Outdoor mobility in old age in two rural regions in Germany*. Unpublished Datareport.

Oswald, F., Hieber, A., Wahl, H.-W., & Mollenkopf, H. (2005). Ageing and person-environment fit in different urban neighbourhoods. *European Journal of Ageing*, 2(2), DOI: 10.1007.s10433-005-0026-5

Oswald, F., & Wahl, H.-W. (2005). Dimensions of the meaning of home. In G. D. Rowles & H. Chaudhury (Eds.), *Coming home: International perspectives on place, time and identity in old age* (pp. 21-46). New York: Springer.

Oswald, F., Wahl, H.-W., Mollenkopf, H., & Schilling, O. (2003). Housing and life-satisfaction of older adults in two rural regions in Germany. *Research on Aging*, 25 (2), 122-143.

Oswald, W. D., & Fleischmann, U. M. (1995). *Nürnberger-Alters-Inventar (NAI).* [The Nuremberg Age Inventory, NAI]. Göttingen: Hogrefe.

Rowles, G. D., Oswald, F. & Hunter, E. G. (2004). Interior living environments in old age. In H.-W. Wahl, R. Scheidt & P. G. Windley (Eds.), *Aging in context: Socio-physical environments (Annual Review of Gerontology and Geriatrics, 2003)* (pp. 167-193). New York: Springer.

Rubinstein, R. L., & Parmelee, P. A. (1992). Attachment to place and the representation of life course by the elderly. In I. Altman, & S. M. Low (Eds.), *Human behavior and environment: Vol. 12. Place Attachment* (pp. 139-163). New York: Plenum Press.

Salthouse, T. A. (1985). Speed of behavior and its implications for cognition. In J. Birren, & K. W. Schaie (Eds.), *Handbook of the psychology of aging* (2 ed., pp. 400-426). New York: van Nostrand.

Schaie, K. W. (1996). Intellectual development in adulthood. In J. E. Birren, & K. W. Schaie (Eds.), *Handbook of the psychology of aging* (4 ed., pp. 266-286). San Diego, CA: Academic Press.

Slangen-De Kort, Y. A. W. (1999). *A Tale of two adaptations.* Eindhoven University of Technology: University Press.

Smith, J., Marsiske, M., & Maier, H. (1996). *Differences in control beliefs from age 70 to 105.* Unpublished manuscript; Max Planck Institute for Human Development, Berlin.

Staudinger, U. M., Freund, A. M., Linden, M., & Maas, I. (1999). Self, personality, and life management: Psychological resilience and vulnerability. In P. B. Baltes & K. U. Mayer (Eds.), *The Berlin aging study: Aging from 70 to 100* (pp. 302-328). New York: Cambridge University Press.

Wahl, H.-W., Heyl, V., & Schilling, O. (2002). The role of vision impairment for the outdoor activity and life satisfaction of older adults: A multi-faceted view. *Visual Impairment Research, 4,* 143-160.

Watson, D., Clark, L. A., & Tellegen, A. (1988). Development and Validation of Brief Measures of Positive and Negative Affect: The PANAS Scales. *Journal of Personality and Social Psychology, 54* (6), 1063 - 1070.

Wechsler, D. (1958). *The measurement and appraisal of adult intelligence.* Baltimore: Williams & Wilkins.

Chapter 8
Social Relations and Mobility

Stephan Baas, Csaba Kucsera, Heidrun Mollenkopf and Zsuzsa Széman

8.1   Introduction

Social relationships are important elements not only for the quality of life of older adults, but also for their outdoor mobility. Social relationships can either support mobility or be a motive for mobility; wanting to visit one's friends or children is one such motivation. Although social relationships in older age are complex (Wagner, Schütze, & Lang, 1999), they are not the main focus in today's research on social relationships, which tends to concentrate on the exchange of material and nonmaterial goods between the different generations (Attias-Donfut, 1995; Bengtson, Schaie & Burton, 1995; Künemund & Rein, 1999).

In the past, the social situation of older persons has been characterised in terms of disengagement (Cumming & Henry, 1961), activity theory (Havighurst, Munnichs, Neugarten & Thomae, 1969; Tartler, 1961), desocialization (König, 1965), and the lack of their roles (Rosow, 1967), as retirement, departure of the children, and later on widowhood, which has been defined by role loss in older age. On the other side, the importance of a social network has been stressed, which not only provides support when help or care is needed (Baltes & Silverberg, 1994), but also has an impact on the everyday mobility of elderly people.

Recent research has not only focused on the loss of roles, but also the changes in social relations (especially family structures) in modern societies due to 'modernisation'. A classic example is retirement: elders retire and are thus excluded from a central sphere of societal life. This loss of the working role is not only connected with a reduction of income, but also with a change in social relationships (Kohli, 1992). Although Rosenmayr (1983) interpreted retirement as a liberation from responsibilities, offering the chance to form new relationships and intensify old ones, building up new relationships after retirement could become very difficult, due to the loss of collegial relationships. For this reason, relations to members of one's own family, such as one's own children, are of special importance. Since Parsons described the structural isolation of the nuclear family, many studies have shown that different generations remain in frequent contact despite living in separate households (Rossi & Rossi, 1990). Moreover, a German study carried out by the German Youth Institute proved that elderly people do not have to travel far to meet their children (Bien & Marbach, 1991; Marbach, Bien, & Bender, 1996): usually different generations like older parents and their middle-aged children live close to one another. In addition, the birth of grandchildren can lead to new relationships and new tasks for grandparents, such as looking after their grandchildren.

As mentioned earlier, family structures might change also, becoming more fragile in modern societies. Due to the decline of birth rates, the later born generations are becoming smaller and smaller, childlessness is on the rise. Therefore, sibling relationships have become very important, especially for single and widowed elderly people in older age (Brubaker, 1990). Despite possible sibling relationships, maintaining social relationships can become more difficult, resulting in loneliness and isolation. In addition, non-familial relationships lose their importance with increasing age (Field & Minkler, 1988; Wagner, Schütze, & Lang, 1999), especially for men. Moreover, while getting older, elderly shift their attention to "significant others", to those persons to whom they feel closest. "Core social network ties (those that involve close friends and family members) remain stable, where more peripheral ties undergo pruning" (Rook, 2000: 177). With widowhood and childlessness comes a greater risk of loneliness and isolation: widowhood might lead to the loss of many roles and therefore to social isolation. However, this was not observed in the Berlin Aging Study: Social networks of widowed persons did differ slightly from those of married persons (Wagner, Schütze, & Lang, 1999). As also shown in a former study widowed persons intensify their contact with relatives and spend more time with friends (Cantor, 1979). The risk of social isolation seems to be higher for childless persons, as they have fewer role relationships in older age when compared to those with children; for instance, the number of personal relationships increases due to the presence of grandchildren (Wagner, Schütze, & Lang, 1999). Childless persons were more isolated than those with children (Ishii-Kuntz & Seccombe, 1989). Moreover they have fewer friends and neighbour contacts (Rempel, 1985).

Up to now, many of the studies focussing on social relationships examined the functions of these relationships, for example in terms of exchange theories. Exchanging instrumental and emotional help (House & Kahn, 1985) are two important processes examined in social research. According to theory, social relationships follow a universal reciprocity norm, assuming that any change of material and nonmaterial goods should be fair and equally advantageous for each interaction partner (Wagner, Schütze, & Lang, 1999), although not every action always requires an immediate reaction. Secondly, socializing is another important function of social relationships. Thirdly, the Berlin Ageing Study pointed out that affection as a dimension of social interaction is often neglected in social relationship research (Wagner, Schütze, & Lang, 1999).

As yet, research has not examined the relation between social networks and the outdoor mobility of elderly people, or, in terms of the theories described above, the function or impacts that social networks might have for outdoor mobility and vice-versa. In the following chapter the relations between older persons and an important part of their social network is investigated, namely the older individual's contact to persons who are important for personal and emotional reasons. Is there any relation between the social situation of elderly people and important mobility patterns, namely visiting and meeting together? The analyses presented in this chapter serve as the basis for further analyses: Are elderly persons more often away from home when they are closely tied into a network of family, friends or other important persons? Thus, it should be possible to investigate possible relations between the quality of the respondents' social network and their everyday mobility.

This chapter is twofold and concentrates on social relations inside and outside the household. In the first part, we provide an overview of the social situation of older people in six European regions (household size, composition of household, number of children), and the overall social relations outside the household. As already known from other studies, the most important reference person is the partner (Diewald, 1993). Therefore, we concentrate on important persons living outside one's household. We asked about various categories of possible confidants (relatives, friends, colleagues, professional helper, etc.), who were not living in the same household with the respondent. In the second part of this chapter, we concentrate on the two most important persons in the social network living outside the respondents' households. Their living distance will be analysed, which can be an important prerequisite for any contact frequency. In the end, difficulties in meeting this part of the older persons' social networks will be analysed.

8.2   Characteristics of the household

8.2.1   Average household size

Examination of the average household size affords an interesting picture: we found the average household size is much larger, by almost one person, in Italy compared to the other countries investigated (see Table 8.1). Analysis of variance (using One-Way ANOVA) showed this difference to be statistically significant when compared to the household size in all other countries.

Table 8.1:   Average size of household (mean)

	Sex		Age		Settlement		Total
	male	Female	<=74	75+	urban	rural	
Finland	2.0	1.6	2.0	1.7	1.7	2.0	1.8
Eastern Germany	2.0	1.8	2.0	1.8	1.7	2.1	1.9
Western Germany	1.9	1.6	2.0	1.5	1.6	1.9	1.8
Hungary	2.1	1.8	2.0	1.9	2.1	1.8	1.9
Italy	2.7	2.6	2.8	2.5	2.5	2.8	2.7
The Netherlands	1.9	1.7	1.9	1.7	1.7	1.9	1.8
Total	2.1	1.8	2.1	1.8	1.9	2.1	2.0

Note. MOBILATE Survey 2000; weighted data, N = 3942

The comparison is even more informative if we include the composition of the household and the number of children. Based on the following considerations, Italy showed especially marked differences, although in many cases Hungary, too, differed substantially from the other countries.

8.2.2   Composition of household

The persons living in the same household with elderly people play a decisive role in their social relations. On the basis of the household members listed in the questionnaire, we classified our interviewees into three groups.

- The first group comprises those who live alone. In their case, staying in a household on their own can be most difficult, both physically and financially (Széman, 1996; Széman & Utasi, 1996) Moreover, a possible isolation of the elderly can cause psychological problems.
- The second group consists of those who live together with person(s) of the same age or older. We placed persons having at least one other person living in their household in this group, whether the spouse or partner of the interviewee, father,

mother, sibling, mother-in-law and/or father-in-law. Although these households have only elderly members, the tasks can be shared to a significant extent.

- The third group comprises those with at least one person in their household who is at least one generation younger than the interviewee (such as a daughter, son, daughter-in-law, son-in-law, and/or grandchild). In this living arrangement, the tasks are also spread between cohabitants; however, the elderly person may have a significantly better quality of life since he or she probably does not have to do the heavier work. Moreover, the younger members of the household are probably also able to provide mobility, care and nursing.

- We did not include in this analysis those interviewees who said that they lived together with persons belonging in the 'other' category where it is impossible to estimate the age (a total of 52 cases).

Table 8.2:   Composition of household by countries (%)

	Finland		Eastern Germany		Western Germany		Hungary		Italy		The Netherlands		Total	
	Urban	Rural	Urban	Rural	Urban	Rural	Urban	Rural	Urban	Rural	Urban	Rural	Urban	Rural
Living alone	40	23	30	22	38	31	28	36	18	15	40	27	32	26
Only elderly persons	51	60	67	59	52	51	48	46	41	34	56	62	53	52
Also younger persons	8	18	4	19	10	18	24	18	41	51	4	11	14	22
Total Column %	100	100	100	100	100	100	100	100	100	100	100	100	100	100

Note. MOBILATE Survey 2000; weighted data, N = 3900

There were sizeable differences in the composition of the households in the different countries. Examining the breakdown by country, we find that the proportion of elderly persons living alone was the lowest in Italy (16%), which is a particularly substantial difference, considering that this rate exceeded 30% in four countries (western and eastern Germany, the Netherlands, Finland, and Hungary) (Table 8.2).[1]

The proportion of households consisting only of elderly persons was the highest in the eastern German city where more than two thirds of the elderly lived in such households. This type of household composition was least characteristic of the Italian regions studied. In fact Italy is the only country in the sample where this was not the dominant type of living arrangement. Consequently, the ratio of the third type of arrangement, elderly persons living in multi-generation households, was the most widespread here (46%). In Hungary this type of arrangement represents over one fifth (21%) of the households assessed, but even this is less than half the Italian level. This proportion was the lowest in the Netherlands (7%), while in the two parts of Germany and Finland it was between 11 and 14%.

Examining the distribution of the three household types by country, the most balanced structure (with the least variation) was found in Hungary and Italy, while the greatest extremes were found in the Dutch and even more in the eastern German household structures.

---

[1] Few elderly persons lived alone in Italy, and many said they do not need outside help from the various social service systems (home help, district nurse, meals). Obviously, the family members bear the main burden of caring for the elderly. See also the part on family relationships in Italy in Chapter 2.

It was characteristic of all countries that a higher percentage of older women than men lived alone. This can be attributed to a number of factors. In all the developed countries, women live somewhat longer than men; in the age group examined marriage customs dictated that men generally married women a few years younger than themselves and in some cases even married much younger women, increasing the chance that the women would become widows. The most disproportionate ratio of independent households by gender was found in the Netherlands and western Germany.

In comparisons of rural vs. urban areas, it is only in Hungary that the proportion of elderly persons living alone was higher in the rural area; in all other countries this proportion was lower in rural areas when compared to the urban areas. The type of settlement (rural vs. urban) is a real dividing line between persons who live together with younger household members and those who do not. In the eastern part of Germany, for example, the rate is 4.9 times higher for those in rural areas (19% vs. 4%). This ratio is 3.4 in the Dutch regions, and in western Germany and Finland too, more than twice as many elderly persons in the rural areas live together with younger household members compared to those in urban areas.

The age of 75 years represents a marked dividing line separating those who lived alone from those who lived with others. This was clearly evident among western Germans and the Italians. In the western German regions, the proportion of those living alone among the 75-years-and-over group was 2.4 times higher than in the below-75-years group (60% vs. 25%). This ratio was similarly high in Italy (2.3). In Hungary it was only 1.3 (36% vs. 27%), and in the Netherlands 1.7.

The highest proportion of persons over 75 living together with persons of a younger generation was found in Italy (38%), and these family relations are very important because they can strongly influence the social care network and the mobility of older persons both inside and outdoors (e.g., there is someone to take them out). The Hungarians ranked second in this respect (23%), lagging far behind the Italians. The proportion of persons over 75 years living together with younger household members (compared to those under 75 years of age living with younger household members) was higher in eastern Germany and Hungary (1.2-fold), while in the other countries it was lower.

Comparing household composition and marital status, we find that three-quarters to four-fifths of the widowed and divorced live alone (Table 8.3). Not surprisingly, a large proportion of persons who were never married live alone. However, 23% of the widowed live together with a younger household member, while this is the case for fewer than 10% of the divorced persons. This is perhaps related to the fact that the divorced are probably younger than the widowed (over the course of the 20th century, it became progressively easier in both the legal and moral senses to obtain a divorce), and it is principally the elderly who move back to live with family members when this becomes necessary to ensure their care. Four times more divorced women than men live with a younger household member (12% vs. 3%). This is a general phenomenon: since the child usually stays with the mother after a divorce, they probably have better relations.

The largest group in our sample, comprising half the full sample (50%), were married elderly persons who live together with their spouse or parents, but without relatives in the younger generation. Elderly persons living in a multi-generation household and with their spouse make up one tenth of the full sample (11%). One fifth of the sample (20%) are widows living alone, and women make up the great majority (83%) of this latter group.

Table 8.3:   Marital status and household composition (%)

	Lives alone	Only elderly HH members	With younger HH members	Total
Married, living with partner	0	82	18	100
Married, permanently separated	45	35	20	100
Widowed	75	3	23	100
Divorced	79	12	9	100
Never married	82	13	5	100
Total	29	53	18	100

Note. MOBILATE Survey 2000; weighted data, N = 3895

8.3   Number of children

A comparison of the different countries shows that the Dutch and Finnish interviewees had the most children, an average of 2.4(Table 8.4). Statistical examination (One-Way ANOVA) also confirms this result; the difference was significant. The Italians had an average of 2.0 children compared to 1.8 in eastern and 1.7 in western Germany. The Italian figure did not differ significantly from the average number of children among Hungarians.

Table 8.4:   Average number of children (mean)

	Sex		Age		Settlement		Total
	male	female	<=74	75+	Urban	rural	
Finland	2.3	2.4	2.3	2.8	2.0	2.8	2.4
Eastern Germany	1.8	1.8	1.9	1.6	1.7	2.0	1.8
Western Germany	1.7	1.7	1.8	1.6	1.6	1.9	1.7
Hungary	1.8	1.8	1.8	1.8	1.6	2.0	1.8
Italy	1.9	2.1	1.9	2.2	1.9	2.2	2.0
The Netherlands	2.3	2.4	2.3	2.7	2.4	2.4	2.4
Total	2.0	2.0	2.0	2.1	1.8	2.2	2.0

Note. MOBILATE Survey 2000; N = 3935

Those living in rural areas had more children except for the Netherlands. However, they may not necessarily live in the same settlement given the general trend of migration from rural to urban areas in the younger age groups. Living in the same locality, of course, increases the chances of meeting often and providing mutual help.

The proportion of those with children was the highest in Hungary and Italy and the lowest in the Netherlands, where roughly one elderly person out of five had no children (Table 8.5). It is worth noting that the average number of children was the highest in the Netherlands despite the fact that this country had the lowest proportion of those having parent status (in calculating the number of children the figure '0' indicated no children).

Table 8.5:   Respondents with children (%)

	Sex		Age		Settlement		Total
	male	female	<=74	75+	urban	rural	
Finland	87	88	87	87	86	89	87
Eastern Germany	88	87	87	89	87	87	87
Western Germany	87	81	85	82	80	88	84
Hungary	92	91	93	86	91	92	91
Italy	87	91	89	90	90	89	89
The Netherlands	81	83	82	83	83	81	82
Total	87	87	87	86	86	87	87

Note. MOBILATE Survey 2000; N = 3935

8.4   Social relations outside the household

The composition of households as theoretically described above and the size of the social networks outside one's household are largely unrelated, as can be seen from Figure 8.1. In other words, who the elderly person lives with has little influence on how many important persons are available outside the household. Obviously, those who live together with children or grandchildren (third column) mentioned the fewest persons regarded as 'important' for emotional and personal reasons outside the household because those closest to them live within the household. Instead, the size of the social network appeared to vary considerably between different countries. Because of the subcategories used (counted from a list of possible categories) the results show the variety of the contacts, but not the number of contacts or important persons. The figures are an underestimation because they were obtained by adding up the 'important person' subcategories mentioned (daughter, friend, neighbour, etc.) and do not represent the absolute number of persons in the individual categories. Nevertheless, 'variety' of important persons and 'number' of important persons will be used synonymously in the following.

A comparison by country shows that the Hungarians reported the biggest variety of important persons. The second greatest variety of important confidants outside the respondents' households was mentioned in Finland: around six persons, which is more than one fewer than the Hungarian figure. The Italians and the Dutch named roughly the same size of their social network. The social contacts of the Italian elders were strongly underestimated because the household size was by far the highest here. The network of social contacts was the same size in the two parts of Germany and the lowest among all the countries examined (less than half the size for Hungary).

Figure 8.1:   Average number of important persons outside the household by composition of
              households

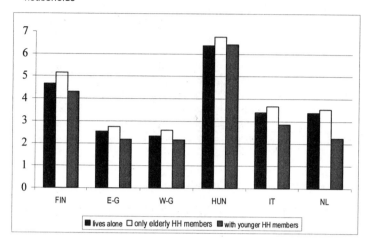

Note. MOBILATE Survey 2000; weighted data, N = 3900

8.4.1   Overview about the important persons outside the household

In a crosstabulation, we summed up the important persons outside the household. As we have
already noted, it would be more precise to describe the table as summing up the heterogeneity
of social contacts because we do not know how many people there are in the different
categories (e.g., how many neighbours or co-workers). The table contains all categories
named by the interviewee (see Table 8.6). In the case of Finland, the data was overestimated
due to problems associated with missing data and inconsistent data collection at that site.

As already presented, the Hungarians reported the greatest number of important
persons. The Hungarian result stands out particularly in the case of the importance of
grandchildren, daughters-in-law and sons-in-law; these persons were mentioned an average of
two to two and a half times more often than in the other countries. The difference is even
more striking for godchildren, clearly pointing to the significance of cultural, traditional - not
religious-based - differences, because in the case of Italy, also a Catholic country, only 1% of
the respondents named a godchild as an important person. German respondents did not
evaluate relatives as being important compared to the elders of the other countries.
Neighbours were mentioned by every second older Hungarian respondent, whereas 30% of
the Finns did so. This is important because the neighbours can indirectly or directly influence
the outdoor mobility of older people (e.g., take them out, shop for them if necessary, handle
official matters for them, etc.) and good relations with the neighbours can help to prevent
isolation. The proportion of co-workers was also relatively high among the Finns and the
Hungarians. In both German samples, more than one tenth of the interviewees did not
mention an important person outside the members of the household.

Table 8.6:   Persons considered as important, by country, multiple responses, urban areas

	Finland		Eastern Germany		Western Germany		Hungary		Italy		The Netherlands	
	% of responses	% of cases	% of responses	% of cases	% of responses	% of cases	% of responses	% of cases	% of responses	% of cases	% of responses	% of cases
partner who doesn't live in the same household	2	6	0	0	1	3	1	3	0	1	1	2
daughter	12	51	20	49	20	43	12	56	13	48	16	51
son	13	53	23	57	21	46	11	52	14	52	14	43
daughter-in-law	4	16	7	18	4	8	7	32	5	20	6	19
son-in-law	4	15	5	12	3	7	7	33	4	15	7	20
grandchild	9	37	12	30	8	18	15	71	15	57	9	29
godchild	3	12	0	0	1	2	4	18	0	1	1	5
brother	7	29	4	10	3	6	5	24	9	33	6	20
sister	8	34	5	11	5	11	7	32	10	40	8	26
mother	3	12	2	5	1	2	1	6	3	12	0	1
father	1	4	0	0	0	1	0	1	1	3	0	1
other relatives	8	33	6	15	6	13	8	39	9	33	5	16
good friend	13	56	5	11	11	23	8	38	9	36	10	32
neighbour	6	25	3	6	4	10	9	45	5	18	5	15
co-worker	5	20	1	4	2	5	2	11	2	8	1	4
household helper	1	2	0	0	1	1	0	1	0	0	2	5
District nurse	1	3	0	0	0	0	1	2	0	0	0	0
Church/preacher/priest	1	3	1	1	1	1	1	6	3	3	2	5
paid helper	0	2	0	0	0	0	0	1	0	0	1	1
other person	1	6	0	1	2	4	0	1	1	3	2	6
only people living in household are important	1	3	5	12	4	9	1	2	0	2	1	4
there is no important person	0	2	2	5	3	7	1	4	0	1	2	7
Total	100		100		100		100		100		100	
N	308	420	389	247	368	217	304	479	298	384	285	312

Note. MOBILATE Survey 2000; weighted data, N = 1952

Table 8.7: Persons considered as important, by country, multiple responses, rural areas

	Finland		Eastern Germany		Western Germany		Hungary		Italy		The Netherlands	
	% of responses	% of cases	% of responses	% of cases	% of responses	% of cases	% of responses	% of cases	% of responses	% of cases	% of responses	% of cases
partner who doesn't live in the same household	0	1	0	1	0	0	1	3	1	1	2	8
daughter	13	58	19	45	19	47	12	59	28	51	12	43
son	13	58	23	55	19	48	12	60	23	43	12	46
daughter-in-law	6	25	5	11	7	17	8	40	2	4	7	25
son-in-law	4	20	5	11	6	14	8	39	2	3	6	21
grandchild	11	48	8	20	11	28	13	68	7	12	9	35
godchild	2	10	0	1	1	2	6	30	0	0	2	7
brother	6	29	3	8	3	9	5	25	5	10	6	23
sister	9	42	3	8	4	11	6	32	8	14	9	33
mother	1	5	1	2	1	3	0	2	3	5	1	4
father	0	1	0	0	1	2	0	1	1	1	0	0
other relatives	8	34	7	16	8	20	7	35	5	9	5	20
good friend	11	49	5	13	4	11	5	25	7	14	11	41
neighbour	8	35	11	26	5	13	11	54	4	8	7	25
co-worker	2	10	3	7	1	2	3	13	0	0	1	4
household helper	1	4	0	0	1	1	1	4	0	0	2	7
District nurse	1	5	1	2	0	1	1	3	0	0	0	1
Church/preacher/priest	2	9	2	4	1	2	2	10	0	0	3	10
paid helper	0	1	0	0	0	0	0	1	0	0	0	1
other person	2	7	0	0	1	1	0	0	1	2	1	4
only people living in household are important	1	4	5	11	5	13	1	3	3	6	3	11
there is no important person	0	1	1	3	3	7	1	6	2	4	2	6
Total	100	455	100	243	100	254	100	512	100	186	100	372
N	301		379		382		300		300		281	

Note. MOBILATE Survey 2000; weighted data, N = 1943

8.5 Further aspects about older persons' social networks outside the household

The respondents were asked questions regarding persons living outside the household who were particularly important for emotional and personal reasons. We first asked for the person being most important to the respondent, afterwards for another important person, and at least for further important persons from a list of possible categories. An overview of the size and composition of this part of the respondent's social network has already been presented above. We assume the sequence in which such persons were named reveals the importance and meaning of these persons. The first two persons regarded as being most important for personal and emotional reasons will be defined as the first and second important person in the following. For them we gathered further information, such as how far away they lived, how frequently the respondent came into contact with them, and how difficult it is to meet these persons. Due to the special attention given to these two confidants outside the household, at first it will be analysed who these persons are, because their living distance and the contact frequency with them can be highly dependent from the question who the first and second important persons is.

Who are the most important persons in the elders' networks outside of their households? One's own children are the most important to those living in the urban areas: In all European cities under investigation, respondents most often mentioned their daughters and sons as being most important to them for personal and emotional reasons; in the urban areas of Finland, western Germany, and the Netherlands, this was followed by a friend. In Italy, a sister and in Hungary, a grandchild were very often reported to be an important person. Contrary to all other urban areas, in the Dutch city, a son was only very important to 15% of the respondents.

On the other side, about 16% to 17% of the older persons in both urban parts of Germany and in the Netherlands reported having no important person at all outside their household. In the other, under a sociological point of view less modernized countries, the percentage of respondents without any important person outside their household varied between 3% and 6%. This pattern differed only slightly when distinguishing between respondents living alone, those living only with elderly household members (e.g., one's partner) and those elders living together with younger household members (e.g., one's children): There were no differences among urban respondents in the structure of these relationships, regardless of whether they lived alone or with others. Moreover, the share of respondents without any important confidant outside their household was not affected by the living situation of the respondents. Only those respondents living together with younger persons differed in their social network: because they most often lived together with their children, these elders named good friends, grandchildren or relatives like a sister as important persons outside the household. In eastern Germany and the Netherlands, more respondents living together with younger persons reported no important person outside their household.

While a daughter was the first important person in all regions under investigation, the distribution of the second important person was different: In most countries, this was a son. In addition, a friend was very often reported as being the second important person. In Italy and Hungary, however, grandchildren, and in eastern Germany, a daughter-in-law were mentioned more often as important than friends. Again, older people living in the urban areas of eastern and western Germany, the Netherlands and Hungary most often reported that there was no further important person outside their households (up to 44%), while in Finland and Italy, the social networks were larger. Similar to the relationships with the first important person, this structure differed only slightly between respondents living alone, those living with elderly household members, and those who live together with younger household members. Those persons who live alone or together with their partners did not have different social networks compared to the other respondents. Those who live together with a younger person again, as a result of living together with their children, mentioned other persons such as a sister or a friend as important.

Rural areas showed a similar structure in the social network outside the older people's households (see Table 8.8): In all rural areas, most respondents reported their children as the first and second most important confidants. Respondents in Finland and Italy also mentioned a friend. In addition, some older persons in the rural areas of both parts of Germany and Hungary regarded a neighbour as the most important person, while for many respondents in Finland and Italy, a good friend was the most important confidant outside the household. As regards the second important person, the pattern was more diversified than in the cities: though a friend was often the second important person in Italy, the Netherlands and Finland, grandchildren, other relatives or daughters-in-law were also frequently mentioned.

Similar to the urban areas, respondents living in the rural areas of both parts of Germany and the Netherlands most often reported having no person outside of their household who was important to them (between 14% and 25%). Between 24% and 44% of the respondents living in the rural areas did not have a second important person, which is a pattern also observed in the urban areas, especially in western Germany and the Netherlands.

Like in the urban areas, this network structure differed only slightly for those living alone or with elderly household members (e.g., their partner) in the rural areas. Again, only those living together with younger persons differed in their social network when compared to all respondents: in addition to their own children these persons mentioned often good friends as well as relatives (e.g., a brother) as being important to them. Moreover, especially in both parts of Germany and the Netherlands, many respondents living together with younger generations did not have important social contacts outside their household.

Summing up the analyses on the two most important persons outside the older people's households, it turned out that children were the most important persons for most of them, regardless of whether they were living in an urban or rural area. Friends and neighbours (especially in rural areas) were also very important persons to our respondents. On the other hand, some elders, especially those living in both parts of Germany and in the Netherlands, often reported not having a social network outside their households or just a very small social network consisting of one important person. The existence of such a limited network was not influenced by the living situation of the respondents: those respondents living alone or together with elderly household members (mainly their partners) did not differ in this respect. The situation was different for persons living together with younger generations, both in the urban and rural areas: because they most often lived together with their own children, besides their own children also other people became important to them. Moreover, a substantial number of respondents living together with younger generations in both parts of Germany and the Netherlands didn't have important persons outside their households.

Table 8.8: Important persons in urban and rural areas (%)

	Finland	%	Eastern Germany	%	Western Germany	%	Hungary	%	Italy	%	The Netherlands	%
Urban areas, first important person												
	Daughter	31	Daughter	37	Daughter	35	Daughter	36	Daughter	38	Daughter	34
	Son	22	Son	35	Son	26	Son	36	Son	33	Son	15
	Friend	16			Friend	6	Grandchild	6	Sister	8	Friend	10
No important person available		3		17		15		6		3		16
Urban areas, second important person												
	Son	19	Son	28	Son	22	Grandchild	21	Son	27	Son	23
	Daughter	18	Daughter	17	Daughter	12	Daughter	20	Daughter	16	Daughter	10
	Friend	14	Daughter in law	7	Friend	6	Son	13	Grandchild	14	Friend	10
No important person available		10		34		44		27		6		31
Rural areas, first important person												
	Son	26	Son	35	Daughter	33	Daughter	38	Daughter	37	Daughter	22
	Daughter	25	Daughter	32	Son	31	Son	35	Son	28	Son	16
	Friend	13	Neighbour	5	Neighbour	4	Friend	5	Friend	7	Sister	11
No important person available		4		14		20		8		10		2510
Rural areas, second important person												
	Son	24	Son	25	Son	21	Daughter	24	Daughter	20	Son	13
	Daughter	21	Daughter	18	Daughter	18	Son	19	Son	19	Daughter	10
	Sister/Friend	12	Other relatives	5	Daughter in law	5	Grandchild	15	Friend	7	Friend	9
No important person available		8		31		36		24		27		44

Note. MOBILATE Survey 2000; Weighted data, N = 3950

8.6   Living distance to the most important persons

The living distance to important persons in the social network is an important premises for personal contact with them. In the following section, we distinguish between important persons living within a range of 15 minutes and those living further away. Living inside a range of 15 minutes means that the important person is living either in the same house as the older person (but not in the same household) or in the same neighbourhood/community and can be reached within 15 minutes. Living further away means that the person is living in the same neighbourhood or community but can be reached between 15 minutes up to 1 hour or that he or she is living further away than 1 hour, independent of the means of transportation used

In the urban areas under investigation, important persons generally lived further away from the respondents than is the case in rural areas (see Table 8.9). Moreover, both in urban and rural areas under investigation, the most important persons generally lived closer to the respondents than the second important persons.

In the *urban areas* of Finland, western Germany and Hungary, only about one third of the respondents had their most important person living within a range of 15 minutes of the their home, but about two third lived further away, while especially in Italy and the Netherlands, the most important persons lived more often in the immediate neighbourhood of the respondents (about 50%) or in the same house. The second important person lived further away than the most important, especially in Finland, western Germany and Hungary, but also in eastern Germany: only between 20% and 30% of these important persons lived within the immediate neighbourhood of the respondent's home. On the other hand, in Italy and the Netherlands, more than 40% of the second important persons lived within a range of 15 minutes from the respondent's home.

Table 8.9:   Living distance of important persons, urban and rural areas (%)

	Urban area				Rural area			
	Person1		Person2		Person1		Person2	
	Up to 15 minutes	More than 15 minutes	Up to 15 minutes	More than 15 minutes	Up to 15 minutes	More than 15 minutes	Up to 15 minutes	More than 15 minutes
Finland	34	66	23	77	39	61	33	67
Eastern Germany	39	61	20	80	59	41	41	59
Western Germany	31	69	22	78	66	34	45	55
Hungary	33	67	29	71	45	55	37	63
Italy	51	49	43	57	63	37	57	43
The Netherlands	52	48	47	53	59	41	43	57

Note. MOBILATE Survey 2000; Weighted data, N (Person1) = 3450, N (Person2) = 2848

In the *rural areas*, the most important persons lived closer to the respondents compared to the urban areas. This was especially true in both parts of Germany and in Italy. Except for Finland and Hungary, up to two-thirds of the respondents reported that their most important confidant lived within their immediate reach. Conversely, in Finland about 61% and in

Hungary about 55% of the most important persons lived further away than 15 minutes. As in the urban areas, the second important person lived further away from the elders' homes than the most important person. However, between 33% (Finland) and 46% (western Germany) of these important persons - and in the Italian rural area 57% - lived within a range of 15 minutes, which is much closer when compared to the urban areas.

Summing up the findings on living distance to the most important persons outside the older persons' households, those living in the *rural areas* lived closer to important persons than those living in the urban areas. In addition, the most important person lived closer to them than the second important person. The distance to a person might therefore influence whether or not he or she is regarded as important. In addition, when distinguishing between those most important persons being family members and those who do not belong to the family, family members lived further away than friends and neighbours.

In the *urban areas*, especially in the Italian city, but also in the Dutch urban area, the most important persons lived very close to the older people, although the social networks differed between Italy and the Netherlands. While in Italy, the most important persons were family members such as children or in some cases a sister, in the Netherlands, friends were mentioned much more often as important persons. Also in the rural area of Italy, the social network was located particularly close to the elders' homes: about 60% of the most important persons lived in the immediate neighbourhood or even in the same house as the respondent. In the Finnish rural areas, the distances were largest.

In both urban and rural regions of the Netherlands, most of the elderly people lived very close to important persons. The differences between urban and rural areas found in the other European regions were not found in the Dutch areas under investigation, which might be due to the suburban character of the Dutch rural area.

The living distance to the most important persons outside the elders' households differed only slightly when distinguishing between persons living alone, those living only with elderly household members and those living together with younger household members. Those who lived alone lived closer to persons who are important to them for personal and emotional reasons, especially in the Italian sample. One possible explanation for this is that those who lived alone (many of whom were widowed) needed more support from their children. Respondents living together with elderly household members such as their partners lived further away from important persons. Possibly, those persons did not require support and could therefore live further away from their children compared to singles. Finally, with regard to elders who lived together with younger household members (e.g., children), the pattern described above was not found: While in the urban areas under investigation, the social network outside the respondents' households lived much further away when compared to all other respondents, those respondents in the rural areas living together with younger generations lived much closer to their social network when compared to the other respondents in the rural area.

8.7   Intensity of contact and used means of transportation

The intensity of personal contact (i.e., meeting one's children or friends) seems to be dependent upon the living distance between the respondent and important persons, at least in the urban areas under investigation.

In the Finnish and eastern German *urban areas*, where the most important confidants lived further away from the older persons' homes than 15 minutes, personal contact was less frequent compared to those countries with a closer living distance like for example Italy and the Netherlands. Only 56% of the respondents in Finland or eastern Germany met the person who is most important to them at least weekly, whereas in Italy (83%) and the Netherlands (73%), there was more frequent personal contact).

Given that the second important person in most urban regions under investigation lived even further away, it is unsurprising that personal contact became even less frequent. Between 30% and 40% of the Finnish and eastern German elders met this person at least weekly, whereas in Italy and the Netherlands, more older people had frequent personal contact (about two third of them at least weekly).

The exception to this rule was Hungary: although few older Hungarians lived close to the most important persons in their social network, they met each other relatively often compared to the other countries. A similar situation can be found in western Germany: despite the greater distance between the older people and important persons, personal contact between these persons was high in the urban area of this country.

The relationship between distance and frequency of personal contact was not that strong in the *rural areas* under investigation: except for Finland, where most of the older people reported great distances to important persons combined with low personal contact (at least weekly: 49% with the first important person and 41% for the second important person), there is no clear relation between living distance and personal contact in rural areas. Although rural elders lived closer to this part of their social network compared to their urban contemporaries, the former met their confidants less often. This was true for most of the regions under investigation, except for Hungary and western Germany.

When distinguishing between persons living alone, those living together with their partner and those living with members of younger generations, it turned out that those living alone met this part of their social network more often when compared with other people (especially in the rural areas), while those elders living together with members of the younger generations (i.e., in most cases their own children) met important persons less often (especially in the urban areas) than for example those living together with their partners. Those living together with younger persons in rural areas reported no differences in the frequency of meeting important persons.

Table 8.10: Means of transportation for reaching first important person by their living distance, urban and rural areas (%)

	Finland		Eastern Germany		Western Germany		Hungary		Italy		The Netherlands	
	< 15 min	15+ min	< 15 min	15+ min	< 15 min	15+ min	< 15 min	15+ min	< 15 min	15+ min	< 15 min	15+ min
Person 1 – urban areas												
By foot	51	9	85	16	62	10	81	8	54	2	44	9
By bike	9	6	1	0	4	6	2	0	0	0	13	6
By car/driver	23	35	5	39	21	47	6	18	27	49	19	26
By car/passenger	9	15	5	24	4	14	6	13	14	26	17	25
Other	1	3	0	0	4	0	0	3	0	2	1	9
Public transport	0	22	1	18	0	15	4	55	2	17	5	19
Get picked up	7	9	4	4	4	9	0	3	4	5	2	8
Person 1 – rural areas												
By foot	39	0	73	6	93	15	55	1	53	2	47	3
By bike	18	4	16	6	3	1	39	23	0	0	12	1
By car/driver	21	42	5	50	2	56	2	15	25	56	23	55
By car/passenger	14	26	4	19	1	21	2	10	17	35	13	13
Other	0	10	1	0	0	0	0	0	2	0	2	2
Public transport	0	13	0	9	1	3	0	43	0	5	2	14
Get picked up	9	6	1	9	1	4	1	9	2	2	2	12

Note. MOBILATE Survey 2000; Weighted data, N = 3950, living distance: important person is either living within a range of 15 minutes or living further away from the respondents' households than 15 minutes, independent from the used means of transportation

8.7.1   Used means of transportation

The distance between older people and important persons not only determines contact frequency, but also the means used to bridge such distances (see Table 8.10). No differences were found between the regions regarding how elders reach important persons living nearby: important persons living in the immediate vicinity of their homes (i.e., within 15 minutes reach) were mainly reached by foot, irrespective of the country or region they lived in. This is especially true for both parts of Germany and Hungary; in the rural areas, however, sometimes a bicycle was used to meet the most important persons. Older Finnish, Italian and Dutch persons more often drove a car to meet their confidants.

Due to the longer distance to those important persons living further away than 15 minutes, different means of transportation had to be used. Except for Hungarian elders, driving one's own car was the transport mode most often used to meet important persons living further away in all countries, and in both urban and rural areas. The second most frequent mode of transportation used for this purpose was riding in a car as a passenger. Because few Hungarian respondents had a car available, in the urban region public transportation was the transport mode of choice. In the Hungarian rural area, public transportation as well as a bicycle were very often used for that purpose.

8.7.2   What does the frequency of personal contact depend on?

Up to now, we have suggested that contact with important persons, especially in the urban areas, is related to the distance between the older people and the other persons outside the household, which is a somehow expected result. What other factors does personal contact depend on? We used a logistic regression model to explain whether the elders meet persons which are important for emotional and personal reasons at least once a week or less often.[2]

Besides the plausible relation between distance and contact frequency, a number of other variables can influence contact frequency. Health is an important prerequisite; those with better health might have fewer problems or hindrances meeting other people. Moreover, having a car can support social contact in most of the countries under investigation. The living situation might be influential also: we have already reported that persons living alone have more contact, especially when compared to people living together with younger generations. Whether or not the confidant is the older person's daughter or son might also influence contact frequency. Finally, demographic characteristics like age, gender and living region are included in the model in order to analyse the influence of such living circumstances.

Results of the logistic regression model did not confirm all of our hypotheses (see Tables 10.11 and 10.12). In particular, there was no evidence that (self-estimated) health status influenced mobility and by this the ability to meet other persons. Also having a car did not systematically support personal contact: Only Finnish elders with a car met such persons more often, while their western German and Dutch contemporaries without a car reported

---

[2] The dichotomous dependent variable has a value of 1 if the important person was met at least one time a week or more often and the value of 0 if the important person was met less often than that. The explanatory variables in a logistic regression estimate the odds that one meets important persons more frequently. The odds ratios show the average change in the contact frequency for a change of one unit in the value of the explanatory variable, while values of other independent variables remain unchanged.

more frequent contact with important persons outside their household (all results not significant). The living situation was not linked with contact frequency in most countries under investigation either: only in the Italian sample those not living together with the younger generations met important people more often. If the most important confidant was the older person's daughter or son, personal contact did take place more often. This was true for all countries except for both parts of Germany and the Netherlands. As already seen in the foregoing analyses, in the urban areas, personal contact seemed to take place more often when compared to the rural areas: except for the Finnish and Hungarian regions, this could not be verified by the logistic regression. For eastern German elders living in the rural area, the probability of meeting important persons was higher when compared with those living in the East German city under investigation.

Table 8.11: Logistic model for contact frequency (first important person)

	Finland	Eastern Germany	Western Germany	Hungary	Italy	The Netherlands
	Odds ratios	Odds ratios	Odds ratios	Odds ratios	Odds ratios	Odds ratios
Gender (1=male, 2=female)	0.96	1.00	1.76	1.15	1.20	1.33
Age	1.01	1.00	0.98	0.99	0.97	1.01
Region (1=urban, 2=rural)	0.52**	1.55	1.23	0.48**	0.69	1.04
Satisfaction with health (0=unsatisfied, 10=satisfied	1.10	1.04	0.99	0.98	0.96	1.10
Living distance (0<15 min, 1= 15+min.)	0.07***	0.04***	0.03***	0.09***	0.08***	0.13***
Car available (0=no, 1=yes)	1.26	0.80	0.58	0.68	1.56	0.49
Living alone (0=no, 1=yes)	1.55	1.40	0.89	1.26	1.32	0.74
Living with younger generation (0=no, 1=yes)	0.73	0.86	0.80	1.14	0.22***	1.15
Important person=child (0=no, 1=yes)	1.96**	1.19	0.93	2.71***	2.87***	1.69
Pseudo R^2 (R_L^2 = G_M/D_0)	0.26	0.44	0.39	0,20	0.34	0.16
N	570	637	608	545	556	456

Note. MOBILATE Survey 2000
**=p<0.01, ***=p<0.001
Dependent variable: 1 = important person is met at least once a week or more often /
0 = important person is met less often than at least one time a week.

Table 8.12: Logistic model for contact frequency (second important person)

	Finland	Eastern Germany	Western Germany	Hungary	Italy	The Nether-lands
	Odds ratios	Odds ratios	Odds ratios	Odds ratios	Odds ratios	Odds ratios
Gender (1=male, 2=female)	1.05	0.67	1.51	1.41	0.65	0.85
Age	1.01	0.98	0.98	0.99	0.97	1.00
Region (1=urban, 2=rural)	0.94	2.51***	1.08	0.52**	0.90	0.91
Satisfaction with health (0=unsatisfied, 10=satisfied)	1.03	1.02	0.98	0.99	0.99	0.92
Car available (0=no, 1=yes)	2.08	0.69	0.57	0.60	0.93	0.56
Living alone (0=no, 1=yes)	1.82	1.31	0.64	1.07	2.05	0.86
Living with younger generation (0=no, 1=yes)	1.02	0.65	0.51	0.75	0.89	1.92
Living distance (0<15 min, 1= 15+min.)	0.11***	0.05***	0.03***	0.06***	0.13***	0.21***
Important person=child (0=no, 1=yes)	0.75	0.70	0.89	1.11	1.62*	1.07
Pseudo R² (R_L² = G_M/D_O)	0.18	0.39	0.34	0.21	0.17	0.07
N	530	508	443	426	496	354

Note. MOBILATE Survey 2000
**=$p<0.01$, ***=$p<0.001$
Dependent variable: 1 = important person is met at least once a week or more often / 0 = important person is met less often than at least one time a week.

Regression analyses confirmed that the distance between the respondents and important persons had the strongest impact on contact frequency: the closer the social network, the more often the elderly persons had contact with persons who are important to them.

8.8   Difficulties in meeting important persons

As already shown, contact frequency between older people and the two most important persons outside their households mainly depended on the distance between their homes. Nonetheless, some people were not able to leave their house or apartment for various reasons or reported difficulties in leaving their surroundings. What are the reasons for difficulties or the inability to leave one's own house or apartment to meet important confidants?

Table 8.13: Difficulties in reaching important persons outside the household (%)

	Finland		Eastern Germany		Western Germany		Hungary		Italy		The Netherlands	
	Urban	Rural	Urban	Rural	Urban	Rural	Urban	Rural	Urban	Rural	Urban	Rural
No difficulties at all	89	75	79	85	81	90	77	70	70	71	91	92
Difficulties to meet important persons	10	22	17	12	15	6	16	24	30	29	8	7
Important persons (at least one) cannot be met	1	3	4	3	4	4	7	6	0	0	1	1

Note. MOBILATE Survey 2000; weighted data; N = 3357

The most difficulties in meeting important persons outside one's own home were reported by Italian elders, the least difficulties, by the Dutch (Table 8.13). Distinguishing between urban and rural areas, the least difficulties in meeting important persons in urban areas were reported by older people in Finland and the Netherlands (about 10%). In both parts of Germany and in Hungary, between 15% and 17% of the elders reported that they had problems meeting important persons. The most difficulties were reported by Italian respondents: about 30% had problems in meeting the most important persons, although in the urban area they had the highest contact frequency to their social network. In the rural areas under investigation, the pattern of international differences changes. The least difficulties were reported by older people in western Germany and the Netherlands, the most difficulties by those living in Finland, Hungary and again, Italy.

Some older persons were not even able to leave their house or apartment in order to maintain social contact: up to 7% were not able to meet important persons outside their own home. The highest rates of such immobility were reported by older Hungarians, the lowest by older persons living in Italy and the Netherlands.

Reasons for difficulties or being unable to maintain social contacts outside the own home among elders in the urban areas in Finland, Hungary and Italy included:

- the important persons lived too far away,
- the respondent had general health problems, or
- the trip was too expensive.

In addition, general health problems were the reasons given most often for difficulties in meeting other people in the eastern and western German cities.

Older people living in the rural areas reported slightly different reasons for difficulties in outdoor mobility. Again, the reasons for difficulties given most often, were:

- the important persons lived too far away, and
- the older person had general health problems (especially in Hungary and Italy).

But in addition to the urban areas, many older people in the countryside reported difficulties meeting persons in their social network because of

- bad connections, no available public transportation, or
- having no car (especially in eastern Germany).

Again, we used logistic regression analysis to uncover what factors predict difficulties in meeting important persons.[3] In addition to the considerations above, we expected problems with mobility to correlate with the financial situation of the respondents and the availability and quality of public transport. For these reasons, satisfaction with income and with public transportation were added to the regression analysis as potential predictors.

Results of logistic regression confirmed that impairments in health or even a bad health condition may create problems in maintaining social contacts (Table 8.14). Moreover, having no car did have a large impact on meeting important persons outside one's own household. This was true for all countries under investigation except for Hungary, where only a minority of older people have a car available. As expected, the distance between the elders and this part of their social network might cause problems in meeting such important persons, especially in Finland where distances are greater, in particular in the Finnish countryside (not significant). The model also explained most of the difficulties or the inability to get in contact with

---

[3] The dichotomous dependent variable has a value of 1 if the respondent had difficulties in meeting at least one important person or if the respondent was unable to meet at least one important person outside his or her household. The dichotomous variable has a value of 0 if the respondent reported no such problems.

important persons in the Italian sample: Italian elders reporting problems in meeting their social network were mostly older and in poor health, and had no car available.

Table 8.14: Logistic model for difficulties or inability in meeting important persons outside one's home

	FIN	GER (E)	GER (W)	HUN	IT	NL
	Odds ratios	*Odds ratios*	*Odds ratios*	*Odds ratios*	*Odds ratios*	*Odds ratios*
Gender (1=male, 2=female)	1.17	1.44	1.54	1.60	2.33**	1.26
Age	1.00	1.04	1.04	1.05	1.11***	0.99
Region (1=urban, 2=rural)	2.98***	0.63	0.38	0.75	0.95	3.69
Living distance 1st important person (0<15 min, 1=15+min.)	2.69**	2.03	1.68	0.79	1.39	3.53
Living distance 2nd important person (0<15 min, 1=15+min.)	2.31	1.12	2.03	6.61***	2.85***	0.33
Car available (0=no, 1=yes)	0.30***	0.41**	0.19***	0.67	0.23***	0.12**
Living alone (0=no, 1=yes)	1.24	1.23	1.58	0.75	0.83	2.04
Living with younger generation (0=no, 1=yes)	1.31	1.78	0.81	0.57	1.83	3.00
Important 1st person=child (0=no, 1=yes)	1.36	1.21	0.72	0.83	0.88	1.79
Important 2nd person=child (0=no, 1=yes)	0.84	0.64	1.28	0.83	1.56	1.95
Satisfaction with health (0=unsatisfied, 10=satisfied)	0.77***	0.82**	0.65***	0.78***	0.77***	0.57***
Satisfaction with public transport (0=unsatisfied, 10=satisfied)	0.94	0.93	0.86	0.93	0.94	1.03
Satisfaction with financial situation (0=unsatisfied, 10=satisfied)	0.90	1.01	0.86	0.92	1.00	1.12
Pseudo R^2 ($R_L{}^2 = G_M/D_0$)	0.14	0.13	0.58	0.19	0.36	0.24
N	500	473	437	332	497	301

Note. MOBILATE Survey 2000
**=$p<0.01$, ***=$p<0.001$
Dependent variable: 1 = important persons can only be met with difficulties or cannot be met outside one's home / 0 = important persons can be met without any problem.

8.9   Summary and conclusions

We showed that among the countries participating in the research project, the average size of households was largest in Italy. There was close to one person more in Italian households (2.7 persons) than in the other countries (1.8 - 1.9 persons). Italian elders seem to be the most integrated into their families: the lowest proportion of persons living alone was found here, less than half that of people living alone in the other countries. We drew attention to the practical and emotional advantages of living with one or more other persons, and to the disadvantages of living alone.

The older Italians were most likely to live in multi-generation households, which also has many practical and emotional advantages. For all countries, the proportion of living alone in old age was much higher for older women than for men, due principally to their higher life expectancy. The two age dimensions (below 75 years and over 75 years) represent a marked dividing line mainly in Germany and Italy; a much higher proportion of the older group (2.3 - 2.4 times more) lived alone compared to the younger group. In breakdown by settlement (rural vs. urban areas), only Hungary had a proportion of persons living alone that was higher in the rural environment than in the urban areas; in the other countries, the opposite pattern occurred, although to varying degrees. The rural environment also favoured multi-generation households.

The average number of children was much higher among older persons in the Netherlands and Finland than in the other countries. The Hungarian interviewees reported the highest variety of important relationships outside the household. This statistic was the lowest in the two parts of Germany; the older people in Italy and the Netherlands had an average number of important relationships, and the Finns an above average number.

The elders' social networks outside their households consist mainly of close relatives, namely their children. The two most important persons outside their households were children in all countries under investigation, regardless of whether the older people lived in an urban or a rural area. If they were already living with children, then they reported other persons like friends or neighbours as being important. In rural areas, important persons lived closer to the elders than was the case in urban areas. In addition, the most important person lived closer to them than the second important person. In the Italian regions, the most important persons lived very close to the older people, while in the Finnish, western German and Hungarian regions, the most important persons lived further away. In the Italian countryside, the social network was located very closely to the older people's homes, while the distances were very large in the Finnish and Hungarian rural areas. In both Dutch areas of investigation, most of the elders lived very close to important persons compared to the other European regions. This might be due to the suburban character of the Dutch rural area. Older people living alone lived even closer to important persons in their social network, especially in the Italian sample.

The intensity or frequency of personal contact to important persons was dependent upon the distance between the older people's homes and this part of their networks, especially in the urban areas. Thus, the elders living in the Dutch and Italian cities reported a very high frequency of personal contact with the persons important to them. Surprisingly, in the Hungarian rural area, despite the relatively great distance between older people and their social networks, personal contact was high. In the other rural areas under investigation, the relationship between distance and contact frequency was not that strong: although older people in the rural areas lived closer to their social networks, they met each other less often compared with the urban areas under investigation (again, except for the Hungarian urban area). Those older persons living alone met their confidants outside their homes more often (especially in the rural areas), and those living together with younger generations met important persons less often (especially in the urban areas).

Those important persons who lived within the immediate reach of the older people (less than 15 minutes away), were mainly reached by foot; this finding did not vary with regards to country or region. If the important persons lived further away than 15 minutes, they were mainly reached by car, except for the Hungarian elders: because only few of them had a car available, they mainly used their bicycles or public transportation.

Logistic regression analyses confirmed most of the results presented above: The distance between older people and their social networks had the strongest impact on personal contact frequency: the closer the elders lived to important persons, the more frequently they met each other. Meetings took place more often if the important person was a son or daughter. However, the health status or the availability of a car did not have any influence on the frequency of personal contact. Moreover, regression analyses did not confirm that the probability of personal contact was higher in the urban areas compared to the rural areas under investigation.

With regards to problems meeting important people outside the home, the most difficulties were reported by older Italians, the least difficulties by older persons in the Netherlands. In addition to difficulties reaching important persons outside the home, older people in Hungary, in particular, were not able to meet these persons outside their households, while Italian and Dutch elders did not report being unable to meet important confidants. A low satisfaction with health and lack of a car (except among older Hungarians) were most often responsible for problems in maintaining social contacts. Again, the distance to these important reference persons seemed to cause problems in meeting them, especially in rural Finland where the distances between persons were very great. Italian elders who had problems in maintaining social contacts were predominantly older women in poor health, living together with members of the younger generations without a car.

These results can provide the basis for further analyses: is there any relation between the social network of older people and their outdoor mobility? In further analyses the following hypothesis should be proven: do older people due to the docility-thesis adapt their decreasing competencies to their environment (Lawton & Nahemow, 1973), does one's own home become more important (Saup, 1999) and do older people shift their attention to those persons to whom they feel closest (Carstensen, 1991)? As a consequence, there should be a coincidence between the reduced range of outdoor mobility due to advancing age and a satisfying social network. It is also possible, however, that elderly persons are more often away from home when they are closely tied into a network of family, friends or other important persons, as theories of attachment assume that a satisfying social network encourages older persons to expand their mobility (Bien, 2001) or at least to maintain their outdoor mobility. Our data suggest that this is the case in a cross-sectional observation, but longitudinal studies are necessary to prove whether this holds also in the long term process of ageing.

References

Attias-Donfut, C. (1995). *Les solidarités entre générations: vieillesse, familles, état* [Solidarity between generations: old age, families, state]. Paris, Nathan.

Baltes, M. M., & Silverberg, S. (1994). The dynamic between dependency and autonomy: Illustrations across the life span. In D. L. Featherman, R. M. Lerner, & M. Perlmutter (Eds.), *Life-span development and behavior* Vol. 12 (pp. 41 - 90). Hilldsdale, NJ: Erlbaum.

Bengtson, V. L., Schaie, W. & Burton, L. (1995). *Adult Intergenerational Relations. Effects of Societal Change*. New York: Springer Publishing Company.

Bien, W. (2001). Aktionsraum und soziales Netzwerk: Reichweite und Ressourcen der Lebensführung im Alter [Space of action and social network: Distance and resources of living in old age]. *Zeitschrift für Gerontologische Geriatrie*, 34, 319-326.

Bien, W. & Marbach, J. H. (1991). Haushalt - Verwandtschaft - Beziehungen: Familienleben als Netzwerk [Household - family relations - relations: Family life as social network]. In H. Bertram (Eds.), *Die Familie in Westdeutschland. Stabilität und Wandel familialer Lebensformen [Family in western Germany: stability and change of familiar living arrangement]* (pp. 3-44). Opladen: Leske + Budrich.

Brubaker, T. H. (1990). *Later Life Families*. Newbury Park/London: Sage Publications.

Cantor, M. H. (1979). Neighbors and friends: An overlooked resource in the informal support system. *Resarch on Aging*, 1, 434-463.

Carstensen, L. L. (1991). Socioemotional selectivity theory: Social activity in life-span context. *Annual Review of Gerontology and Geriatrics*, 11, 195-217.

Carstensen, L. L. (1992). Social and Emotional Patterns in Adulthood: Support for Secioemotional Selectivity Theory. *Psychology and Aging, 7*(3), 331-338

Cumming, E., & Henry, W. E. (1961). *Growing old, the process of disengagement*. New York: Basic Book Inc.

Diewald, M. (1993). Netzwerkorientierungen und Exklusivität der Paarbeziehung. Unterschiede zwischen Ehen, nichtehelichen Lebensgemeinschaften und Paarbeziehungen mit getrennten Haushalten [Orientations towards networks and exclusive couple relations]. *Zeitschrift für Soziologie, .22*, 279-297.

Field, D., & Minkler, M. (1988). Continuity and change in social support between young-old and old-old or very-old age. *Journal of Gerontology: Psychological Sciences*, 43, 100-106.

Havighurst, R.J., Munnichs, J.M., Neugarten, B.L. & Thomae, H. (1969). *Adjustment to retirement. A cross-national study*. Oxford: Royal Vangorcum.

House, J. S., & Kahn, R. L. (1985). Measures and concepts of social support. In S. Cohen & S.L. Syme (Eds.), *Social support and health* (pp. 83 - 105). New York: Academic press.

Ishii-Kuntz, M. & Seccombe, K. (1989). The impact of children upon social support networks throughout the life course. *Journal of Marriage and the Family*, 51, 777-90.

König, R. (1965). *Die strukturelle Bedeutung des Alters in den fortgeschrittenen Industriegesellschaften* [The structural meaning of age in industrialised societies]. Köln: Kiepenheuer & Witsch.

Kohli, M. (1992). Altern in soziologischer Perspektive [Ageing in a sociological point of view]. In P. B. Baltes, & J. Mittelstraß (Eds.), *Zukunft des Alterns und gesellschaftliche Entwicklung* [The future of ageing and social development] (pp. 231-259). Berlin: de Gruyter.

Künemund, H., & Rein, M. (1999). There is more to receiving than needing: theoretical arguments and empirical explorations of crowding in and crowding out. *Ageing and Society, 19*, 93-121.

Lawton, M. P., & Nahemow, L. (1973). Ecology and the aging process. In C. Eisdorfer, M. P. Lawton (Eds.), *The psychology of adult development and aging* (pp. 619-674). Washington: APA.

Marbach, J. H., Bien, W., & Bender, D. (1996). Vergleich der Lebensformen in den alten und neuen Bundesländern zwischen 1988 und 1994 [Comparison of living arrangements in eastern and western Germany 1988 - 1994]. In W. Bien (Eds.), *Familie an der Schwelle zum neuen Jahrtausend - Wandel und Entwicklung familialer Lebensformen* [Family at the turn of the millennium - change and development of familiar living arrangements] (pp. 28 - 37). Opladen: Leske + Budrich.

Rempel J. (1985). Childless elderly: Why are they missing? *Journal of Marriage and the Family*, 47, 343-348.

Rook, K. S. (2000). The Evolution of Social Relationships in Late Adulthood. In S. H. Qualls & N. Abeles (Hrsg.), *Psychology and the aging revolution: how we adapt to longer life* (pp. 173-191). Washington, DC: American Psychological Association.

Rosenmayr, L. (1983). *Die späte Freiheit: Das Alter - ein Stück bewusst gelebtes Leben* [Late freedom: Old age - living a life of awareness]. Belin: Severin & Siedler.

Rossi, A. S. & Rossi, P. H. (1990). *Of human bonding: Parent-child relationships across the life course*. Hawthorne, New York: de Gruyter.

Rosow, I. (1967). *Social integration of the aged*. New York: Free Press.

Saup, W. (1999). Alte Menschen in ihrer Wohnung: Sichtweise der ökologischen Psychologie und Gerontologie [Older adults in their home: point of view of environmental psychology and gerontology]. In H.-W. Wahl, H. Mollenkopf, & F. Oswald (Eds.), *Alte Menschen in ihrer Umwelt: Beiträge zur Ökologischen Gerontologie* [Older adults in their environment. Contributions to environmental gerontology] (pp. 43-51). Opladen: Westdeutscher Verlag.

Széman, Z. (1996). The Elderly in a Society of Transition. Report on Hungary. In Z. Széman, & V. Gáthy (Eds.), *Ageing and technology. Exploring European Old Age in East and West* (pp. 33-41). Saarijärvi: Gummerus Kirjapaino Oy.

Széman, Z., & Utasi, Á. (1966). The Role of the Budapest Centre in the Hungarian Maltese Charity Service in the Lives of the Elderly. In Z. Széman, & V. Gáthy (Eds.), *Ageing and Technology. Exploring European Old Age in East and West* (pp. 41-57). Saarijärvi: Gummerus Kirjapaino Oy.

Tartler, R. (1961). *Das Alter in der modernen Gesellschaft* [Old age in modern society]. Stuttgart: Enke.

Wagner, M., Schütze, Y., & Lang, F. R. (1999). Social relationships in old age. In P. B. Baltes, & K. U. Mayer (Eds.), *The Berlin Aging Study. Aging from 70 to 100* (pp. 282-301). Cambridge, U.K.: Cambridge University Press.

Enhancing Mobility in Later Life
H. Mollenkopf et al. (Eds.)
IOS Press, 2005

Chapter 9
Mobility and the Built-Up Environment

Fiorella Marcellini, Heidrun Mollenkopf, Zsuzsa Széman,
Sabina Ciarrocchi, Csaba Kucsera, Andrea Principi, and Liana Spazzafumo

9.1   Introduction

It is not possible to consider mobility without considering also the sourrounding environment. According to the psychologist Kurt Lewin, behaviour is both a personal and environmental function (Lewin, 1951). On this basis M. Powell Lawton developed the ecological model of adaptation and aging and applied it to a variety of different person-environment situations, related to the macro-environment, the micro-environment, the context of populations and the context of the individuals (Lawton, 1986). The less competent an individual is (competence being full possession of certain inherent characteristics regarding health, functional and cognitive ability, and self-esteem), the greater the impact of environmental factors on the individual himself (Lawton, Windley, & Byerts, 1982).

Moreover, even if many elderly are healthy and can perform their activities of daily living without help and can therefore be considered as active citizens and new consumers in the future, it is at the same time important to consider the needs of the increasing oldest population, especially the impaired ones (Marcellini et al., 2000). Health is closely linked to elderly mobility, so for better ageing it is necessary to encourage and facilitate mobility in the elderly population by intervening on the relationship between environment and ageing (Lawton et al., 1982; Cvitkovich & Wister, 2001). Disability, that is the limitation or loss of capacity to perform an activity, does not affect only the person but again involves an exchange between that person and the surrounding environment (Verbrugge & Jette, 1994), because due to the progressive deterioration of health and psychophysical factors with age, the elderly person can become more vulnerable to environmental pressure (Heikkinen, 1997). Hence, the characteristics of the area lived in are important prerequisites for mobility.

Obstacles in the environment (spatial and technical conditions) can affect mobility and thus autonomy, creating further problems in the management of daily life and social activities (Mollenkopf & Flaschenträger, 2001). These obstacles can be overcome also with the help of technology (Cullen & Moran, 1991), with good practice in using the 'information society' for the benefit of older people and disabled ones (Promise Consortium, 1998). The progressive inability to carry out activities of daily living can create a vicious circle of immobility, where the passive state has a negative effect on health which in turn leads to isolation and passivity. The motivation to remain active can thus be greatly reduced (Passuth & Bengtson, 1998). The problem of overcoming architectural barriers, of improving access for disabled people to both public and private areas, is imminent due to the increase of the elderly population and social awareness that the phenomenon is likely to grow substantially in the future. This means that an increasing number of elderly and disabled persons will continue to use dwellings, urban spaces, and public transport (OECD, 1996). Therefore, the environment will have to be modified in relation to their needs because at present, it is often unsuitable, sometimes inaccessible, and even dangerous (Marcellini et al., 2000). This way interaction between the elderly person and the environment would lead to an improved quality of life for the whole older population (Krause, 2004).

9.2   Housing conditions in urban and rural areas

On the one hand we can suppose that the less well equipped a person's household is, the more frequently he or she will be forced to leave it. It is also likely that the older a person is and, parallel with this, the shorter the time that person has been living in the given household, the more probable it is that the move was motivated by reasons of comfort. The person may have moved in with family members because he or she was no longer able to care for him/herself, had limited outdoor mobility, etc. At the same time it must also be taken into account that these are also influenced by numerous other factors acting against mobility; such factors include the different types of welfare systems, the norms characteristic of the given society, regional differences, the cultural background, traditions, etc. The meaning of housing in old age for outdoor mobility can have a positive or negative influence on all this and the extent of mobility in the given case is a function of the combined effect of all these elements.

9.2.1   Duration of residence

Substantial differences can be found between different countries in the duration of residence in a given place. The Finnish respondents lived in their respective locality for a significantly shorter period (45 years) than the respondents from other countries. The Italian older people in the sample spent the longest period (54 years) in their current locality, followed by the Hungarian older people (52 years); besides, the Finnish, the Dutch and the western German respondents differed considerably from the Italians in this respect (48 years). The duration of residence also varied by locality (urban or rural settings). In the urban areas, duration of residence in the same locality was longest in eastern Germany, Italy and the Netherlands, while the shortest was in Finland. In rural areas, this figure was well above the average in Hungary and much lower in the Netherlands.

   Another aspect taken into consideration is the change of the house since five years earlier (Table 9.1). With the highest figure, one quarter of elderly persons living in the eastern German urban region had moved into their present home in the last five years. They had moved from home to home within the same city. The considerable differences between eastern and western Germany are in accordance with findings on a societal level (Kohli & Künemund, 2000). These findings are at least partially related to the reunification and to processes in the domain of housing, such as high proportions of (only partially voluntary) relocation in the former German Democratic Republic (GDR). In addition, reconstruction of the notorious 'Plattenbau' apartment houses was especially widespread in these regions.

Table 9.1: Proportion of persons who have been living in the same home since 1995, urban and rural areas (%)

House	URBAN		RURAL		N
	before 1995	1995, or later	before 1995	1995, or later	
Finland	78	22	89	11	603
Eastern Germany	75	25	92	8	767
Western Germany	93	7	95	5	750
Hungary	88	12	94	6	605
Italy	90	10	95	5	600
The Netherlands	84	16	88	12	609

Note. MOBILATE Survey 2000; weighted data, N = 3934

9.2.2 Type of home and ownership

The housing conditions in general are important factors determining the quality of life. For elderly people, ownership of the home can be an especially important factor; whether or not one must devote declining income (compared to the economically active stage of life) on rent, or 'only' pay for the maintenance and overhead costs that arise for all types of housing. Moreover, ownership in countries in transformation such as Hungary (Hegedüs & Tosics, 2001), where this is a part or the only part of property, also represents a form of capital which can be used when entering into a maintenance contract or moving into a home for the aged. Home ownership also protects older persons from anxiety arising from insecurity (at least in those countries where rented apartments are not the general norm). Being a tenant can give some freedom of choice and lower the housing-related responsibilities. In other countries (e.g., Germany) ownership might be a less important factor.

In general, rented houses or flats are more frequent in urban than in rural areas. There was a strikingly high proportion of rented apartments or houses in the eastern and western German cities; in both places it exceeded 70%. Eastern and western Germany had high proportions of renters (urban: ca. 73%, rural: ca. 18%) and low, or at least in comparison with other countries, lower proportions of owner/occupiers (urban: ca. 26%, rural: ca. 82%). Unlike many other European countries, most people in Germany are not owners but live in privately rented apartments (Scharf, 1998). Besides Germany, the proportion of elderly persons living in rented homes also exceeded 50% in the Netherlands. The proportion of rented apartments or houses reaches one fifth even in the rural areas in the Netherlands, but both parts of Germany also approached this level. At the other extreme we find Finland with only 11% of the respondents living in rented apartments or houses, and Hungary and Italy, where the number of rented apartments was less than 10%.

The proportion of elderly persons living in their own homes varied most along the settlement or locality variable in Hungary (in favour of rural Jászladány in comparison with the city of Pécs). Around the 1990ies the proportion of privately owned apartments was much lower in the former socialist countries, especially in the cities, compared to western countries. Socialist ideology allowed only very limited private ownership. At the beginning of the systematic change, housing policy was given a stronger market orientation (Hegedüs & Tosics, 2001). In Hungary at the time of the systemic change many could obtain a rented apartment relatively cheaply, but since then housing prices have risen at an accelerating pace. In this country it is especially important for the elderly person (or a family member) to be the main owner of the home; it is not an uncommon practice for elderly people to enter into a contract with someone who will provide care and support in return for inheriting the apartment/house.

Equipment of the apartment or house

A comparison of the equipment of homes showed that Hungarian households have less basic amenities, especially in the case of rural areas, whether compared to western rural areas or the urban Hungarian area (Figures 9.1-9.2).

Figure 9.1:   Equipment of the home among urban elders (%)

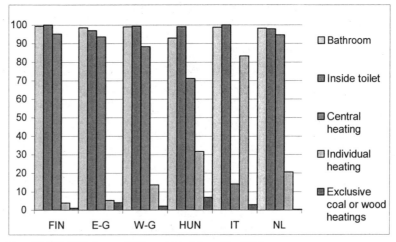

Note. MOBILATE Survey 2000; weighted data, N = 3916

Figure 9.2:   Equipment of the home among rural elders (%)

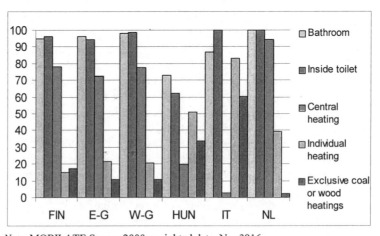

Note. MOBILATE Survey 2000; weighted data, N = 3916

In Germany, although significant improvements have undoubtedly taken place since reunification in 1990, some differences in housing quality have remained to the disadvantage of elderly persons in the eastern rural regions, especially for the older age groups; conversely, living arrangements in urban regions have achieved some level of parity.[1] A similar situation could be observed in the Hungarian regions.

The provision of telephones was almost total in the participant countries, regardless of settlement type (locality) and age. However, in Hungary, the possession of a telephone fell significantly in the rural area, and was especially low in the older age group, of whom only 54% had a telephone.

Satisfaction with apartment or house

The variance regarding housing satisfaction was very small; there is hardly any significant difference between groups divided along the basic demographic variables (sex, settlement type, or age). The values were also quite high (between 8 and 9. Interviewees answered the question with the help of an 11-point scale, where 0 indicated complete dissatisfaction and 10 indicated complete satisfaction).

The interviewees were then asked to rate, on a scale from 0 (not important at all) to 10 (very important), how important their home is for them. In all countries, there was a strong tie between the elderly respondents and their home, with a slightly lower value in the Netherlands, both for the urban and rural areas (Table 9.2). There were, however, significant differences between urban and rural areas in eastern Germany, Hungary and Italy.

Table 9.2:   Indoor Place Attachment (means)

	URBAN		RURAL		
	Mean	Std. Dev	Mean	Std. Dev	T
Finland	9.7	0.6	9.7	0.7	-0.73
Eastern Germany	8.8	1.4	9.1	1.2	-3.59*
Western Germany	9.0	1.7	9.3	1.3	-1.93
Hungary	9.5	0.9	9.2	1.4	2.92*
Italy	9.5	1.3	8.6	1.6	7.52*
The Netherlands	7.9	2.0	8.0	1.6	-0.84

Note. MOBILATE Survey 2000; weighted data; N = 3941
Scale from 0 (not important at all) to 10 (very important).
*p<0.01

9.3   Neighbourhood conditions in urban and rural areas

As has already been mentioned, the reciprocal relationship between space and individual can become even stronger in the elderly as they tend to passively experience the environment rather than dominate it. An environment with few social and relational possibilities can lead to immobility (Heikkinen, 1997). That is why the residential area assumes special importance: it represents not only the physical space but also an area of interests and stimulation with

---

[1] It is possible that more refined methods might reveal the quality differences between households in East and West Germany mentioned above. This would be possible by measuring the qualitative level of the existing home equipment instead of the quantitative (yes/no) measurement.

emotional value. Thus, personal autonomy in a broad sense is connected to the structures, facilities, and opportunities presented to the elderly person. For this reason the residential area around the dwelling, the presence of services potentially useful to the elderly, certain characteristics of the resident population, and feeling safe in the area, are all extremely important factors linked to personal autonomy.

Besides the family, neighbours can play an important role in the lives of the elderly who, as they grow older and possibly less mobile, require more human contact and support in constantly diminishing social circles (Van Tilburg, Aartsen, & Knipscheer, 2000). In rural areas, one might assume that due to low density settlement types, neighbours live quite far away from the elderly person. We therefore asked the interviewees where their neighbours live. For most of the subjects in the rural areas of all countries the neighbours lived either in the same house or less than 100 meters away. Exceptions were Hungary, where 16% of neighbours lived over 2 km away, and Finland, where 29% of neighbours lived between 100 and 500 meters away.

The outdoor environment was generally quite important for the outdoor mobility of elderly people (Table 9.3). In this case we asked the respondents to rate the importance of going out on a scale from 0 (not important at all) to 10 (very important). The highest values were obtained from the elderly Finns (8.9 in the urban area and 8.8 in the rural area), who not only felt the strongest tie with their home, but were also the ones who liked to go out most. The lowest values were found among Hungarians living in the rural area (6.1), followed by the Italians in the rural area (6.7) and by western Germans living in the urban area (6.9). Attitude differences between the urban and rural areas were found in eastern and western Germany, Hungary and Italy (see also Chapter 7).

Table 9.3: Importance of being out (means)

	URBAN		RURAL		
	Mean	Std. Dev	Mean	Std. Dev	t
Finland	8.9	1.2	8.8	1.6	0.67
Eastern Germany	7.4	2.4	7.9	2.3	-3.02*
Western Germany	6.9	2.7	7.4	2.6	-2.62*
Hungary	7.3	2.5	6.1	2.6	5.71*
Italy	7.4	2.4	6.7	2.7	3.26*
The Netherlands	7.8	1.7	8.1	1.3	-2.31

Note. MOBILATE Survey 2000; weighted data, N = 3940
Scale from 0 (not important at all) to 10 (very important).
*p<0.01

9.3.1   The use of services

Being able to get to and reach shops, cultural facilities, medical services etc. is a fundamental precondition for maintaining an independent way of life. The interviewees were asked to give the following information: which services are available in the residential area (i.e., easily reached within 15 minutes regardless of the means of transportation used), and which of them are considered important? In this way it is possible to have a subjective quantification of what services they need, how they get there, and what obstacles they encounter along the way. The unavailability is crucial, if these facilities are important for elderly persons.

Table 9.4: Satisfaction with local services in urban and rural areas (means)

| | URBAN | | RURAL | | |
	Mean	Std. Dev	Mean	Std. Dev	t
Finland	7.4	2.2	7.1	2.7	1.64
Eastern Germany	7.3	2.1	5.7	2.7	9.24*
Western Germany	7.7	2.1	7.2	2.4	3.29*
Hungary	7.9	2.4	7.3	2.3	2.96*
Italy	6.7	2.7	6.2	2.8	1.97
The Netherlands	6.7	1.9	7.2	1.2	-3.64*

Note. MOBILATE Survey 2000; weighted data, N = 3922
Scale from 0 (very unsatisfied) to 10 (very satisfied).
*p<0.01

Results (Table 9.4) show a sufficient degree of satisfaction with services in the urban area of each country. Regarding the rural areas, eastern Germany stands out with its mean value of 5.7, and had the lowest level of satisfaction on a scale ranging from 0 (very unsatisfied) to 10 (very satisfied).

Available services

Elderly people in Hungary appeared to be the most satisfied with services and facilities in their area out of the whole sample, both in the urban and rural area. Italians were among the least satisfied, which might indicate that in spite of the existence of many important services (see Figures 9.3-9.6), their quality is probably low. Analysing the differences between the urban and rural areas of the various countries (Table 9.4), we found significant differences in eastern and western Germany, in Hungary and in the Netherlands. In the Netherlands, satisfaction was higher in the rural (non-urban) area than in the city, while the greatest difference between the urban and rural areas were found in eastern Germany. What then, does satisfaction depend on? These results should be read on the basis of the data described below.

The availability of certain services is assumed to be very important in order to evaluate the quality of life of elderly people. In our study, availability means the possibility of reaching fundamental services (food store, pharmacy, doctor, bank, post office, bus or tram stop, church, cemetery, hairdresser/barber, library; more green areas only for the urban areas) by whatever means of transport, within a time range of 15 minutes. To answer this question, we chose to represent the data using the following structure: services available for a range of 1 to 19% of the elderly respondents, from 20 to 39%, from 40 to 59%, from 60 to 79% and from 80 to 100% (Figures 9.3 and 9.4)

Ranking (Figure 9.3) shows that in the urban areas, the western German city was the one with the greatest number of services (9 out of 11) which can be reached within 15 minutes by more than 80% of the interviewees. It was followed by Italy and the Netherlands with 8, Hungary and eastern Germany with 7 and then Finland with only 5 services.

Figure 9.3:   Ranking of available services in urban areas

	FIN (N = 309)	GER (E) (N = 389)	GER (W) (N = 368)	HUN (N = 305)	IT (N = 300)	NL (N = 302)
80% - 100%	Food store Green areas Bus/Tram stop Church Hairdresser / Barber	Food store Pharmacy Doctor Bank Post office Bus/Tram stop Hairdresser / Barber	Food store Pharmacy Doctor Bank Post Office Green areas Bus/Tram stop Church Hairdresser / Barber	Food store Pharmacy Doctor Post office Green areas Bus/Tram stop Hairdresser / Barber	Food store Pharmacy Doctor Bank Post Office Bus/Tram stop Church Hairdresser / Barber	Food store Pharmacy Doctor Bank Post office Bus/Tram stop Church Hairdresser / Barber
60% - 79%	Pharmacy Doctor Post Office Library	Green areas	Cemetery Library	Bank Church	Green areas Cemetery	Green areas
40% - 59%	Cemetery Bank	Church Cemetery		Library		Cemetery Library
20% - 39%		Library		Cemetery		
0% - 19%					Library	

Note. MOBILATE Survey 2000; weighted data, N = 1973
From the bottom to the top: services available for a range between 1 and 19% of the elderly respondents, from 20 to 39%, from 40 to 59%, from 60 to 79% and from 80 to 100%.

The two most available services in all the cities were the food store and bus or tram stop, while cemetery and library (with the exception of Italy and western Germany) were among the less present ones. In case of library a large difference was found between the Finnish (73%) and western German cities (68%) on the one hand, and the remaining cities on the other, with Italy scoring lowest (14%). One difference regards the churches, which were found in great numbers in the Italian, Dutch, western German and Finnish urban areas, and much less in the other countries, especially Hungary and eastern Germany, where the churches became less important during the socialist regimes.

Generally speaking the most difficult situation seems to appear in Finland, with a limited presence of fundamental services such as the doctor (available for only 67% of the interviewed elderly), pharmacy, bank and post office. This can be explained by the longer distances within cities (urban development is more diffuse than in other countries) and also because the most frequent mode of transport is walking; it thus takes longer than 15 minutes to reach the service facilities in question.

The situation changes in the rural areas. According to ranking (Figure 9.4), the availability of services for more than 80% of the elderly interviewees decreased sharply in Finland (4 services less than in the urban area), in eastern Germany (4 services less) and in Hungary (5 services less). Italy and western Germany were the countries with the most services in the rural areas studied.

Figure 9.4:   Ranking of available services in rural areas

	FIN (N = 301)	GER (E) (N = 379)	GER (W) (N = 382)	HUN (N = 300)	IT (N = 300)	NL (N = 315)
80% - 100%	Bus/Tram stop	Bus/Tram stop Church Cemetery	Food store Pharmacy Doctor Bank Post Office Bus/Tram stop Church Cemetery Hairdresser / Barber	Food store Bus/Tram stop	Food store Pharmacy Doctor Bank Post Office Bus/Tram stop Church Cemetery Hairdresser / Barber	Food store Doctor Bank Bus/Tram stop Church Cemetery
60% - 79%	Food store Pharmacy Doctor Bank Post Office Church Cemetery Hairdresser / Barber Library	Food store Doctor Post Office Hairdresser / Barber		Pharmacy Doctor Bank Post Office Church Hairdresser / Barber	Library	Pharmacy Post Office Hairdresser / Barber
40% - 59%		Pharmacy Bank	Library	Cemetery Library		
20% - 39%		Library				Library
0% - 19%						

Note. MOBILATE Survey 2000; weighted data, N = 1977
From the bottom at the top: services available for a range between 1 and 19% of the elderly respondents, from 20 to 39%, from 40 to 59%, from 60 to 79% and from 80 to 100%.

It is fundamental to analyse the importance given to services by elderly population in the various countries, analysing once again the differences between the urban and rural areas. The next step of this study was in fact to ask the elderly respondents what services were important to them, among those that could be reached. We must stress that only those interviewees who had these services available to them were asked to give their opinion.

Important services

Elderly people living in urban areas of all the countries studied considered the food store to be the most important service. In eastern Germany (Figure 9.5), 8 services were fundamental for more than 80% of the interviewees, while not much importance was given to the services in Finland (only the food store and bank were considered of top importance), not even fundamental services such as the pharmacy and doctor. The limited presence of these services in Finland found before is in agreement with the data regarding importance. Indeed Table 9.4 indicates that in spite of everything, satisfaction for services in Finland was quite high.

Figure 9.5:   Ranking of important services in urban areas

	FIN (N = 309)	GER (E) (N = 389)	GER (W) (N = 368)	HUN (N = 305)	IT (N = 300)	NL (N = 302)
80% - 100%	Food store Bank	Food store Pharmacy Doctor Bank Post office Green areas Bus/Tram stop Hairdresser / Barber	Food store Pharmacy Doctor Bank Post Office Green areas Bus/Tram stop	Food store Pharmacy Doctor Post office Green areas Bus/Tram stop	Food store Pharmacy Doctor Post Office Church	Food store Pharmacy Doctor Bank Post office
60% - 79%	Pharmacy Doctor Post Office Green areas Bus/Tram stop Hairdresser / Barber Library		Church Cemetery Hairdresser / Barber	Bank Cemetery	Bank Green areas Bus/Tram stop Cemetery Hairdresser / Barber	Green areas Bus/Tram stop Hairdresser / Barber
40% - 59%	Church Cemetery	Cemetery Library	Library	Church Hairdresser / Barber		Church Cemetery Library
20% - 39%		Church		Library	Library	
0% - 19%						

Note. MOBILATE Survey 2000; weighted data; N = 1973
From the bottom at the top: services important for a range between 1 and 19% of the elderly respondents, from 20 to 39%, from 40 to 59%, from 60 to 79% and from 80 to 100%.
The number of interviewees is the same as before, as each person replied 'yes" at least once when asked about the 11 services studied.

The greatest difference in the comparison between urban and rural areas within a country were found in Hungary and eastern Germany, where in the rural areas there were three services less in the highest ranking (Figure 9.6) than in the urban areas. The services which were considered by nearly all rural interviewees to be fundamental are the food store, the pharmacy and doctor.

An open question which cannot be answered using these data, is whether people have adapted their evaluations to the limited availability of local services in the areas they live, or whether they truly do not consider these services to be important.

Figure 9.6: Ranking of important services in rural areas

	FIN (N = 301)	GER (E) (N = 379)	GER (W) (N = 382)	HUN (N = 300)	IT (N = 300)	NL (N = 315)
80% - 100%	Food store Pharmacy Doctor Bank	Food store Pharmacy Doctor Bank Post Office	Food store Pharmacy Doctor Bank Post Office Church Hairdresser / Barber	Food store Pharmacy Doctor	Food store Pharmacy Doctor Post Office Church Cemetery	Food store Pharmacy Doctor Bank Post Office
60% - 79%	Post Office Church Cemetery Hairdresser / Barber	Cemetery Hairdresser / Barber	Cemetery	Post Office Bus/Tram stop Church Cemetery	Bank Hairdresser / Barber	Bus/Tram stop Church Cemetery Hairdresser / Barber
40% - 59%	Library	Pharmacy Bus/Tram stop	Bus/Tram stop	Bank Hairdresser / Barber Library		Library
20% - 39%	Bus/Tram stop	Church	Library		Bus/Tram stop	
0% - 19%		Library			Library	

Note. MOBILATE Survey 2000; weighted data , N = 1977

From the bottom at the top: services important for a range between 1 and 19% of the elderly respondents, from 20 to 39%, from 40 to 59%, from 60 to 79% and from 80 to 100%.

The transport modes for reaching services

In order to evaluate the degree and patterns of everyday mobility of the elderly, it is necessary to find out what modes of transport they normally use to reach services, and particularly those they feel are important. Elderly interviewees able to reach fundamental services were asked what means of transport they used among the following: on foot, by bicycle, by car as driver, by car as passenger, by moped or scooter, by bus, taxi, special transport, or wheelchair. In order to summarize the data clearly, an estimation procedure was used, as shown in the following figures, for the urban and rural areas (Figure 9.7). Single cases (that are the sum of all the services reached, calculated for each means of transport used by all the interviewees) within each country were considered in order to create variables describing the means of transport used (for reaching any service) with the intention of no longer talking about single services but 'services' in general (for more detailed explanation see example in note of Figure 9.7).

In the urban areas, the elderly interviewees in all countries mainly reached important services on foot. The highest percentage can be found in Hungary (90%), which is also the country with the lowest percentage of car drivers (1%) and car passengers (2%). Elderly Italians used a car more often than the others, with the highest values both as car drivers (18%) and as passengers (11%). Use of the car as a driver was also quite diffused in Finland and Germany, less so in the Netherlands. The highest value regarding the use of bicycles was in the Netherlands (13%), and for the bus/tram in Hungary.

Figure 9.7: Transport mode for reaching services in urban and rural areas in each country

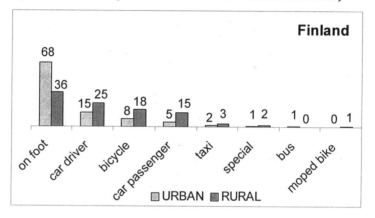

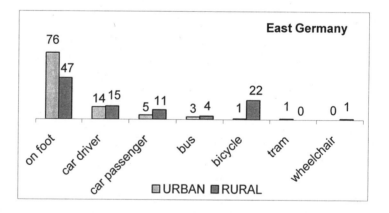

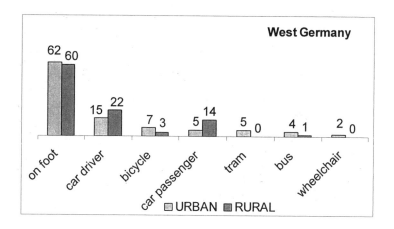

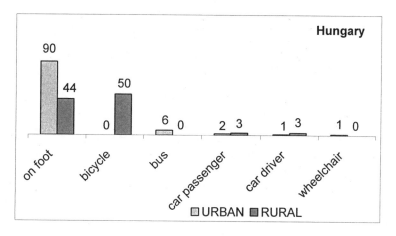

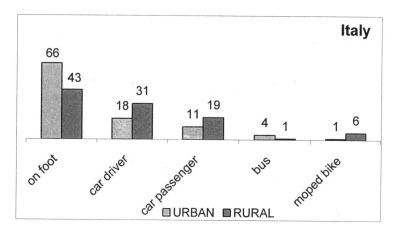

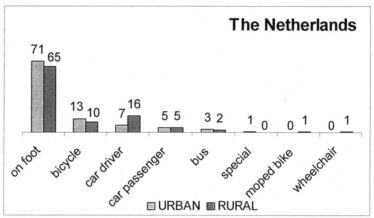

Note. Mobilate Survey 2000; weighted Data; N = 1973;
Estimation procedure. Example: country=Finland; area=urban.
Means of transport=foot: counted cases of services reached =1165; Means of
transport=bicycle: counted cases of services reached =132; Means of transport=etc.;
Total counted cases of services reached=1165+132+etc. =1717; Estimated percentage
Finland urban by foot = counted cases of services reached by foot/ total counted cases
of services reached x 100=1165/1717x100=68 (see Figure 9.7, Finland urban on foot,
Finland urban by bicycle = etc.).

In the rural areas, elders less often travelled on foot, but walking still remained the mode of
transport most used in all countries, with the exception of Hungary (47%), where the bicycle
was used more (50%). The bicycle was also used quite a lot in Finland and eastern Germany.
Another interesting data for all countries except Hungary was the increased use of the car both
as driver and as passenger (data referring to the driver were always higher than for the
passenger, as in the case of the urban area), and the most determined drivers were the Italians
who also reported the highest use of the moped-scooter (6%). The tram and bus were
generally not used often, except by a rather small percentage of elderly eastern Germans.

As for more detailed comments about single services, it must be stressed that
percentages regarding going to places on foot were lower in all the rural areas, and especially
in Finland and eastern Germany, to the food store, pharmacy, doctor and bank. This is
probably due to the greater distances from home to these services in rural areas.

The car was the second most important mode of transport used in all countries except in
Hungary and in the Dutch urban areas, but with lower values than going by foot. In the
Netherlands this may be due to good public transport. In Hungary, cars were available only to
a small proportion of older persons. When elderly people used the car, they generally did so
as drivers. In the urban areas, the Italian and Finnish elderly drove most. In the rural areas, the
values rose in all countries (even for those who used cars as passengers).

The Hungarian data stands out regarding the bicycle as it was used much more than in
other countries. In the rural area, it was the mode of transport most used to reach fundamental
services (pharmacy, doctor, bank, post office). However, Hungarians living in the urban area
hardly used it at all; as already seen they go predominantly by foot. In general, the bicycle
was used more often in the rural areas (with the exception of Italy and western Germany).
Italy is the country where the bicycle was used the least and this depends on the fact that the
urban as well as the rural areas are very hilly. Residents in the urban areas might also be

dissuaded from using the bicycle due to the difficulties of getting about in busy traffic, or to land conformation.

Generally speaking, the bus was not used much, and hardly at all in the rural areas. This corresponds with the previous result showing the scarce importance given to this service, even if bus stops are widespread. The elderly Hungarians living in the urban area used it more than the others, above all to reach cemetery, church and hairdresser/barber. In the rural area in Finland, no elderly person took the bus to reach any kind of service, mainly because distances were great and due to the limited number of bus lines in spite of the many bus stops.

Access to local services

Another important factor that possibly affects mobility regards the possible difficulties elderly people might have in reaching services. In order to study this, the elderly interviewees were asked if they could reach important services without difficulty, with difficulty or not at all. This was done both in the urban and rural areas. Tables 9.5 and 9.6 were created by summing the options 'with difficulty' and 'no access'.

Table 9.5: Access to local services in urban areas with difficulty or no access (%)

| | URBAN | | | | | | |
	FIN (N = 309)	GER (E) (N = 389)	GER (W) (N = 368)	HUN (N = 305)	IT (N = 300)	NL (N = 302)	χ^2
Food store	7	12	10	11	9	2	41.67*
Pharmacy	8	14	10	10	7	2	45.24*
Doctor	8	12	9	12	7	2	40.11*
Bank	4	14	8	6	5	4	40.17*
Post office	3	13	10	10	4	5	36.25*
Green areas	5	8	8	11	8	2	19.30
Bus or tram stop	4	8	7	10	10	3	28.47*
Church	7	15	8	13	8	2	19.79
Cemetery	7	7	9	10	10	4	7.29
Hairdresser/Barber	7	8	6	9	8	1	17.58
Library	6	4	3	3	-	2	4.63

Note. MOBILATE Survey 2000; weighted data; N = 1973
      *p<0.01

Table 9.6: Access to local services in rural areas with difficulty or no access (%)

| | RURAL | | | | | | |
	FIN (N = 301)	GER (E) (N = 379)	GER (W) (N = 382)	HUN (N = 300)	IT (N = 300)	NL (N = 315)	χ^2
Food store	12	11	9	22	12	4	72.71*
Pharmacy	12	12	8	24	11	5	68.37*
Doctor	10	11	9	26	13	3	71.98*
Bank	11	13	8	16	8	3	37.06*
Post office	11	12	8	16	11	2	38.88*
Bus or tram stop	6	4	11	13	2	3	30.93*
Church	13	7	10	19	15	4	67.76*
Cemetery	11	7	10	25	14	4	72.31*
Hairdresser/Barber	11	11	9	17	12	2	23.18*
Library	5	-	15	15	-	4	12.26

Note. MOBILATE Survey 2000; weighted data, N = 1977; *p<0.01

Most of the older adults in all the countries had no difficulty reaching the services that are important to them, but when investigating the negative cases (elderly who are unable, or have difficulty accessing them, Table 9.5 and 9.6) the most difficult situation can be found in the Hungarian rural area for essential services such as the food store (22%), pharmacy (24%) and doctor (26%), and in the eastern German urban area. Difficulties also existed in the rural areas of Italy and Finland (for about 10% of the interviewees). The best situation was found in the Netherlands, with very low percentages of difficulties in reaching services.

Elderly people who have difficulties or are unable to reach services were asked to give the main reasons for this. The main reason given in nearly all countries, both in the urban and rural areas was poor health (with the exception of eastern Germany and the urban area of the Netherlands, where large distances were most important). As shown in Figure 9.8, the situation was always worse in the rural areas except in Italy. The country with the highest percentages regarding the difficulties 'for general health reasons' was Finland (51% in the urban area and 64% in the rural area), while the lowest were eastern Germany (29%) and the Netherlands (36%).

Figure 9.8:　The reasons mentioned by older persons with problems in accessing services by country and area (%; multiple answers possible)

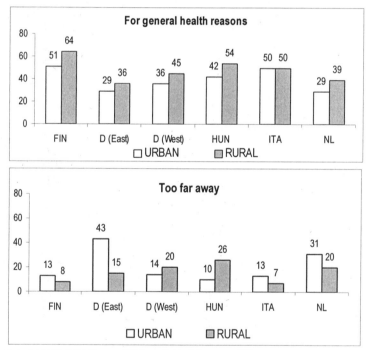

Note. MOBILATE Survey 2000; weighted data, n = 449

After 'general health reasons' the next most common reason for difficulty was that the destination was 'too far away'. In the urban area of eastern Germany, the percentage of respondents endorsing this statement (43%) was actually higher than the percentage of respondents citing health reasons in the same country (29%). 'Too far away' was the main reason of difficulty in the Netherlands (31%) and also has a certain weight in the rural areas of Hungary (26%) and western Germany (20%).

The difference between the two previous reasons and the others is quite large, but it is interesting to note that in Italy, Hungary and the urban area of western Germany, the problem of bad road conditions was quite relevant. While the reason 'I don't have a car' was chosen by 12% of the Hungarians living in the urban area, it was not reported in the rural area. The opposite pattern of response occurred in western Germany, with 10% in the rural area and 2% in the urban area. 'Badly connected' was the most commonly mentioned difficulty (after health and/or distances) in the urban areas in the Netherlands (14%), in western Germany (10%) and Italy (7%), and in the rural areas in the Netherlands (7%) and in Finland (6%).

9.3.2 Feelings of security

The usability of the residential area is not only influenced by the accessibility of services or the presence of neighbours, but also by the sense of security or insecurity experienced by the elders. Fear can become a psychological barrier which influences mobility-related decisions and inhibits outdoor behaviour.

Table 9.7: Feeling of security in the living area during the day (%)

	URBAN		RURAL		
	Insecure	Secure	Insecure	Secure	χ^2
Finland	3	97	3	97	0.003
Eastern Germany	10	90	6	94	2.92
Western Germany	13	87	2	98	36.88*
Hungary	12	88	34	66	40.87*
Italy	14	86	25	75	9.49*
The Netherlands	7	93	2	98	11.11*

Note. MOBILATE Survey 2000; weighted data, N = 3946
χ^2 Urban-Rural, p<0.01

Table 9.8: Feeling of security in the living area during the night (%)

	URBAN		RURAL		
	Insecure	Secure	Insecure	Secure	χ^2
Finland	9	91	4	96	5.52
Eastern Germany	39	61	22	78	27.36*
Western Germany	32	68 .	6	94	78.36*
Hungary	18	82	41	59	38.02*
Italy	37	63	38	62	0.007
The Netherlands	22	78	9	91	22.46*

Note. MOBILATE Survey 2000; weighted data, N = 3930
χ^2 Urban-Rural, p<0.01

Most of the respondents in all the countries, and especially in Finland, seemed to feel secure (very secure and rather secure) in the area they live in both during the day (Table 9.7) and night (Table 9.8). The Finns seemed to be the most secure during the day and during the night in urban and rural areas. As expected, the feeling of insecurity (rather insecure and very insecure) showed a higher amount at night, both in the urban and rural areas. The level in insecurity increased at night in the urban areas in all countries, with the highest values in eastern Germany (39%), western Germany (32%), and Italy (37%).

The chi-square test applied between the urban and rural areas of each country showed significant differences during the day in Italy, Hungary, eastern Germany and the Netherlands. At night time instead, significant differences were found in eastern Germany, western Germany and the Netherlands. It must be noted, though, that the most insecure respondents by day were the Italians and Hungarians, with higher percentages in the rural areas (34% Hungary, 25% Italy). The same pattern occurred in these two countries at night, only with even higher values.

It is interesting to understand the reasons of insecurity felt by the interviewees. Of course, only elderly interviewees who had previously stated they felt very or quite insecure during the day and/or during the night were asked to give reasons for their feeling of insecurity. As already mentioned, most elderly respondents said they felt secure, and this must be taken into consideration.

The main reasons for feeling insecure given were 'I'm afraid to leave the house/apartment when it is dark', 'I'm afraid of being mugged when it is dark', 'I'm afraid of burglars during my absence', and 'Presence of unwanted people or groups', both in the urban and rural areas. In the urban areas the most important result regarded eastern Germany and the item 'I'm afraid to leave the house/apartment when it is dark' (42%). This was also the main reason for feeling insecure in western Germany (21%). Instead the main reason in Italy (31%), the Netherlands (23%) and Finland (21%), was 'I'm afraid of being mugged when it is dark'. Hungarian elderly were particularly insecure with the 'Presence of unwanted people/groups' (16%), which also has the highest percentage for the rural area of that same country (20%).

9.3.3   Environmental features

The decision to live in a certain area or not can depend on environmental characteristics (e.g., whether the residential area is quiet, clean, and has good access to shops and services, etc.). Elderly interviewees were asked their opinion on the importance of certain characteristics, choosing from among three options: 'very important', 'less important' and 'not important'. We also examined whether the characteristics mentioned by the elders were actually present or not in the living area in question.

Considering the ratings of importance and availability in the urban areas, in many cases the respondents stated that in their living area the features rated as very important are not available. These include 'a quiet residential area' (very important for all respondents, but especially for those in Finland, eastern Germany, Italy and Hungary) and 'clean environmental conditions' (also generally very important, but especially for the Italians).

Also in the rural areas, the features considered to be most important were 'a quiet residential area' and 'clean environmental conditions'. With regards to a quiet residential area, both 'supply and 'importance' accord well with one another in Finland (96% residential areas are quiet and 91% of the respondents regard this feature to be important), in West Germany (90% and 89%) and Italy (91% and 83%). With regards to a clean residential area, only in eastern Germany is the supply (87%), higher than the importance (84%). The other countries therefore feel the lack of 'clean environmental conditions'.

The rural areas also had greater difficulties regarding being 'well connected' (especially in the Netherlands) and having 'good access to shops and services' in all countries except

Hungary. Also the situation for 'good medical care in the vicinity' was unsatisfactory in all countries, especially in Italy, Finland, eastern Germany and the Netherlands. Compared to the urban areas, the rural situation improves for 'a pleasant neighborhood'. The greatest differences between supply and demand were found for the environmental feature 'cultural opportunities in the vicinity'. We found, both in the urban and rural area, a sufficient presence faced with a poor demand in western Germany. Also in Finland and Hungary this feature has a greater presence than importance, contrary to the situation in the Netherlands, but especially to Italy where cultural opportunities were considered very important only by a minority of elderly respondents, but were present for an even lower number of them.

Finally, elderly respondents were asked to rate their satisfaction with their living area on a scale from 0 (lowest satisfaction) to 10 (higher satisfaction). In all the countries, both in the urban and rural areas, they were well satisfied with the area they live in (Table 9.9). The highest ratings (8.9) were found in the rural area in western Germany, while the lowest is in the rural area in Hungary (6.9). The t-test showed significant differences between the urban and rural areas in western Germany, Hungary and the Netherlands. It must be stressed that in western Germany and the Netherlands, satisfaction with the living area was significantly higher in the rural than in the urban areas.

Table 9.9:   Satisfaction with living area (means)

	URBAN		RURAL		
	Mean	Std. Dev	Mean	Std. Dev	T
Finland	8.7	1.3	8.6	1.4	0.57
Eastern Germany	8.0	1.8	8.1	2.2	-0.70
Western Germany	7.7	2.4	8.9	1.5	-9.27*
Hungary	7.9	2.5	6.9	2.6	4.39*
Italy	8.3	1.9	7.9	2.1	2.29
The Netherlands	7.4	1.7	8.1	1.3	-5.30*

Note. MOBILATE Survey 2000; weighted data, N = 3934
Scale from 0 (lowest satisfaction) to 10 (higher satisfaction)
*$p<0.01$

9.4   Summary and conclusions

In conclusion, even if the respondents were all quite satisfied with their living areas, some environmental obstacles to outdoor mobility were found. They were more present in rural than in urban areas. The relation between mobility and environment was clear, for example, regarding the transport modes used for reaching services. In rural areas, distances from homes to services were generally (and obviously) bigger. So here the car becomes more important than in urban places, with the exception of Hungary, where there was a widespread use of bicycle due to the low income that didn't allow elderly to own a car.

The home, especially after retirement, becomes the environment of life privileged by older people. The level of infrastructure in Hungarian homes - especially in the rural area - was much lower than in homes in the Western countries. On the other hand, the proportion of home ownership was the highest in Hungary.

Our study showed that the elderly people mainly lived in the same building or less than 100 meters from their nearest neighbour. This means that elders could usually rely on others for help or a simple interaction. The Finnish and Italian older persons were most strongly tied to their homes and neighbourhoods while Dutch elderly people showed the weakest tie to a particular place, although generally speaking, indoor place attachment was quite high in all countries. The tie was weaker between the older persons and their outdoor environment. In Hungary, the difference between the tie with the home and the importance of going out was the highest among all the countries studied (both for the rural and urban areas). Finland had the highest values both for the urban and rural areas in both cases, that is regarding the attachment to the home and the outdoor environment.

Most of the older persons in all the countries had good access to fundamental services (which can be reached in 15 minutes) such as food store, doctor, pharmacy, bank, post office, bus or tram stop, etc. (except for Finland). The services which were rated the most important by elderly people were food store, pharmacy, doctor and (except Hungary and Italy) bank. This shows that above all the elderly look after their primary needs: food, health and savings. Still regarding services, the presence of a bus or tram stop, which is the most widespread service of all (together with the food store) both in the rural and urban areas, was also one of the least important ones. This indicates that the availability of a bus/tram stop is not equivalent to a service meeting the needs of older people.

The Hungarians were the most satisfied with their services, both in the urban and rural areas, even though in the latter case they were not always frequently available, except for the food store. Why were they nonetheless satisfied? Is it most likely due to cultural reasons and to a lesser demand of quality in the services? Generally, elderly Hungarians, especially those living in the rural area, do not attach great importance to services, but it is not clear if this is really so, or if they have resigned or adapted their expectations to the situation.

The most unsatisfied were older people living in the rural area of eastern Germany. This findings seems due to the lack or infrequent presence of services rated by the respondents as fundamental, such as food store, pharmacy, doctor, bank and post office. The Italian interviewees did not seem greatly satisfied either, even though the important services are usually well diffused. As emphasized previously, the reason could lie in the poor quality of Italian services. Finally, despite the poor availability of services (compared to other countries), the Finns showed a good degree of satisfaction.

It is interesting to analyse those services which elderly people consider of secondary importance, as they can give some idea, or indications, of the dominant cultural characteristics in the various countries. A strong religious feeling can be found in Italy, while it was very weak in eastern Germany. Elderly persons who felt the library is important were the Dutch, Finns and Hungarians living in the rural areas. An open question is why libraries are of scarce importance to those living in urban areas.

The mode of transport most often used in all countries to reach services was walking. The car was fundamental in Italy. In the rural areas, going on foot was most common in the Netherlands and western Germany, while use of the car was very important in Italy, Finland and western Germany. The bicycle was used most in Hungary followed by eastern Germany, Finland and the Netherlands. Public transport such as bus or tram was not used much, either in the urban or rural areas. The worst situation observed with regard to means of transportation was in Hungary. This is confirmed by the infrequent ownership of a car, and by the greater use of bicycles and buses. The more frequent use of the bus in the Hungarian city is due to the free travel for persons above 65 years. Nonetheless, Hungarian elders had the greatest difficulty reaching services. Even if most elderly people did not have difficulties in reaching services, it is interesting to note that the reasons which prevent accessing services were mainly linked to health conditions. Also great distances were considered a difficulty in both urban and rural areas.

Security, generally speaking, was not a problem for most elderly respondents. The elderly people in Finland feel most secure. The highest percentages of insecurity were found in the Hungarian rural area, both by day and night. Also the Italians generally feel less secure than the Dutch and Finnish elders. Other problems arose when analysing the characteristics of certain conditions of the environment which were felt to be important. In both urban and rural areas, many elderly felt they lacked important conditions, such as a quiet living area and a clean environment.

In spite of the mobility-related problems of today's elders uncovered by the study, it seems that the elderly interviewees were all quite satisfied with their living area. It can be assumed that this is also due, at least in part, to the strong emotional bond created by the elderly people with their environment over the years. Nevertheless, the environment should be improved in function of needs of older persons, especially in rural areas and for the oldest and impaired ones, because it is often unsuitable and in some cases felt as unsafe.

References

Cullen, K., & Moran, R. (1991). *Technology and the elderly. The role of technology in prolonging the indipendence of the elderly in the community care context*. Dublin: Work Research Centre and EKOS.

Cvitkovich, Y., & Wister, A. (2001). The importance of transportation and prioritization of environmental needs to sustain well-being among older adults. *Environment & Behavior*, 33(6), 809-829.

Hegedűs, J., & Tosics, J. (2001). Transition of the housing sector in the East Central European Countries. In G. Lengyel & Z. Rostoványi (Eds.), *The Small Transition* (pp.233-287). Budapest: Akadémiai Kiadó.

Heikkinen, E. (1997). Background, design and methods of the project. In E. Heikkinen, R-L. Heikkinen, & I. Ruoppila (Eds), Functional capacity and health of elderly people - The Evergreen project. *Scandinavian Journal of Social Medicine*, Suppl 53, 1-18.

Kohli, M., & Künemund, H. (2000). *Die zweite Lebenshälfte - Gesellschaftliche Lage und Partizipation im Spiegel des Alters-Survey* [The second half of life - Societal position and participation from the ageing survey perspective]. Opladen: Leske + Budrich.

Krause, N. (2004). Neighborhoods, health, and well-being in late life. In H.-W. Wahl, R. J. Scheidt, & P. G. Windley (Eds.), *Focus on aging in context: Socio-physical environments* (Annual Review of Gerontology and Geriatrics, Vol. 23) (5th ed., pp. 272-294). New York: Springer Publ.

Lawton, M. P, Windley, P.G., & Byerts, T. O. (1982). *Aging and the Environment*. New York: Springer Publishing Company.

Lawton, M. P. (1986). *Environment and Aging*, New York: CSA, Albany.

Lewin, K. (1951). *Field theory in social science*. New York: Harper & Row.

Marcellini F., Gagliardi C., Leonardi F. (2000). The Ageing Population and Transport: A new balance between demand and supply. In European Conference of Ministers of Transport (ECMT), *Transport and Ageing of the Population* (pp. 143-176). Paris: OECD Publications Service.

Mollenkopf, H., Marcellini, F., Ruoppila, I., & Tacken, M. (Eds.) (2004). *Ageing and Outdoor Mobility. A European Study.* Amsterdam: IOS Press.

Mollenkopf, H., & Flaschenträger P. (2001). *Erhaltung von Mobilitat im Alter* [Maintaining mobility in old age]. (Vol. 197 - Schriftenreihe des Bundesministeriums für Familie, Senioren, Frauen und Jugend). Stuttgart: Kohlhammer.

OECD (1996). *Caring for frail elderly people. Policies in evolution.* Social Policy Studies No. 19. Paris: OECD.

Passuth, P. M., & Bengtson, U. L. (1998). Sociological theories of aging: current perspective and future directions. In J. E. Birren, & U. L. Bengtson (Eds.), *Emergent theories on aging* (pp. 333-355). New York: Spinger Publishing Company.

Promise Consortium (Eurolink Age, European Disability Forum, Stakes Finland, Work Research Centre Ireland) (1998). *Promoting an Information Society for Everyone*, Promise Project, www.stakes.fi/promise/index.html.

Schaie, K. W., & Pietrucha, M. (Eds.). (2000). *Mobility and transportation in the elderly.* New York, NY: Springer.

Scharf, T. (1998). *Ageing and Ageing Policy in Germany.* Oxford, New York: Berg.

Verbrugge, L. M., & Jette, A. M. (1994). The disablement process. *Social Science & Medicine, 38*, 98, 1-14.

Van Tilburg, T., Aartsen, M. J., & Knipscheer, K. (2000). Effect of changes in physical capacities upon personal social network in aging people. *Tijdschr Gerontol Geriatr 2000* Oct; 31(5), 190-7.

Enhancing Mobility in Later Life
H. Mollenkopf et al. (Eds.)
IOS Press, 2005

Chapter 10
Main Issues of Older People's Out-of-Home Mobility

Mart Tacken and Heidrun Mollenkopf

10.1   Introduction

In the MOBILATE study, the main research aims were the description and explanation of mobility behaviour of elderly people, and application of results. At this place we want to indicate how far we succeeded in clarifying older people's out-of-home mobility and to what extent we met these aims. We do this in two steps: First, we take up and integrate the main issues dealt with in the foregoing chapters, and discuss the following more detailed research questions:

- How mobile are elderly people?
- Is this mobility in line with their needs?
- What are the hindrances and barriers they encounter?
- How do they cope with these problems?
- What can be done to improve the mobility of elderly people?

Thus, in the first sections of this chapter we summarise how far we came in answering the first four questions. Based upon the answers, we ask for possible improvements to enhance older people's out-of-home mobility in the last section.

10.2   Older people's actual mobility

A central question of this project involves how to measure mobility. Traditionally mobility is expressed in the number of trips undertaken over a given period of time. But as explained in Chapter 1.2, we attempted to find a concept that is broader than trip making and reflects quality of life. We have introduced a concept of mobility that consists of the variety of outdoor activities, variety of transportation means, and the number of movements (see also Chapter 11).

Further methodological questions concern whether or not one can establish a new metric or ordinal variable or must rely on categorical descriptions (e.g., immobile vs. mobile). Must we use these characteristics separately or can they be combined, and how? We expect that:

- people who make no or a few trips also cover little or no distance, use less different modes and have a smaller mix of outdoor activities; whereas

- people who make many trips also cover long distances, use many different modes of transportation and pursue a great variety of activities.

The results of our analysis generally support these expectations, but there is a very large group of respondents for whom these variables are not consistently related. A first elaboration in a correlation matrix shows a high correlation between the mean number of realised trips and distance travelled, as well as low correlations between mean number of trips and variety of activities and transportation modes (Table 10.1).

Table 10.2, which differentiates by country, shows only minor differences with Table 10.1. Distance travelled was left out of the analysis because of its logical relation to number of trips (making no trips means no distance). This table shows that the highest correlations were between variety of outdoor activities and variety of transportation modes. The correlation between the mean number of trips and the variety of outdoor activities or variety of transportation modes is rather low, except in Finland and Italy.

Table 10.1: Correlation matrix of mobility aspects

		mean of trips	distance covered	variety of activities	variety of transport modes
mean of trips	Pearson	1			
	sign.				
distance of trips	Pearson	.61	1		
	sign.	.000			
variety activities	Pearson	.32	.28	1	
	sign.	.000	.000		
variety transport modes	Pearson	.29	.28	.56	1
	sign.	.000	.000	.000	

Note. MOBILATE Survey 2000; weighted; N = 3934

Table 10.2: Correlations between main aspects of mobility in Pearson correlation coefficients

	trip * activities	trip * modes	activities * modes
Finland	0.37	0.38	0.55
Estern Germany	0.30	0.19	0.53
Western Germany	0.31	0.22	0.42
Hungary	0.32	0.27	0.54
Italy	0.45	0.42	0.55
Netherlands	0.24	0.14	0.47

Note. MOBILATE Survey 2000; weighted N = 3934
All coefficients are significant (p <.01)

In a second step, we divided the total sample into a number of subgroups which show a maximal contrast in the number of trips made. A CHAID analysis was used to divide all subgroups of the sample in such a way that the subgroups have a maximal contrast on the dependent variable (Magidson, 1993). For this analysis, 4 variables were split up in 3 or 4 subgroups, depending on the desired number of respondents in each subgroup. Each variable has a subgroup 0, a highest group, and one or two in between (a larger number of subgroups were needed for the variables 'numbers of activities' and 'transportation modes'). Figure 10.1 shows the distribution of the subgroups.

Figure 10.1: CHAID contrasting subgroups divided on the percentages of trip making

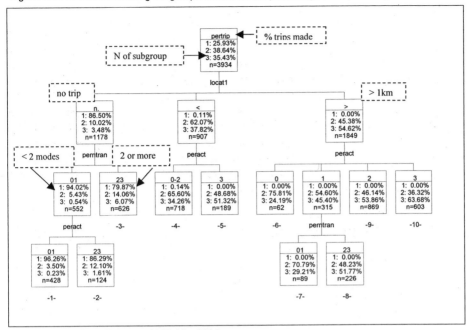

Note. MOBILATE Survey 2000, N = 3934

PERTRIP: percentages of average number of trips per day (0=0, 1=<2, 2=≥2)
PERNTRAN: percentages of numbers of transport modes used (0=0, 1=<2, 2=≥ 2 and <4, 3=≥ 4)
PERACT: percentages of outdoor activities (0=0, 1=<2, 2=≥2 and <6, 3=≥ 6)
LOCAT1: range of trips (0=0, 1=< 1km, 2=> 1km)

The mean number of trips (including trips back home) was chosen as the dependent variable. This variable was used to split up the sample into 3 groups: 1 (no trip), 2 (less than 2 trips), and 3 (2 or more trips).

This group was further split up first by the distance covered (locat1): 87% of the persons who cover no distance made no trip; this group could be further split up by number of transport means and then by number of activities (total 1,178 persons). This results in a subgroup in which 96% made no trip. These respondents have little variety in outdoor activities, few transportation modes available, and travel short distances.

The long distance group was further split up by number of activities: group 9 and 10, both with rather high variety in activities, and consisting of mobile people: 54 - 64% made more than 2 trips (1472 respondents).

There is a rather large group (1300 respondents) in between, with low mobility in terms of number of trips made, but no clear distinction in activities and number of transport modes. This makes it difficult to use these variables together to divide the total group into relevant subgroups. We believe, however, that these characteristics are important to describe the mobility of people, and they are therefore employed separately in our analyses.

10.3   The mobility needs of older people

What are the mobility needs of elderly people? How can we measure or analyse them? Are there any indications of a discrepancy between the needs of the elderly and the level of mobility they are able to achieve?

The variable that comes closest is the satisfaction people have with the different aspects of mobility and the interrelation of these with quality of life. The overview in Table 10.3 shows satisfaction to be generally high, but it also clearly shows differences between urban and rural areas. In all countries the satisfaction in rural areas is lower, except for the Netherlands and western Germany. An evaluation of lower than 6 is a rather negative reaction, and such low satisfaction ratings can be found in several rural areas. In Italy and western Germany, public transport is evaluated very negatively, in Hungary, the possibilities to pursue leisure activities, and in eastern Germany, the availability of services and facilities don't seem to correspond to older people's needs. These findings can be seen as an indication of a discrepancy between what people expect and what is available to them in rural areas.

Table 10.3: Mean satisfaction[1] scores for mobility related aspects per country

URBAN	Finland	Eastern Germany	Western Germany	Hungary	Italy	The Netherlands
	Mean	Mean	Mean	Mean	Mean	Mean
Satisfaction leisure activities	8.4	7.0	7.3	7.8	7.8	7.5
Satisfaction services and facilities	7.4	7.3	7.7	7.9	6.7	6.7
Satisfaction mobility	8.5	7.6	7.8	7.9	8.1	7.5
Satisfaction public transport	8.2	7.1	7.7	7.5	6.4	6.3
Satisfaction travelling	8.0	8.6	8.2	8.2	8.4	8.1

RURAL	Finland	Eastern Germany	Western Germany	Hungary	Italy	The Netherlands
	Mean	Mean	Mean	Mean	Mean	Mean
Satisfaction leisure activities	7.8	6.1	7.5	5.9	6.8	7.5
Satisfaction services and facilities	7.1	5.7	7.2	7.3	6.2	7.2
Satisfaction mobility	8.1	7.7	7.6	6.0	7.0	7.8
Satisfaction public transport	6.2	6.6	5.3	6.6	4.9	6.4
Satisfaction travelling	8.2	8.0	8.7	7.2	9.9	8.6

Note. MOBILATE Survey 2000, weighted, N = 3950
[1] Assessed on an 11-point scale (0 = completely unsatisfied: 10 = completely satisfied)

Satisfaction is always a relative measurement. People judge the present situation against some personal means of reference. This could be a situation in the past, or the situation of friends or peers. A positive value means that they have positive feelings about the subject related to their point of reference. This does not mean that they have no unfulfilled needs, but they can cope with them or have come to terms with the facts as they are. Moreover, there is no absolute reference point. Standards of reference can be different per country and will be different per person.

Travelling got, on average, rather high scores, perhaps because older people no longer go on long trips and are happy with what they can do. Conversely, perhaps elders use travel opportunities much more extensively than they could in their younger years and therefore are satisfied (see also section 6.3.6 on this issue).

Public transport got the lowest values, especially in Italy. This means that people experience the most shortcomings in this mode of transportation. In short, public transportation does not offer what people expect of it.

With regards to *services and facilities*, older people are dissatisfied in eastern Germany, Italy, and the Netherlands, but this is not necessarily in line with the availability of such services. Dissatisfaction could be related to comparisons made with past service delivery or comparisons with other residential areas.

In general, this approach does not show large discrepancies between expectations and the existing environment, except for public transport and the accessibility of services. Pervasive problems are probably indicated when respondents report a rather low satisfaction score across many domains. Further analyses showed that 19 persons had a score of 4 or lower on the satisfaction scales for mobility, public transport, travelling, services, and leisure. Only one person out of five (86 persons) had an average score of 5 or lower on these five aspects and only 2% had an average score of 4 or lower. For these people one may expect that they feel a rather serious discrepancy between their needs and what the environment can offer (see also the chapter on the 'Mobility rich' and 'Mobility poor').

10.3.1   Barriers and hindrances in the mobility of people of old age

What are the main barriers and hindrances to mobility? In our view, mobility is needed to realise specific activities at different places and originates in an interrelation between a person (with certain personal, physical and psychological characteristics) and the environment (with spatial and social dimensions). Mobility serves a purpose; it facilitates a desired action. Therefore, we collected information on:

- spatial environment: housing conditions, services and facilities: available and accessible, spatial context: urban-rural;
- social context: network as drive or support;
- transport conditions: available means of transport, public transport, distances to relevant destinations;
- physical conditions: actual and experienced physical conditions such as walking, vision, hearing, ADL;
- mental or psychological background, and
- personal background: marital status, socio-economical conditions, education, age, gender.

For reaching services and social networks, distance is very often the critical factor. The transportation system offers good or bad conditions for reaching destinations, sometimes enforced by the spatial environment. Basic personal factors also play a role: the physical mobility and ability to perform the activities of daily living (ADL) are resources for pursuing out-of-home activities, and the psychological characteristics of the individual influence his or her needs and drive to cope with worsening conditions. We do not address these issues in this inventory of the hindrances experienced by people of old age. Instead, we focus in this section on the external hindrances and barriers experienced by older people (see also Chapter 9; for psychological influences, see Chapter 7).

10.3.1.1   Hindrances in the spatial environment

An important factor in the spatial context concerns the availability and accessibility of services. Wachs (1979) argued that "Observed behaviour represents the interaction of the supply of available services with the demand for travel" (p. 212). This report offers support for this claim, since more trips (2.2) were made in urban areas than in rural ones (1.9).

The availability of services has been measured in the survey as accessibility: a service is available if it is accessible within 15 minutes by normal transport means.

Table 10.4:   Accessibility of services and facilities in the spatial environment

service	Urban	Rural
food store	95	85
pharmacy	90	70
doctor	87	76
bank	80	73
post office	83	74
park, green area	85	81
bus stop	97	93
church	80	86
cemetery	54	84
hairdresser	85	73
library	45	50

Note. MOBILATE Survey 2000; weighted, N = 3950

The list of services in Table 10.4 has been taken from former research initiatives (see again Chapter 9). It comes as no surprise that services are more accessible in the urban context. Only the church and cemetery (and strangely, the library) are more available in the rural areas. In urban areas, the services are accessible within 15 minutes for more than 85% of the older people; in the rural area this percentage falls to about 70%. These people may have difficulty reaching essential services such as food store, pharmacy or medical doctor.

Distance is usually the most important hindrance to accessibility. When questioned regarding difficulties, respondents usually first mention their bad health and second the distance. Both can be seen as interrelated: longer distances need more effort to cover.

In other parts of the survey, further spatial aspects were mentioned as hindrances. Car drivers avoid darkness and bad roads. Cyclists and pedestrians also report difficulty travelling in the dark. Pedestrians are most sensitive to problems that arise in the spatial context, such as bad roads, lack of pedestrian crossovers, and busy roads without sidewalks.

People also reacted to statements on the present traffic situation. Some of these statements concern spatial elements, such as: lack of pedestrian crossings (72% true or partly true), too narrow sidewalks (73%), mix of cyclists and pedestrians (51%), and not enough cycle lanes (84%).

Respondents also suggested how the transportation system might be improved. The improvements they listed included:

more benches,	44%
more control in public spaces,	40%
more cycle paths are important,	36%
more pedestrian crossings,	30%

more shops and services nearby,   30%
better access to public buildings (no stairs),   30%
more special parking places,   25%
more meeting points at big bus stations   11%.

This overview affords an idea about the spatial problems older people experience. The distance to services is the main hindrance. In other cases, the circumstances of the route and conditions at the destination play a major role: lighting, pedestrian crossings, well-tended and clearly designated pedestrian routes, rest areas, parking, and easy access to public buildings.

10.3.1.2   Hindrances in the social context

The social context can be both a stimulus and a form of support for mobility. Having a partner with a car makes it easier to go out, particularly for people who don't have a driving license. However, living together or having children were not very decisive for outdoor mobility. There were no differences between people living alone and those living with others regarding trip-making behaviour, even when controlling for age. With increasing age the mean number of trips made decreased, but across all groups, the number was quite similar (see Chapter 8 on Social Relations). Children could support elder mobility by driving the car or by acting as companion, but also having children made no difference in the mean numbers of trips undertaken. This shows clearly that living with other people or having children is not decisive for the number of trips made.

Nonetheless, the social context obviously influences trip-making behaviour. Individuals with a social network outside the own household made more trips (trip mean of 2.2 a day) than people without important persons living outside the household (trip mean 1.8). Hence, the presence of an out-of-home social network was in fact a stimulus to go out.

Table 10.5: Most important obstacles to meeting the most important person outside of the household, differentiated by living situation(%)

Obstacles	total	Living together	living alone
General health reasons	65	60	74
Relatives and friends live too far away	27	28	26
No car available	10	10	9
No one to go with	8	8	9
Too expensive	7	7	8
Difficulty in using public transport	6	6	6
Bad connected	5	5	6
I have to care for a family member	4	7	1
Bad road conditions	4	4	4
No public transportation	4	5	3
Have to take stairs to get into the flat	4	4	4
There isn't anyone who could pick me up	3	2	4
I feel insecure when it is dark	3	2	4
Have to cross difficult/broad streets	2	2	2
No parking	1	2	0
Not enough time	1	2	0
Other reasons	10	10	11

Note. MOBILATE Survey 2000

In general, hindrances cannot be found in the social context. Table 10.5 shows that poor health was the most important obstacle to meeting persons out of home. Distance is the second reason, and the relation to health or physical mobility is obvious. Lack of a car or household composition were less important, even when one examines the items that are directly related to this issue (e.g., 'There isn't anyone who could pick me up.') The most important difference between those who live alone and those who do not, concerns their health, which must be viewed in light of the fact that most of the oldest people live alone.

10.3.1.3 Hindrances in the transport system

The greater the variety in available modes of transportation, the better the conditions for mobility. The older generation typically has problems using various modes of transportation. Therefore, the variety of modes used serves as an indicator of mobility. The respective figures (see Chapter 5 on Transport Behaviour and Realised Journeys and Trips) show clearly that the private modes of transportation, i.e., walking, cycling and riding a car, are the most preferred ones. Among the present generation of older people, not everyone has a driver's licence, especially older women. They also seem to have more problems in handling the complex task of driving.

Public transport could be an alternative, but the figures suggest that this mode is chosen only when there are no other options or when service is excellent, as is the case for example in urban areas where bus stops are everywhere and the buses run frequently. Older people have more problems than others using and accessing public transportation. These findings confirm the statement of Rosenbloom (2003) that it is necessary to debunk the myth that elderly people first lose the ability to drive, and then use public transport, after that walk and finally go to special transport. Long before they lose the ability to drive they are unable to board and ride public transportation.

The present study examined what kind of hindrances elders typically encounter using three different approaches:

1.   The elders' opinions regarding what made a trip comfortable or uncomfortable offer one kind of insight into the problem. Note that only persons who actually made a trip could be assessed regarding comfort, and very poor transportation conditions could have prevented some from making any trips at all. For those who did make a trip, the comfort of a trip was enhanced by:

     19%   light traffic,
     18%   broad and plain sidewalks,
     13%   traffic calmed areas,
     9%   good parking places near destinations.

The small group who mentioned discomfort of the journey, mentioned most:

     21%   heavy traffic,
     12%   problems with health,
     7%   parking problems,
     6%   too many people.

Hence, the amount of traffic was important, as well as the availability of parking places and good sidewalks. Regarding personal factors, health played a role.

2.   The respondents' reactions to the present traffic situation provides further information. We summarise only the percentages of statements directly related to the functioning of the traffic system:

46%	doors of buses and trams close too fast,
43%	problems in reading timetables and route maps,
41%	problems in getting in or out a bus,
38%	traffic lights go too fast to red,
32%	frequency of buses is too low,
27%	not enough seats or shelters at bus stops.

Virtually most of these items deal with riding the bus. Traffic lights, which change quickly to red, made elderly traffic participants nervous.

3.   We also asked all of the respondents to look to the future and select the three most important ways of improving traffic situations for them personally (see Table 5.28 in Chapter 5). Interestingly, the respondents did not give highest priority to typical kinds of traffic improvements such as more pedestrian crossings or technical improvements; rather, courtesy and help from passerbys, as well as the economical situation and the costs of travelling were rated as being most important. Among the more typical traffic items, bus design that is adapted to the needs of older people received the highest score. Two items concerning public safety follow these items. From these findings, it is evident that the social context of trip making has the highest priority and that typical transport items have a relatively lower one. This can be traced back to the lack of some basic conditions for the elderly traffic users. However, regardless of the approach used, the result is the same: the context of travelling is rather important: public safety, courtesy, shelter for bad weather, no darkness, and economical aspects.

10.3.2   Coping behaviour of elderly people

Older people have many problems with outdoor mobility. How do they cope with these problems? As early as 1985, the OECD (1985) published a report on the traffic safety of elderly road users. In this report they mention the performance of elderly people in traffic and the ways they cope with the personal changes. They mention that older people drive much less kilometres compared to younger people. Changes in driving behaviour include reduction of speed, less driving at peak hours, shorter distances and less driving at night (also found by others, e.g. Schlag, 1990). In the most recent report of the OECD (2001), the same coping strategies were mentioned: reducing car driving, only taking local trips, avoiding bad weather, night time, rush hour, and unfamiliar places. We summarise here several solutions reported by our respondents:

Avoiding unwanted or complicated situations

The OECD findings can be confirmed and deepened by our research. In the survey we gave a list of situations which one could avoid to car drivers, cyclists and pedestrians, asking them for their own behaviour. In the transport chapter these items are extensively summarised in tables. Here we only report the most striking findings:

Older people tried to avoid situations which they experience as hindrances and which they have mentioned before as situations that should be changed. These concern bad weather, long distances, darkness, and unsafe public routes or places. The weather and public safety may be more critical for cyclists and pedestrians, whereas for car drivers, rush hour was avoided, as can be seen in the graph of the time expenditure (see Chapter 12).

Immobility

As mentioned earlier, age is accompanied by health problems, which affect the mobility of older people. By dividing the ADL scale into three categories, we see that people without any ADL problem made 1.15 journeys a day, while people with serious ADL problems made 0.63 journeys a day. For self-reported physical mobility, the same relation was found: people with very good physical mobility made 1.18 journeys a day whereas people with very poor mobility made only 0.31 journeys a day. Health problems are reported more often by older people, and in all analyses, older respondents made fewer trips than younger ones. This is the most obvious way of coping with mobility problems.

Adaptation of the trip making behaviour

The graphs with the distribution of activities during the day show clearly that older respondents more often stay at home during the day and after 18:00 than young respondents do (Figures 10.2, 10.3).

People in worse physical condition travel also shorter distances. Only 17% of people with self-reported very poor physical mobility travelled more than 1 km compared to 65% of people with very good physical mobility. 63% of people with no ADL problem travelled more than 1 km, whereas only 33% of those with many ADL problems did so.

Figure 10.2: People active outdoors from 6:00 - 21:00, age group 55 - 74

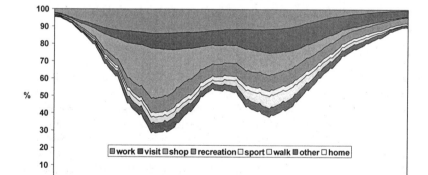

Note. MOBILATE Survey 2000, N = 2175

Figure 10.3: People active outdoors from 6:00 - 21:00, age group 75+

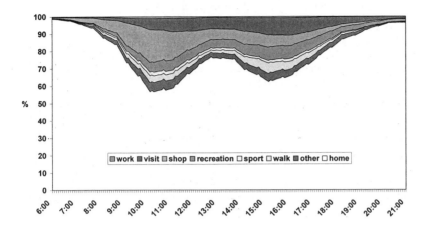

Note. MOBILATE Survey 2000, N = 1775

People adapt to old age and poor health by making different choices. One way to cope with impediments to mobility could be to select a different mode of transportation. Surprisingly, health problems led elders to travel by foot: 35% of the trips made by elders with no ADL problem were by foot compared to 56% in the frailest group. The same can be found for age: in the youngest group, 43% of the trips were made by foot, while this figure is 60% for those in the oldest group. This does not mean that older people made more trips, but only that the share of pedestrian trips increased. This pattern of behaviour may be due to a decrease of car trips or the lack of good alternatives, i.e., it could be a forced choice situation. Several licensed car drivers stopped driving, mostly for health reasons. Wachs (1979) mentioned that a decline in drivers' licenses is due to the process of ageing. Some people give up driving, others forego driving because of physicians' instructions or because they become unable to qualify for a license.

The availability of a car was the main reason for not using public transport. The use of the main transport modes shows clearly that older people went less by car and walking was the most common mode of transportation. This is not always by free choice, but often due to a lack of alternatives: elders can not always use a car (health reasons, too expensive), they may not be used to public transport, or be unable to access it. The decision to walk explains the short distances covered on the average trip. Elders often go to nearby shops and services and they more often go by foot. But the decision to travel more often by foot is more often made by the frailest group of elderly, who are faced with no alternatives. They are forced to choose a dangerous mode of transportation; most traffic victims are pedestrians, and the very old run considerable physical risk given their generally frail state of health.

Social support in trip making

Company can also be a solution for feelings of insecurity or for a lack of self-confidence based on a bad health condition. 46% of the trips taken by the oldest age group were made alone, whereas this figure was 55% for the younger age group.

Another indication of social support could be found in the change of transportation mode. The first change one would expect is the move from driver to passenger. In the group of people with no ADL problem, 42% of the trips were made as a car driver and 8% as a car passenger. In the group with serious problems, these figures were 16% and 15% respectively, which confirms this expectation.

10.4   Improvement of the mobility conditions

How can mobility be improved? What obstacles can be removed or ameliorated? To answer this question, elders' reactions to the current traffic situation, information on transport alternatives, or the tailor-made, demand-responsive transport system used in the Netherlands might be used. Potential improvements also offer better conditions for other mobility-impaired groups: the handicapped, children or people travelling with children.

One might begin by accepting the fact that private modes are the first choice, not only of older people. If age-related circumstance reduces the use of fast modes of transportation, walking becomes a very important transport mode, especially for the oldest age group, and perhaps the last available option. This means that the residential environment of older people should offer the most important services within walking distance. Moreover, these places and routes must be designed in accordance with the present findings on avoidance behaviour, the elderly individual's evaluation of the present traffic situation, the wanted desired improvements in the traffic situation, and the conditions that make a trip comfortable or uncomfortable.

Technology can be used to remove or to lighten some of the mobility problems experienced by the elderly traffic user. The OECD (2001) is rather optimistic about the role of technology for elderly people; they espouse the view that vehicles and road infrastructure can be improved by better information and communication systems (ICT). ICT can also reduce the need for transportation, because of the increasing role of tele-activities. This is a two-edged sword, however, because older people should be encouraged to maintain their mobility, especially their physical mobility, as a matter of principle.

The analysis of the use of new technologies shows that older people do use automatic teller machines and ticket machines. Elders are sometimes forced to use technologies for lack of alternatives, but our data clearly show that the users very often are happy with the new situation. This confirms what other research shows: older people need some practice, a good introduction to the technology, and must have a clear need to use the new equipment, but then they also will be happy users (see also Tacken, Marcellini, Mollenkopf et al., 2005) .

Two new opportunities for using ICT to improve the lives of the elderly present themselves. ICT can bridge distances and bring services and facilities, which are located far from the residences (teleshopping, telebanking, telelearning, telelibrary, etc...) within reach. On the other hand new technology can make the mobility easier by improving in-vehicle technology (cruise-control, anti-collision equipment, way-finding etc.), intelligent infrastructure (dynamic route information, warning for icy or slippery roads) and better information on the available alternatives in public transport (location of nearest stops, travel information, arrangement of journeys; OECD, 2001; Docampo Rama, 2001; Technieuws, 1991).

One of the possibilities related to the more common introduction of ICT is the tailor-made or demand responsive transport. This type of transport relies on ICT for the organisation, the functioning of the system, and the communication between users and vehicle operators. The Dutch case shows that it works, that it can be a useful alternative for the specific mobility problems of older people. For the specific groups, e.g., older women, those with a low income or no car and no good public transportation alternatives, this type of service can be worthwhile. Unfortunately, the present figures show this service did not become a relevant part on the transportation market for older people. In the Dutch sample, only a small group of respondents actually used the service. The present service can be criticised on several grounds; it has become clear that the introduction of a new service should be very well prepared, user-friendly, and provide up-to-date information on the system.

References

Docampo Rama, M. (2001). *Technology generations handling complex user interfaces.* Eindhoven: Technical University of Eindhoven (TUE).

Magidson, J. (1993). *SPSS for Windows CHAID Release 6.0.* Illinois: SPSS inc.

OECD (1985). *Traffic safety of elderly road users.* Paris: OECD, Road Transport Research.

OECD (2001). *Ageing and Transport, Mobility needs and safety issues.* Paris: OECD.

Rosenbloom, S. (2003), *The mobility needs of older Americans: implications for transportation reauthorisation.* The Brookings Institution Series on Transformation Reform, Centre on urban and metropolitan policy. Washington. www.brookings.edu/urban

Schlag, B. (1990). Empirische Untersuchungen zur Leistunsfähigkeit älterer Kraftfahrer [Emperical Research of Older Drivers' Capacity]. *Zeitschrift für Gerontologie*, 23, 300-306.

Tacken, M., Marcellini, F., Mollenkopf, H., Ruoppila, I., & Széman, Z. (2005). Use and acceptance of new technology by older people. Findings of the international MOBILATE survey: 'Enhancing mobility in later life'. *Gerontechnology* (3), 3, 126-137.

Technieuws Washingtoon (1991*).* Intelligente Autos en snelwegen [Intelligent cars and highways]. In *Technieuws, 's Gravenhage: Ministry of Economical Affairs.*

Wachs, M. (1979). *Transportation for the elderly, Changing lifestyles, changing needs.* Berkeley: University of California Press.

Enhancing Mobility in Later Life
H. Mollenkopf et al. (Eds.)
IOS Press, 2005

Chapter 11
A New Concept of Out-of-Home Mobility

Heidrun Mollenkopf, Stephan Baas, Fiorella Marcellini, Frank Oswald, Isto Ruoppila,
Zsuzsa Széman, Mart Tacken, and Hans-Werner Wahl

11.1   Introduction

One main objective of the MOBILATE project was to provide a comprehensive and detailed description and explanation of the actual out-of-home mobility of older people. In this chapter, we take up again our concept of mobility as a complex phenomenon, based on motives and transport options, and realised in everyday trips. In other words, flexibility regarding different transport modes and a wide range of leisure time interests as motives for out-of-home mobility are taken into consideration.

Figure 11.1: The MOBILATE Model of Out-of-home Mobility

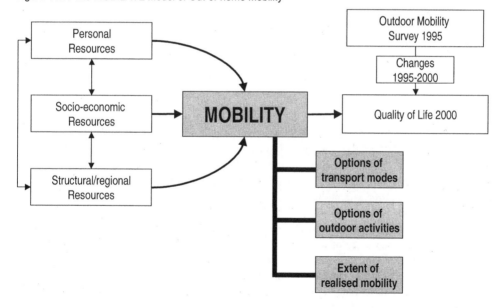

Accordingly, descriptive analyses of these three indicators of out-of-home mobility are presented. In a second step, the different aspects of out-of-home mobility are explained in bivariate analyses. The comprehensive model of out-of-home mobility employed is related to the model introduced in the introduction to this book and includes three parts (see Figure 11.1; see also Figure 1.1):

- The number of *transport modes used* covers the variety of transport options available to a person.
- The number of options of *outdoor activities performed* shows the variety of activities that may lead a person to become mobile.
- The *extent of realised mobility* per day and person is based on the mobility diaries (number of realised trips per day and per person).

11.2   Mobility indicators

11.2.1   The options of transport modes

The reported number of transport modes used was calculated from the following list:
- on foot,
- bicycle,
- private car as driver,
- private car as passenger,
- moped/motorcycle,
- bus,
- tram (not assessed in Finland),
- train,
- taxi,
- shuttle taxi,
- special driving service,
- plane,
- ship (only assessed in Finland),
- and other means of transportation.

A mobility index based on transport options can be calculated by aggregating the number of transport modes used; the index ranges from 0 (immobile) to 13 (use of every mode of transportation). Using a large number of transport modes does not necessarily mean that the person in question is more mobile; rather, it indicates that the person uses a larger variety of modes and thus has more mobility options at his or her disposal.

The greatest variety of transport modes was reported by older Finnish people, both in the urban and rural areas, when compared to all respective regions (Table 11.1). Moreover, both urban and rural Dutch elders reported a comparatively broad range of transport modes available. The smallest range of transport modes was reported by older Hungarian and Italian people, especially those living in the rural Italian area, which is possibly due to differences in the infrastructure and to mobility habits in different cultures. For example, public transportation is less available in the Italian rural area, and Hungarian elders reported the lowest availability of private cars compared to all other respondents.

In all participating countries, older urbanites had significantly more transport modes available than their contemporaries living in the countryside, which is an expected result due to the higher availability of public transport in city areas. When distinguishing between genders, it became obvious that in all countries, men reported more transport options than women (although the difference reached statistical significance only in four sites). This is probably due to the fact that more men drive.

Table 11.1: Options of transport modes used[1] in different countries (mean of sumscores)

0-13	Finland		Eastern Germany		Western Germany		Hungary		Italy		The Netherlands	
	Mean	SD	Mean	SD	Mean	SD	Mean	SD	Mean	SD	Mean	SD
Region												
Urban	5.4	2.4	4.0	1.9	4.9	2.3	3.3	1.5	4.0	1.7	4.5	2.1
Rural	4.1	1.9	3.5	1.4	3.1	1.4	2.9	1.6	2.7	1.1	4.1	2.0
Difference between regions	***		***		***		***		***		**	
Gender												
Male	5.2	1.9	4.1	1.5	4.1	1.8	3.4	1.5	3.9	1.4	4.3	2.0
Female	4.5	2.5	3.6	1.9	3.9	2.4	2.9	1.6	3.0	1.6	4.2	2.1
Difference between genders	***		***		n.s.		***		***		n.s.	
Age												
55-74	5.3	2.5	4.2	1.7	4.4	2.6	3.3	1.9	3.7	1.8	4.6	2.3
75+	3.4	1.5	2.5	1.2	2.7	1.5	2.3	1.0	2.5	1.0	3.3	1.5
Difference between age-groups	***		***		***		***		***		***	

Note. MOBILATE Survey 2000; weighted, N = 3950; **=$p<0.01$, ***=$p<0.001$
[1] Sumscore ranging from 0 (no transport mode used, respondent is immobile) to 13 (all transport modes are used)

Also as expected, younger elders (aged 55 to 74 years) used significantly more transport modes than people aged 75 or older in all countries under investigation. The biggest difference between the age groups was found for Finland, whereas the smallest difference was found for Hungary. Regardless of age, Hungarian elders were deprived in terms of available transport modes.

11.2.2 Options of outdoor activities

The second indicator shows the variety of outdoor activities a person pursues. In order to also include information on activities that are not part of the everyday routine, the diversity of outdoor activities was calculated from the following list:

- meeting friends, relatives or acquaintances (outside one's home),
- going to a café, restaurant or bar,
- going out for a walk / strolling through the town,
- making small trips or journeys,
- gardening,
- hiking / riding a bicycle,

- dancing / bowling,
- actively pursuing sports,
- watching sporting events (not on TV),
- visiting theatre / opera / concerts / movies,
- visiting a library,
- taking courses and further education,
- religious events / attending church,
- fishing
- hunting
- picking berries and mushrooms,
- activities in clubs or associations,
- activities for retired people,
- travelling (at least one week).

Again, a high outdoor activity sum score does not necessarily mean that the person in question is more active or mobile; rather, it indicates that he or she can and does pursue a large diversity of activities. The range differed between the regions under investigation due to the fact that one or several modes were not assessed, i.e., were not common in the respective country. Therefore, the sum scores of outdoor activities were standardised to the number of activities assessed in each country. Due to this standardisation, the range of this index was between 0, which means that a person pursued no outdoor activity at all and 1, which means that a person pursued all of the outdoor activities assessed.

Older people in the Netherlands pursued the most activities, and western German and Finnish elders also pursued a large number of different outdoor activities (Table 11.2). Older Hungarians and Italians had the lowest level of outdoor activity. When distinguishing the urban and rural areas under investigation, no clear pattern was visible: in the Finnish, Hungarian and Italian regions, more outdoor activities were reported in the cities, whereas virtually no rural-urban differences were found in the German regions. In the Dutch rural area, more activities were reported compared to the urban area. One might expect that the opportunity to perform different outdoor activities is larger in cities - which seems to be evident in the findings from the Finnish, Hungarian and Italian regions. On the other hand, this assumption does not appear to be true for elders living in rural western Germany. They perform about the same number of outdoor activities as those living in the urban areas, although the opportunity structure for outdoor activity surely differs. As already stated, the rural Dutch area was very suburban, which might have led to the fact that Dutch respondents living in the rural area reported significantly more outdoor activities compared to the urban area.

Moreover, differences between men and women in number of outdoor activities were not readily apparent, with the exception of eastern Germany and Italy: in these countries, older men showed a greater variety of outdoor activities than their female counterparts. Italian women reported the lowest level of outdoor activities of all respondents. Though again, a similar level of outdoor activities in all other countries does not automatically mean a similar structure of activities - they again might differ due to gender.

Clear differences were found when analysing the number of activities by age: unsurprisingly, the younger elders in all countries reported a significantly higher level of activity when compared to persons aged 75 years of age and older.

Table 11.2: Options of outdoor activities[1] pursued in different countries (mean of sumscores)

0-1	Finland		Eastern Germany-		Western Germany		Hungary		Italy		The Netherlands	
	Mean	SD	Mean	SD	Mean	SD	Mean	SD	Mean	SD	Mean	SD
Region												
Urban	0.37	0.17	0.26	0.17	0.29	0.18	0.20	0.16	0.21	0.15	0.36	0.21
Rural	0.28	0.17	0.23	0.14	0.30	0.18	0.14	0.11	0.14	0.11	0.40	0.22
Difference between regions	***		*		n.s.		***		***		*	
Gender												
Male	0.31	0.15	0.26	0.14	0.31	0.17	0.17	0.13	0.23	0.14	0.39	0.21
Female	0.33	0.2	0.23	0.17	0.29	0.19	0.17	0.16	0.14	0.13	0.38	0.21
Difference between genders	n.s.		**		n.s.		n.s.		***		n.s.	
Age												
55-74	0.36	0.20	0.27	0.17	0.33	0.19	0.18	0.18	0.21	0.17	0.42	0.24
75+	0.21	0.11	0.14	0.09	0.19	0.12	0.12	0.08	0.12	0.08	0.28	0.15
Difference between age-groups	***		***		***		***		***		***	

Note. MOBILATE Survey 2000; N = 3950, weighted. **=$p<0.01$, ***=$p<0.001$
[1] Standardized sumscore ranging from 0 (no outdoor activity pursued) to 1 (all asked outdoor activities pursued)

11.2.3   Extent of realised mobility

The third indicator of mobility is the number of actual trips taken per day and per person, as reported in the MOBILATE diaries.

International comparisons did not produce a clear picture using this indicator of mobility: The number of trips per day and person was highest for older people in Finland, followed by the older Italians. On the other hand, Dutch respondents reported the lowest level of out-of-home mobility (for details about the out-of-home mobility and differences between the countries under investigation, see Chapter 5). The extent of mobility did not differ between the urban and rural regions in most countries, except for Hungary and the Netherlands. In these countries, older people living in the urban areas reported a significantly higher level of out-of-home mobility compared to those living in the rural area. The same pattern was found for the Italian, eastern German and Finnish elders, although these differences were not significant (Table 11.3).

Actual mobility patterns differed between genders in Finland, eastern Germany and in particular, Italy. In these countries, older men reported a significantly higher number of trips per day and person, while in western Germany, Hungary and the Netherlands, no such differences were found. Younger elders in general reported a higher level of actual out-of-home mobility (measured by the number of trips) when compared to older respondents.

Table 11.3: Extent of realised mobility (mean number of trips per day and person)

	Finland		Eastern Germany		Western Germany		Hungary		Italy		The Netherlands	
	Mean	SD	Mean	SD	Mean	SD	Mean	SD	Mean	SD	Mean	SD
Region												
Urban	3.0	1.8	2.0	1.3	2.0	1.6	2.0	1.4	2.6	1.9	1.7	1.7
Rural	2.7	1.9	1.9	1.5	2.2	1.9	1.2	1.4	2.3	1.9	1.1	1.7
Difference between regions	n.s.		n.s.		n.s.		***		n.s.		***	
Gender												
Male	3.1	1.8	2.1	1.3	2.2	1.6	1.6	1.4	3.2	1.8	1.4	1.8
Female	2.6	1.9	1.8	1.5	2.0	2.0	1.6	1.6	1.9	1.8	1.4	1.6
Difference between genders	***		**		n.s.		n.s.		***		n.s.	
Age												
55-74	3.2	2.3	2.1	1.5	2.3	2.0	1.8	1.8	2.9	2.2	1.5	2.1
75+	1.8	1.1	1.5	1.0	1.5	1.3	1.2	1.0	1.6	1.4	1.0	0.9
Difference between age-groups	***		***		***		***		***		**	

Note. MOBILATE Survey 2000; weighted, N = 3950; $**=p<0.01$, $***=p<0.001$

11.3   Explaining out-of-home mobility

In the following, the out-of-home mobility of older people is explained by means of mobility-related personal as well as environmental factors. As hypothesised in Figure 11.1, out-of-home mobility depends on personal resources (age, gender, health, competencies), socio-economic resources (education, income) and structural/regional resources including the social environment (urban/rural region, living environment, social network). The relation between all out-of-home mobility variables and different types of resources is tested for all three facets of out-of-home mobility using regression analyses.

When interpreting the results of the regression analyses the fact has to be considered that the number of eastern German, Hungarian and Dutch respondents included in the analyses was greatly influenced by listwise deletion. Only between 40% (Hungary) and 52% (eastern Germany) of all respondents were used in the regression analyses which might have led towards a distortion of our results. Income per person, the quality of the near vicinity, the provision of services and facilities, and the psychological test of visumotoric coordination (Digit Symbol Test) all had a high number of missings in the individual national samples as well as in the total sample. These variables are therefore responsible for most of the listwise deletions employed in the analyses.

In order to answer the question of whether the listwise deletion led to a positive, negative, or in fact, non-systematic bias of the regression analyses, the means of the mobility indicators (options of transport modes, options of outdoor activities, and realised mobility) were compared. The respective means of the respondents included in the analyses were compared with means of those who were not included due to listwise deletion of their predictors. As can be seen in Table 11.4, the analyses of the mobility indicators have a systematic distortion or positive bias. The means of respondents included in the regression analysis were significantly higher compared to the missing respondents in most cases: The latter respondents showed a significantly decreased level of out-of-home mobility - in terms of options of transport modes, number of outdoor activities, and actual number of trips taken. Those respondents who were included in the regression analyses were much more mobile. This is true not only for the samples with an insufficient number of respondents (eastern Germany, Hungary, the Netherlands), but also for those with a smaller number of listwise deletions (Finland, western Germany, and Italy). Therefore, the following results have to be interpreted with caution; they are positively biased towards an overestimation of out-of-home mobility in the regions under investigation.

Table 11.4: Means of different mobility indicators by respondents included in the regression analyses and missing respondents

	Finland	Eastern Germany	Western Germany	Hungary	Italy	The Netherlands	All countries
Options of transport modes[1]							
Analysed	4.8	3.8	3.8	3.3	3.3	4.3	4.0
Missing	3.0	3.5	3.8	2.7	2.9	3.8	3.3
Difference between groups	***	***	n.s.	***	**	**	***
Options of outdoor activities[2]							
Analysed	0.32	0.25	0.29	0.19	0.18	0.40	0.27
Missing	0.18	0.21	0.26	0.13	0.15	0.33	0.21
Difference between groups	***	**	n.s.	***	n.s.	***	***
Realised mobility[3]							
Analysed	2.8	2.0	2.2	2.0	2.6	1.6	2.3
Missing	1.9	1.8	1.5	1.2	1.7	1.0	1.5
Difference between groups	***	n.s.	***	***	***	***	***

Note. MOBILATE Survey 2000; **=$p<0.01$, ***=$p<0.001$
[1] Sumscore ranging from 0 (no transport mode used, respondent is immobile) to 13 (all transport modes are used)
[2] Standardized sumscore ranging from 0 (no outdoor activity pursued) to 1 (all asked outdoor activities pursued)
[3] Mean number of trips per person and day

11.3.1   Transport options

Out of the different types of predictors employed in the analysis, the region an individual lives in had the greatest impact on the variety of transport options used in all countries (Table 11.4). This result confirms our assumption that public transport is less available in rural areas in general. Besides region, higher income and education, better functional health, vision and visumotoric coordination were important prerequisites for using a larger variety of transport options as well. This finding confirms that using different transport options requires good health and better socio-economic background. Moreover we had assumed that the social network could offer a reason for taking trips, and could facilitate or actively support out-of-home mobility. This assumption, however, only found partial support in the analyses:

Although older people with a larger social network and those living together with others persons reported a larger variety of transport options, the contribution of having children to this variety was not important. In the following, we examine if the predictors of variety of transport modes remain the same across individual countries.

Detailed analyses for each country reveals that the region an individual lives in had the greatest impact on options of transport modes across all countries. In Finland, western Germany, Italy and the Netherlands, older people in the urban areas reported significantly more options of transport modes compared to those living in the rural areas, indicating that different kinds of public transport are less available in most rural areas under investigation; however, in eastern Germany and Hungary, no such differences were observed between elders living in urban and rural areas.

Aspects of the environment such as the availability of services and facilities or feelings of security when outside during the night did not play a decisive role in the number of transport options used in the individual countries. Besides region, certain socio-demographic characteristics were important and decisive in this respect: In the Finnish, eastern German and Hungarian regions, better educated people used more transport options than those with lower education, while in the Italian, western German and Dutch regions, education did not have any effect on the variety of transport options. Contrary to assumption, age and gender did not show any significant effects on the variety of transport modes used: for example, older individuals reported a smaller variety of transport options compared to younger persons only in the West German areas. Moreover, older Italian men used more transport options than women, which might be due to the fact that men more often drive a car. The elders' income did not show the expected effect on transport options: our assumption was that people with a higher income might be able to use more transport options (e.g., the availability of a car might depend on a person's income). In contrast, no significant relation was found. Concerning environmental aspects, older people in western Germany reported using more options of transport modes when the near vicinity was of higher quality (i.e., when the neighbourhood possessed a number of important features).

Contrary to expectation, a person's health did not have a consistent impact on the number of transport modes used in different countries. Our assumption that certain transport options might depend on one's health (especially walking, or driving a car) could not be proven by the regression analyses: satisfaction with health had no significant impact on transport options in any region. The ability to perform activities of the daily living (ADL) was not a significant predictor either. In fact, out of all health-related predictors, only visual acuity was a significant predictor of the variety of transport modes used among Finnish and Italian elders. Visumotoric coordination was important for ones' options only in Italy: in this country, older persons with higher fluid intelligence (measured by the Digit-Symbol-Substitution) used a greater variety of transport modes.

Table 11.5: Regression analysis of options of transport modes[1], all countries

	All countries	
	Stand. ß-weights	Semi-partial r^2
Socio-structural resources		
Age	-0.1***	0.7
Gender (1=male; 2=female)	-0.04	0.1
Education (years of full-time education)	0.1***	0.6
Income per person	0.14***	1.1
Satisfaction with income[2]	0.03	0.1
Regional resources		
Region (1=urban; 2=rural)	-0.19***	2.9
Satisfaction with area [2]	-0.04	0.1
Feeling secure when being outside during night (0=insecure; 1=secure)	0.02	0
Features of the neighbourhood (10 = high quality to 20 = low quality)	-0.04	0.1
Services within reach (10=all services accessible; 20=no service accessible)	0.07***	0.3
Satisfaction with services[2]	-0.04	0.1
Personal resources		
Visual acuity (0.02 to 1.00)	0.07***	0.4
Visual abilities (1=very poor; 5=very good)	-0.05**	0.2
ADL (10=all ADL possible, 30=no ADL possible)	-0.16***	1
Physical mobility (1=very poor; 5=very good)	-0.02	0
Satisfaction with health[2]	0.04	0.1
Digit-Symbol-Substitution[3]	0.08***	0.4
External control (powerful others) (1=strongly disagree; 5=strongly agree)	-0.02	0
Social resources		
Size of network	0.08***	0.6
Number of children	-0.03	0.1
Living alone (0=no; 1=yes)	-0.11***	0.8
Further resources		
Satisfaction with leisure activities [2]	0.05**	0.2
Indoor/outdoor motivation (0=indoor-type/10=outdoor-type)	0.02	0
Importance of being out (0=not important at all; 10=very important)	0.06**	0.3
N	2330	
Model r^2	0.36	

Note. MOBILATE Survey 2000

Analysis is based on N = 2330 due to listwise deletion of missings; **=p<0.01, ***=p<0.001

[1] Sumscore ranging from 0 (no transport mode used, respondent is immobile) to 13 (all transport modes are used)

[2] Self-evaluation rating on an 11-point rating scale, higher scores indicting higher satisfaction

[3] Range 1-67, higher scores indicate higher visumotoric coordination.

Table 11.6: Regression analysis of options of transport modes[1], differentiated by countries

	Finland		Eastern Germany		Western Germany	
	Stand. ß-weights	Semi-partial r[2]	Stand. ß-weights	Semi-partial r[2]	Stand. ß-weights	Semi-partial r[2]
Socio-structural resources						
Age	-0.03	0	-0.13	0.9	-0.16***	1.5
Gender (1=male; 2=female)	-0.08	0.4	-0.02	0	0.02	0
Education (years of full-time education)	0.16**	1.2	0.2***	2.7	0.08	0.4
Income per person	0.12	0.8	-0.06	0.2	0.05	0.1
Satisfaction with income[2]	-0.07	0.3	0.01	0	0.04	0.1
Regional resources						
Region (1=urban; 2=rural)	-0.14**	1.3	-0.06	0.2	-0.35***	6
Satisfaction with area [2]	-0.04	0.1	-0.05	0.2	-0.01	0
Feeling secure when being outside during night (0=insecure; 1=secure)	-0.01	0	-0.07	0.3	-0.05	0.1
Features of the neighbourhood (10 = high quality to 20 = low quality)	-0.04	0.1	0.05	0.1	-0.11**	0.8
Services within reach (10=all services accessible; 20=no service accessible)	0.09	0.5	0.06	0.3	0.07	0.3
Satisfaction with services[2]	-0.05	0.2	-0.08	0.4	-0.02	0
Personal resources						
Visual acuity (0.02 to 1.00)	0.12**	1	0.05	0.1	-0.06	0.2
Visual abilities (1=very poor; 5=very good)	-0.02	0	-0.1	0.8	-0.04	0.1
ADL (10=all ADL possible, 30=no ADL possible)	-0.15	0.7	-0.13	0.8	-0.09	0.3
Physical mobility (1=very poor; 5=very good)	0	0	-0	0	-0.08	0.2
Satisfaction with health[2]	0.03	0	0.05	0.1	0.07	0.2
Digit-Symbol-Substitution[3]	0.03	0	0.04	0.1	0.05	0.2
External control (powerful others) (1=strongly disagree; 5=strongly agree)	-0.04	0.1	-0.11	0.7	-0.06	0.2
Social resources						
Size of network	0.1	0.8	0.04	0.1	0.09	0.6
Number of children	0	0	-0.03	0.1	-0.15***	1.8
Living alone (0=no; 1=yes)	-0.07	0.3	-0.03	0.1	-0.15**	1.3
Further resources						
Satisfaction with leisure activities [2]	0.04	0.1	0.08	0.4	0.08	0.3
Indoor/outdoor motivation (0=indoor-type/ 10=outdoor-type)	0.1	0.8	-0.01	0	0.08	0.4
Importance of being out (0=not important at all; 10=very important)	0.02	0	0.13	1	0.05	0.1
N	480		400		490	
Model r[2]	0.38		0.28		0.42	

Note. MOBILATE Survey 2000

Analyses is based on recuded N in each country due to listwise deletion of missings,
**=p<0.01, ***=p<0.001

[1] Sumscore ranging from 0 (no transport mode used, respondent is immobile) to 13 (all transport modes are used)

[2] Self-evaluation rating on an 11-point rating scale, higher scores indicting higher satisfaction

[3] Range 1-67, higher scores indicate higher visumotoric coordination.

Table 11.7: Regression analysis of options of transport modes[1], differentiated by countries

	Hungary		Italy		The Netherlands	
	Stand. ß-weights	Semi-partial r^2	Stand. ß-weights	Semi-partial r^2	Stand. ß-weights	Semi-partial r^2
Socio-structural resources						
Age	-0.1	0.7	-0.08	0.3	-0.09	0.6
Gender (1=male; 2=female)	-0.07	0.3	-0.14***	1.3	0.05	0.2
Education (years of full-time education)	0.2**	2.2	0.05	0.1	0.08	0.5
Income per person	0.15	1.5	0.11	0.7	0.1	0.6
Satisfaction with income[2]	0.02	0	-0.08	0.5	0.08	0.5
Regional resources						
Region (1=urban; 2=rural)	0.09	0.5	-0.28***	3.8	-0.22***	4.2
Satisfaction with area [2]	-0.07	0.4	0	0	0.01	0
Feeling secure when being outside during night (0=insecure; 1=secure)	0.02	0	-0	0	0.06	0.3
Features of the neighbourhood (10 = high quality to 20 = low quality)	-0.09	0.6	-0.01	0	-0.05	0.2
Services within reach (10=all services accessible; 20=no service accessible)	0.14	1.1	0.08	0.4	0.03	0.1
Satisfaction with services[2]	0.04	0.1	-0.01	0	-0.11	0.8
Personal resources						
Visual acuity (0.02 to 1.00)	-0.04	0.1	0.11**	0.8	-0.05	0.2
Visual abilities (1=very poor; 5=very good)	-0.03	0.1	-0.01	0	-0.05	0.2
ADL (10=all ADL possible, 30=no ADL possible)	-0.14	0.7	-0.05	0.1	-0.13	0.7
Physical mobility (1=very poor; 5=very good)	0.03	0	0.09	0.3	0.15	0.9
Satisfaction with health[2]	0.09	0.4	-0.04	0.1	-0.01	0
Digit-Symbol-Substitution[3]	0.1	0.5	0.21**	1.2	0.05	0.2
External control (powerful others) (1=strongly disagree; 5=strongly agree)	-0	0	-0	0	-0.1	0.9
Social resources						
Size of network	0.05	0.2	-0.01	0	0	0
Number of children	0.01	0	-0.03	0.1	-0.08	0.6
Living alone (0=no; 1=yes)	-0.24***	3.9	-0.13***	1.3	-0.18**	1.9
Further resources						
Satisfaction with leisure activities [2]	0	0	0.07	0.3	0.06	0.2
Indoor/outdoor motivation (0=indoor-type/ 10=outdoor-type)	0.02	0	0.15***	1.3	0.03	0.1
Importance of being out (0=not important at all; 10=very important)	-0.08	0.5	-0.07	0.2	-0.02	0
N	244		433		278	
Model r^2	0.38		0.53		0.22	

Note. MOBILATE Survey 2000

Analyses is based on recuded N in each country due to listwise deletion of missings, **=p<0.01, ***=p<0.001

[1] Sumscore ranging from 0 (no transport mode used, respondent is immobile) to 13 (all transport modes are used)

[2] Self-evaluation rating on an 11-point rating scale, higher scores indicting higher satisfaction

[3] Range 1-67, higher scores indicate higher visumotoric coordination.

The impact of the social network differed between the countries under investigation. It could be hypothesized that people with a larger social network use a greater variety of transport options; wanting to visit people in one's network affords the individual a reason to go out, and the social network can support the individual's mobility. This hypothesis could not be proven by the data for all countries: children were not important for the variety of transport options used, and the size of a person's social network outside her or his household was not a significant predictor in any area either. Among social network factors, the size of the elders' households had the largest impact: those who lived alone reported a significantly reduced variety of transport options in all countries except for Finland and eastern Germany. Finally, outdoor motivation was not a significant predictor of the variety of different transport modes used (with the exception of Italy, where those persons who evaluated themselves as being an outdoor-type reported using significantly more transport modes).

Our hypothesized model fit best for Italy (53% of explained variance): Being male, living in an urban area, living together with other persons, and having higher visumotoric coordination increased the variety of transport options, while health did not show any impact. The model also explained a sufficient amount of variance in transport modes usage in western Germany (42%), although in this area, the transport options were only dependent on a person's age, the region lived in (urban area) and certain aspects of social relations. In contrast to our assumption, western Germans with fewer children reported a higher variety of transport options compared to others.

The model did not explain much variance among the Dutch and eastern German respondents (22% and 28% of explained variance, respectively). In the Netherlands, the variety of transport options used was higher among elders living in the urban area and living together with others. For eastern Germans, this aspect of out-of-home mobility was only dependent on their education, and contrary to most other countries, no difference was found between the urban and rural regions. Different patterns were found for Finnish and Hungarian elders: in the Finnish regions, the transport options were linked closely to living in the urban area, to education and visual acuity, while in Hungary, the region (urban or rural) made no difference.

11.3.2   Options of outdoor activities

The variety of outdoor activities can be explained to the same degree as the options of transport modes (36% vs. 38%), although outdoor activity depends on different preconditions as can be seen in Table 11.8. Among the socio-economic variables entered into the equation, only income per person had an impact on the variety of outdoor activities, while environment-related predictors were less important (at least compared with their impact on transport modes). This is especially true for the region a person lives in: the urban-rural variable had an impact on transport modes but was not important at all for outdoor activities. This was somewhat surprising: we had assumed that people living in urban areas might be able to pursue a larger variety of outdoor activities, but this hypothesis was not supported by our data. Still the patterns of activities might differ between urban and rural areas while the number of activities does not differ. Among the environment-related predictors, only high quality neighbourhoods supported a variety of activities. An individual's health and his or her visumotoric coordination were much more important for pursuing outdoor activities compared to other predictors, which accords well with the assumption that being able to move is an important prerequisite for being active outdoors.

Although social network had only limited impact on the variety of transport modes used, it did clearly influence outdoor activities: People with larger social networks and those living together with other persons reported significantly more outdoor activities. As expected, outdoor motivation and satisfaction with leisure activities were additional predictors of outdoor activities. Though, this pattern of predictors differed between the individual countries.

Detailed analyses for each country revealed that the region an older person lives in (either urban or rural) did not consistently affect the number of reported outdoor activities. Environmental factors, such as the availability of services and facilities, did not always have an important effect on outdoor activity either. The one exception was the quality of the near vicinity in the western German sample: the higher the quality of the vicinity, the more activities were performed. Socio-demographic aspects were even less important in the prediction of outdoor activity than in the variety of transport modes, except for gender in the Finnish and age in the Italian regions. Finnish women reported more outdoor activities than Finnish men, and young Italian men reported more outdoor activities than their older counterparts. Contrary to expectations, the variety of outdoor activities pursued hardly showed any relation to a person's financial situation when distinguishing by country. Again, it has to be stressed that the pattern of activity may still differ due to socio-structural variables such as age, gender or income; these relations are not visible when considering the level of outdoor activities in terms of the number of different activities pursued.

Health and social network showed slightly more influence on the variety of outdoor activities pursued than on variety of transport modes employed. This was true for all elders as well as for the individual regions. As expected, aspects of health (satisfaction with health, visumotoric coordination, ADL) were significantly positively related to the variety of outdoor activities in most countries. Higher satisfaction with health was associated with a higher number of outdoor activities (especially in western Germany). Higher self-rated physical mobility (Italy), better ability to perform the activities of daily living (ADL) (Finland), and better visual acuity (eastern Germany) were likewise associated with a larger variety of such activities. Finally, better visumotoric coordination went along with more outdoor activities, especially in eastern and western Germany. In sum, the better a person's health, the larger the variety of outdoor activities reported.

In addition, out of the different aspects describing older people's mobility, their social network showed a big impact on the outdoor activities both for all elders and when distinguishing between the different countries: The size of the social network was linked with the variety of outdoor activities (significant in all countries under investigation except for eastern Germany and Hungary): older people perform more outdoor activities when they have a larger social network outside their households. On the other hand, the size of their households was not related to outdoor activities, except for western Germans: those who lived together with other persons had a larger variety of outdoor activities compared to those living alone. Having children, however, did not have any systematic effect on outdoor activities. Another important precondition for the variety of outdoor activities was one's satisfaction with leisure activities: those elders who were more satisfied with their leisure activities reported more activities (especially in eastern Germany and Italy).

Table 11.8: Regressions analysis of options of outdoor activities[1], all countries

	All countries	
	Stand. ß-weights	Semi-partial r^2
Socio-structural resources		
Age	-0.05	0.2
Gender (1=male; 2=female)	0.03	0.1
Education (years of full-time education)	0.06**	0.2
Income per person	0.15***	1.2
Satisfaction with income[2]	0.07***	0.3
Regional resources		
Region (1=urban; 2=rural)	0	0
Satisfaction with area[2]	-0.02	0
Feeling secure when being outside during night (0=insecure; 1=secure)	0.05**	0.2
Features of the neighbourhood (10 = high quality to 20 = low quality)	-0.08***	0.5
Services within reach (10=all services accessible; 20=no service accessible)	0.02	0
Satisfaction with services[2]	-0.04	0.1
Personal resources		
Visual acuity (0.02 to 1.00)	0.02	0
Visual abilities (1=very poor; 5=very good)	-0.02	0
ADL (10=all ADL possible, 30=no ADL possible)	-0.11***	0.5
Physical mobility (1=very poor; 5=very good)	0.03	0.1
Satisfaction with health[2]	0.08***	0.3
Digit-Symbol-Substitution[3]	0.17***	1.7
External control (powerful others) (1= strongly disagree; 5=strongly agree)	-0.04	0.1
Social resources		
Size of network	0.14***	1.5
Number of children	0.03	0.1
Living alone (0=no; 1=yes)	-0.05**	0.2
Further resources		
Satisfaction with leisure activities[2]	0.11***	0.8
Indoor/outdoor motivation (0=indoor-type/10=outdoor-type)	0.06**	0.3
Importance of being out (0=not important at all; 10=very important)	0.08***	0.5
N	2330	
Model r^2	0.38	

Note. MOBILATE Survey 2000

Analyses is based on N = 2330 due to listwise deletion of missings. **=p<0.01, ***=p<0.001

[1] Standardized sumscore ranging from 0 (no outdoor activity pursued) to 1 (all asked outdoor activities pursued)

[2] Self-evaluation rating on an 11-point rating scale, higher scores indicting higher satisfaction

[3] Range 1-67, higher scores indicate higher visumotoric coordination.

Table 11.9: Regressions analysis of options of outdoor activities[1], differentiated by countries

	Finland		Eastern Germany		Western Germany	
	Stand. ß-weights	Semi-partial r^2	Stand. ß-weights	Semi-partial r^2	Stand. ß-weights	Semi-partial r^2
Socio-structural resources						
Age	-0.11	0.4	-0.04	0.1	-0.04	0.1
Gender (1=male; 2=female)	0.12**	0.9	0.01	0	0.05	0.2
Education (years of full-time education)	0.06	0.2	0.09	0.6	0.03	0
Income per person	0.04	0.1	0.07	0.3	0.08	0.3
Satisfaction with income[2]	-0.04	0.1	-0.02	0	0.08	0.3
Regional resources						
Region (1=urban; 2=rural)	-0.1	0.6	-0.07	0.3	0.09	0.4
Satisfaction with area [2]	0	0	0	0	-0.04	0.1
Feeling secure when being outside during night (0=insecure; 1=secure)	-0	0	0.02	0	-0.05	0.1
Features of the neighbourhood (10 = high quality to 20 = low quality)	-0.08	0.5	0.08	0.4	-0.16***	1.8
Services within reach (10=all services accessible; 20=no service accessible)	0.01	0	-0.04	0.1	0.01	0
Satisfaction with services[2]	-0.05	0.2	-0.03	0	-0.02	0
Personal resources						
Visual acuity (0.02 to 1.00)	0.06	0.3	0.17***	2	0.03	0
Visual abilities (1=very poor; 5=very good)	-0.06	0.3	-0.06	0.3	0.02	0
ADL (10=all ADL possible, 30=no ADL possible)	-0.29***	2.5	-0.09	0.4	-0.03	0
Physical mobility (1=very poor; 5=very good)	0.07	0.2	0.03	0.1	0.02	0
Satisfaction with health[2]	0.07	0.3	0.12	0.7	0.16**	1
Digit-Symbol-Substitution[3]	-0.01	0	0.17***	2.1	0.17***	1.9
External control (powerful others) (1=strongly disagree; 5=strongly agree)	-0.03	0.1	-0.04	0.1	-0.04	0.1
Social resources						
Size of network	0.17***	2.2	0.07	0.3	0.25***	4.7
Number of children	-0.01	0	0.02	0	-0.04	0.1
Living alone (0=no; 1=yes)	0	0	-0.03	0.1	-0.13**	0.9
Further resources						
Satisfaction with leisure activities [2]	0.05	0.2	0.21***	2.4	0.04	0.1
Indoor/outdoor motivation (0=indoor-type/ 10=outdoor-type)	0.2***	3.3	0.06	0.2	0.08	0.4
Importance of being out (0=not important at all; 10=very important)	0.03	0.1	0.1	0.6	0.11	0.8
N	480		400		490	
Model r^2	0.41		0.38		0.42	

Note. MOBILATE Survey 2000

Analyses is based on reduced N in each country due to listwise deletion of missings
**=p<0.01, ***=p<0.001
[1] Standardized sumscore ranging from 0 (no outdoor activity pursued) to 1 (all asked outdoor activities pursued)
[2] Self-evaluation rating on an 11-point rating scale, higher scores indicting higher satisfaction
[3] Range 1-67, higher scores indicate higher visumotoric coordination.

Table 11.10: Regressions analysis of options of outdoor activities[1], differentiated by countries

	Hungary		Italy		The Netherlands	
	Stand. ß-weights	Semi-partial r²	Stand. ß-weights	Semi-partial r²	Stand. ß-weights	Semi-partial r²
Socio-structural resources						
Age	0.05	0.2	-0.23***	2.5	-0.12	1
Gender (1=male; 2=female)	0.06	0.3	-0.22***	3.3	0.01	0
Education (years of full-time education)	0.18	1.8	0.01	0	0.13	1.4
Income per person	0.13	1.1	-0.02	0	0.09	0.5
Satisfaction with income[2]	0.05	0.2	0.1	0.7	0	0
Regional resources						
Region (1=urban; 2=rural)	0.06	0.2	-0.03	0	0.03	0.1
Satisfaction with area [2]	0.01	0	0.04	0.1	0	0
Feeling secure when being outside during night (0=insecure; 1=secure)	0.06	0.2	0.04	0.1	-0.07	0.4
Features of the neighbourhood (10 = high quality to 20 = low quality)	-0.09	0.7	-0.04	0.1	-0.1	0.7
Services within reach (10=all services accessible; 20=no service accessible)	0.06	0.2	0.02	0	-0	0
Satisfaction with services[2]	0.01	0	-0.08	0.4	-0.08	0.4
Personal resources						
Visual acuity (0.02 to 1.00)	-0.03	0.1	-0.01	0	-0.08	0.5
Visual abilities (1=very poor; 5=very good)	-0.15**	1.8	0.01	0	0.04	0.1
ADL (10=all ADL possible, 30=no ADL possible)	-0.22	1.7	0.12	0.5	-0.11	0.5
Physical mobility (1=very poor; 5=very good)	0.04	0.1	0.16**	1	0.09	0.3
Satisfaction with health[2]	0	0	0.05	0.1	-0.02	0
Digit-Symbol-Substitution[3]	0.07	0.2	0.17	0.8	-0	0
External control (powerful others) (1=strongly disagree; 5=strongly agree)	-0.09	0.5	-0.02	0	-0.24***	4.8
Social resources						
Size of network	0.13	1.5	0.19***	2.1	0.15***	1.8
Number of children	0.01	0	-0.08	0.5	0.09	0.7
Living alone (0=no; 1=yes)	-0.11	0.8	-0.06	0.2	-0.11	0.7
Further resources						
Satisfaction with leisure activities [2]	0.04	0.1	0.18***	2.1	0.14	1.4
Indoor/outdoor motivation (0=indoor-type/ 10=outdoor-type)	0.14	1.5	0.01	0	0.01	0
Importance of being out (0=not important at all; 10=very important)	0.05	0.2	0.06	0.2	0.07	0.3
N	244		433		278	
Model r²	0.35		0.40		0.30	

Note. MOBILATE Survey 2000

Analyses is based on reduced N in each country due to listwise deletion of missings

**=p<0.01, ***=p<0.001

[1] Standardized sumscore ranging from 0 (no outdoor activity pursued) to 1 (all asked outdoor activities pursued)

[2] Self-evaluation rating on an 11-point rating scale, higher scores indicting higher satisfaction

[3] Range 1-67, higher scores indicate higher visumotoric coordination.

International differences in the amount of total variance explained were observed. Again, our model did not fit the Dutch sample very well (explained variance 30%): The most important predictors of outdoor activity for Dutch respondents were the size of their social network and external control by powerful others: a larger social network supported outdoor activities, while the feeling of being controlled by powerful others hindered outdoor activities. The model did not explain the outdoor activity of Hungarians either. The only significant predictor was visual ability, and the relation was just the opposite of what one would expect. Hungarian elders with poor visual ability performed a larger number of outdoor activities - a result which is not plausible and cannot be explained.

In all other countries under investigation the model seemed better able to explain the range of outdoor activities (explained variance between 38% and 42%), but the patterns of important predictors differ. Aspects of the older people's health and their visumotoric coordination were especially important for explaining outdoor activities of Finnish and German elders. Moreover, the size of the social network was important for older people's level of outdoor activities in Finland, western Germany and Italy. In the Italian regions, socio-demographic aspects were also important predictors of outdoor activities: younger men reported a higher level of outdoor activities compared to women or older persons.

11.3.3   Number of trips/realised mobility

Our model for explaining different aspects of out-of-home mobility which postulated that socio-demographic aspects, health aspects, characteristics of the environment and the social network are important, was not suited to explain the actual number of trips taken over a two-day observation period (Table 11.11). Only 15% of the variance could be explained. Measuring mobility using a trip diary is a feasible idea and common practice in transport research. However, there was relatively low variability in the number of trips in our sample, which may have produced these poor results. Nevertheless, among the different types of predictors examined, socio-economic factors had the biggest impact on actual mobility behaviour: younger and male persons with a higher income reported a higher number of trips, which can be due to the fact that those people were more likely to still be employed. Conversely, aspects of the environment and the health (except visual acuity) were not decisive for one's out-of-home mobility - an unexpected result. Everyday mobility seems to be independent of environmental features of the near vicinity (availability of services, neighbourhood safety) or personal variables (health), which runs contrary to our assumptions.

The amount of variance explained by the model was low in all countries examined. With an explained variance between 12 and 16% the hypothesized model did not fit the Dutch, nor the eastern and western German data: in these countries, everyday mobility did not depend on the elders' health, visumotoric coordination, or social network, which is contrary to our assumptions. We would have expected health to have a particularly strong impact on everyday mobility. Surprisingly, environmental aspects like the region or the availability of services and facilities were not important for out-of-home mobility either. Even the 19% of explained variance observed in the Hungarian sample must be viewed as insufficient. Unlike other countries, the actual mobility behaviour of the Hungarian elders seemed to be highly dependent upon the region lived in: those living in the urban area had much higher everyday mobility in terms of actual trips made.

It should be noted, however, that the model functioned rather well for the Italian elders (explained variance 35%): Men with higher visumotoric coordination reported a particularly high level of realised mobility. The hypothesized model also explained somewhat more variance for Finnish respondents (24%): as in Italy, individuals with higher visumotoric coordination reported more trips.

Table 11.11: Regression analysis of realised mobility[1], all countries

	All countries	
	Stand. ß-weights	Semi-partial r^2
Socio-structural resources		
Age	-0.12***	0.9
Gender (1=male; 2=female)	-0.09***	0.6
Education (years of full-time education)	-0.01	0
Incombe per person	0.07**	0.3
Satisfaction with income[2]	0.04	0.1
Regional resources		
Region (1=urban; 2=rural)	-0.04	0.1
Satisfaction with area[2]	0.02	0
Feeling secure when being outside during night (0=insecure; 1=secure)	0.04	0.1
Features of the neighbourhood (10 = high quality to 20 = low quality)	0.02	0
Services within reach (10=all services accessible; 20=no service accessible)	0.05	0.1
Satisfaction with services[2]	0.01	0
Personal resources		
Visual acuity (0.02 to 1.00)	0.08***	0.4
Visual abilities (1=very poor; 5=very good)	-0.02	0
ADL (10=all ADL possible. 30=no ADL possible)	-0.07	0.2
Physical mobility (1=very poor; 5=very good)	0.06	0.2
Satisfaction with health[2]	-0.03	0
Digit-Symbol-Substitution[3]	-0.01	0
External control (powerful others) (1= strongly disagree; 5=strongly agree)	-0.03	0.1
Social resources		
Size of network	0.13***	1.4
Number of children	-0.03	0.1
Living alone (0=no; 1=yes)	-0.01	0
Further resources		
Satisfaction with leisure activities[2]	0.05	0.2
Indoor/outdoor motivation (0=indoor-type/10=outdoor-type)	0.08***	0.5
Importance of being out (0=not important at all; 10=very important)	-0.01	0
N	2319	
Model r^2	0.15	

Note. MOBILATE Survey 2000
Analysis is based on N = 2319 due to listwise deletion of missings; **=p<0.01, ***=p<0.001
[1] Mean number of trips per person and day
[2] Self-evaluation rating on an 11-point rating scale, higher scores indicting higher satisfaction
[3] Range 1-67, higher scores indicate higher visumotoric coordination.

Table 11.12: Regression analysis of realised mobility[1], differentiated by countries

	Finland		Eastern Germany		Western Germany	
	Stand. ß-weights	Semi-partial r^2	Stand. ß-weights	Semi-partial r^2	Stand. ß-weights	Semi-partial r^2
Socio-structural resources						
Age	-0.08	0.3	0.04	0.1	-0.11	0.8
Gender (1=male; 2=female)	-0.11	0.8	-0.06	0.3	0.02	0
Education (years of full-time education)	-0.05	0.1	0.01	0	-0.03	0
Income per person	0.05	0.1	0.2**	2.3	0.18**	1.7
Satisfaction with income[2]	0.05	0.2	-0.03	0.1	-0.02	0
Regional resources						
Region (1=urban; 2=rural)	0.05	0.2	0.13	1.1	0.17**	1.4
Satisfaction with area [2]	-0.07	0.3	0	0	0.06	0.2
Feeling secure when being outside during night (0=insecure; 1=secure)	-0.01	0	-0.08	0.4	-0.04	0.1
Features of the neighbourhood (10 = high quality to 20 = low quality)	-0	0	-0.07	0.3	-0	0
Services within reach (10=all services accessible; 20=no service accessible)	0.06	0.2	0.01	0	0.04	0.1
Satisfaction with services[2]	0.04	0.1	0.12	0.9	-0.03	0
Personal resources						
Visual acuity (0.02 to 1.00)	0.04	0.1	0.01	0	-0.04	0.1
Visual abilities (1=very poor; 5=very good)	0.09	0.6	0.08	0.5	0.02	0
ADL (10=all ADL possible, 30=no ADL possible)	-0.07	0.1	-0.09	0.4	-0.06	0.1
Physical mobility (1=very poor; 5=very good)	0.03	0	0.05	0.1	-0.05	0.1
Satisfaction with health[2]	-0.09	0.4	-0.11	0.6	0.11	0.5
Digit-Symbol-Substitution[3]	0.21**	1.5	0.07	0.4	0.03	0
External control (powerful others) (1=strongly disagree; 5=strongly agree)	0.03	0.1	-0.26***	3.8	-0	0
Social resources						
Size of network	0.1	0.8	0.12	1	0.12**	1.2
Number of children	-0.1	0.9	-0.03	0.1	0.03	0.1
Living alone (0=no; 1=yes)	-0.04	0.1	-0.06	0.2	-0.09	0.4
Further resources						
Satisfaction with leisure activities [2]	0.12	1	-0.04	0.1	0.05	0.1
Indoor/outdoor motivation (0=indoor-type/ 10=outdoor-type)	0.11	1	0.07	0.3	0.18***	2.1
Importance of being out (0=not important at all; 10=very important)	-0.03	0.1	-0.19**	2.2	-0.02	0
N	**469**		**400**		**490**	
Model r^2	**0.24**		**0.16**		**0.15**	

Note. MOBILATE Survey 2000

    Analyses is based on reduced N in each country due to listwise deletion of missings
    **=p<0.01, ***=p<0.001
    [1] Mean number of trips per person and day
    [2] Self-evaluation rating on an 11-point rating scale, higher scores indicting higher satisfaction
    [3] Range 1-67, higher scores indicate higher visumotoric coordination.

Table 11.13: Regression analysis of realised mobility[1], differentiated by countries

	Hungary		Italy		The Netherlands	
	Stand. ß-weights	Semi-partial r[2]	Stand. ß-weights	Semi-partial r[2]	Stand. ß-weights	Semi-partial r[2]
Socio-structural resources						
Age	-0.01	0	-0.04	0.1	-0.08	0.5
Gender (1=male; 2=female)	0.01	0	-0.25***	4.1	-0.01	0
Education (years of full-time education)	0.04	0.1	-0.01	0	0.13	1.2
Income per person	-0.08	0.5	0.12	0.7	0.07	0.3
Satisfaction with income[2]	0.03	0.1	0.06	0.2	0.01	0
Regional resources						
Region (1=urban; 2=rural)	-0.25***	4	0.07	0.3	-0.23***	4.5
Satisfaction with area [2]	0.04	0.2	-0.02	0	0.08	0.5
Feeling secure when being outside during night (0=insecure; 1=secure)	0.08	0.4	-0	0	0.13	1.5
Features of the neighbourhood (10 = high quality to 20 = low quality)	0.11	0.9	-0.05	0.1	0.08	0.5
Services within reach (10=all services accessible; 20=no service accessible)	0.1	0.5	0.09	0.5	0	0
Satisfaction with services[2]	0.01	0	-0.01	0	0.1	0.7
Personal resources						
Visual acuity (0.02 to 1.00)	-0.01	0	0.06	0.2	-0.04	0.1
Visual abilities (1=very poor; 5=very good)	0.01	0	-0.03	0.1	-0.04	0.1
ADL (10=all ADL possible, 30=no ADL possible)	-0.16	0.9	-0.1	0.4	0.07	0.2
Physical mobility (1=very poor; 5=very good)	0.11	0.5	0.13	0.7	0.08	0.2
Satisfaction with health[2]	-0.05	0.1	-0.05	0.2	-0.02	0
Digit-Symbol-Substitution[3]	0.09	0.5	0.19**	1	0.07	0.3
External control (powerful others) (1=strongly disagree; 5=strongly agree)	0	0	-0.05	0.2	-0.15	2
Social resources						
Size of network	-0.02	0.1	-0.04	0.1	0.03	0.1
Number of children	0.18**	2.6	-0.03	0.1	-0.01	0
Living alone (0=no; 1=yes)	0.15	1.5	0.09	0.7	-0.07	0.3
Further resources						
Satisfaction with leisure activities [2]	0	0	0.03	0.1	-0.04	0.1
Indoor/outdoor motivation (0=indoor-type/ 10=outdoor-type)	0.06	0.3	0.03	0	0.17**	2.5
Importance of being out (0=not important at all; 10=very important)	-0.01	0	0.07	0.3	0.06	0.3
N	244		433		278	
Model r[2]	0.19		0.35		0.12	

Note. MOBILATE Survey 2000

Analyses is based on reduced N in each country due to listwise deletion of missings

**=p<0.01, ***=p<0.001

[1] Mean number of trips per person and day

[2] Self-evaluation rating on an 11-point rating scale, higher scores indicting higher satisfaction

[3] Range 1-67, higher scores indicate higher visumotoric coordination.

11.4   Summary and conclusions

In addition to a high level of actual mobility, a great variety of transport options and outdoor activities can be regarded as modern aspects of mobility such as self-determination, flexibility and variability.

The findings confirm the general tendency that in urban areas, older people can use a greater variety of modes of transportation than their contemporaries living in rural areas. Beside this general trend, an individual's income, education, health and social network were important prerequisites for using a large variety of transport options. However, these variables showed differing impact across the countries under observation.

With regard to outdoor activities, the urban-rural comparison offered no clear pattern. Instead, a high quality of neighbourhood features and an individual's health, income, education and social network contribute significantly to a high diversity of outdoor activities. Outdoor motivation and satisfaction with leisure possibilities were additional predictors. Again, we found diverging impact of these variables when distinguishing between the different countries.

Regarding the third indicator of mobility, that is the actual number of trips made per person and day, there was relatively low variability, and no general pattern could be found except the fact that in all countries younger elders reported a higher number of trips than those aged 75 years or older. Contrary to expectations, health (except visual acuity) and aspects of the environment were not decisive for one's out-of-home mobility.

The three indicators will be considered further – particularly with respect to their impact on older people's quality of life – in the following chapter.

Enhancing Mobility in Later Life
H. Mollenkopf et al. (Eds.)
IOS Press, 2005

Chapter 12
Mobility and the Quality of Life

Heidrun Mollenkopf, Stephan Baas, Fiorella Marcellini, Frank Oswald, Isto Ruoppila,
Zsuzsa Széman, Mart Tacken, and Hans-Werner Wahl

12.1   Introduction

This chapter deals with our main question: How is mobility related to quality of life? Besides a comprehensive and detailed description and explanation of older people's out-of-home mobility, another goal of the MOBILATE project was to identify how subjective well-being depends on outdoor mobility as well as on mobility-related person and environmental factors (see Figure 12.1). We apply structural equation modelling considering a wide range of explanative variables to answer this complex question.

Figure 12.1: The MOBILATE Model, including the quality of life

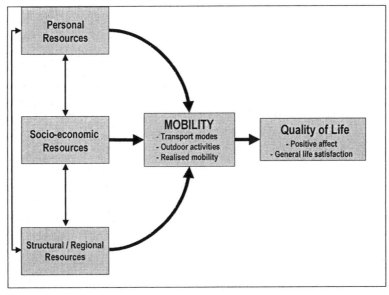

The findings presented in previous sections of this report afford a complex picture of mobility; mobility can be explained by recourse to a wide range of different personal, socio-economic, and structural predictors. However, in the MOBILATE project, outdoor mobility is

understood as an even more complex phenomenon, i.e., it is simultaneously characterised by transport modes, outdoor activities, and realised mobility. Thus, regression analyses do not suffice to explain general outdoor mobility. Subsequently a structural equation model (SEM) is introduced in the next step to calculate multiple influences on mobility (based on our theoretical assumptions) as well as to model outdoor mobility as a latent variable. A path model is necessary in order to consider the theoretical relation between outdoor mobility and quality of life. For methodological reasons, we reduced our extensive set of predictors. . Furthermore, we focus on just one model for the total sample (and not on country-specific solutions) in order to maximize the sample size which is necessary when working with a relatively large number of variables.

Up to now, the results have clearly supported the notion that a whole range of variables play a substantial role in the explanation of outdoor mobility. However, regressions analyses, upon which these findings were based, have limitations. First, interrelations between predictors are not considered. Second, regressions analyses were run for each mobility outcome in a separate manner, thus excluding co-variation between outcomes.

A more complex understanding of outdoor mobility, depicted in Figure 13.6, simultaneously considers the variety of transport modes used, the variety of outdoor activities pursued and realised mobility (actual trip-making). In addition, links between variables in terms of direct and indirect effects must be considered. Finally, quality of life is also explicitly included in this model as a major dependent variable.

To statistically manage a model of this complexity, structural equation modelling (SEM) was used to calculate multiple influences. That is, most of the theoretically relevant variables were treated as latent variables, including the major outcomes, i.e., outdoor mobility and quality of life. In order to keep the model as transparent as possible, we used only a minimum set of substantial indicators for each latent construct. An empirical reason for a slightly reduced set of variables (compared to the regression analyses) was that measurement model pre-tests called for the elimination of some variables.

As mentioned earlier, this analysis is intended to predict mobility in a wide variety of settings, and we thus disregard the country-specific findings, and use the whole MOBILATE sample in the analysis. There are methodological reasons for this as well: with a total number of 97 parameters to be estimated, separate analyses for individual countries would result in unfavourably small parameter-subject ratios.

12.2   The conceptual MOBILATE-model: extension to quality of life

Mobility, as conceptualised by the MOBILATE project, goes beyond the common notion of trip-making behaviour to include the variety of transport modes used and the variety of outdoor activities pursued. In other words, flexibility regarding different transport modes and a wide range of leisure time interests as motives for mobility are taken into consideration.

In general, the MOBILATE project proposes that mobility is determined by socio-structural, health-related and psychological factors as well as environmental conditions and features of the person-environment interaction.

Going into more detail of the conceptual MOBILATE model, person-related aspects span age, gender and socio-economic status. The latter construct comprises education, income per person and overall satisfaction with one's financial situation.

The health-related aspects linked to mobility can be divided into physical functionality and visual capability. Objective measures were used as well as subjective evaluations. The construct 'vision' therefore comprises a measurement of visual acuity as well as the individuals' subjective evaluation of visual ability. Physical mobility was indicated by objective functional capacity (activities of daily living, ADL) and by self-assessed physical agility.

Living in an urban vs. rural area was assumed to affect mobility behaviour. Likewise, aspects of the residential area, such as the availability of services, feelings of security and the overall satisfaction with the area were assumed to do the same. The variety of the social network was also considered to be an important variable that could contribute to mobility.

Psychological determinants of outdoor mobility involve cognition, agency and motivation. Because mobility was thought to depend on basic orientation and coordination skills, the Digit-Symbol Test (DST) was included to measure visumotoric coordination, processing speed and fluid intelligence. External control beliefs, a measure of how elders perceive the influence of powerful others on their behaviour (LOC-subscale) was regarded as another psychological moderator of mobility. With respect to motivational aspects of outdoor mobility, environment-related attitudes that reflect emotional bonds to the residential area were also taken into consideration. The individual importance attributed to being out was assessed as well as the self-assessment of being an Indoor vs. Outdoor Type.

'Quality of Life' forms the final construct within the conceptual MOBILATE model. A high quality of life was hypothesised to impact on individual evaluations of life satisfaction and the experience of positive affect states. Therefore the 'Positive Negative Affect Scale' (PANAS) and a self-assessment of general life satisfaction were used as indicators for the latent dimension 'quality of life'.

The assumed relationships between quality of life, outdoor mobility and their various antecedences and moderators can be summed up to form a comprehensive model. Quality of life is theorized to be directly influenced by physical mobility as well as by socio-economic status. In addition, there are strong arguments for the close relationship between mobility and the quality of life earlier, which we have cited earlier in this report. Mobility may indeed mediate various influences on quality of life. Mobility is modelled to be directly influenced by geographic region, aspects of the residential area, the social network, socio-economic status, visual capabilities and physical mobility, visumotoric coordination, control beliefs and outdoor motivation/orientation. Age, we theorise, moderates aspects of social networks and influences health-related characteristics and cognitive functioning. Gender differences were expected to be found regarding socio-economic status and the social network. Physical mobility may inhibit mobility in a rather obvious and direct way; moreover, it may influence control beliefs and place attachment/outdoor motivation. Finally, living in a rural or urban area may affect one's mobility directly, but may also show effects mediated by several aspects of the residential area.

Figure 12.2: The conceptional MOBILATE Model

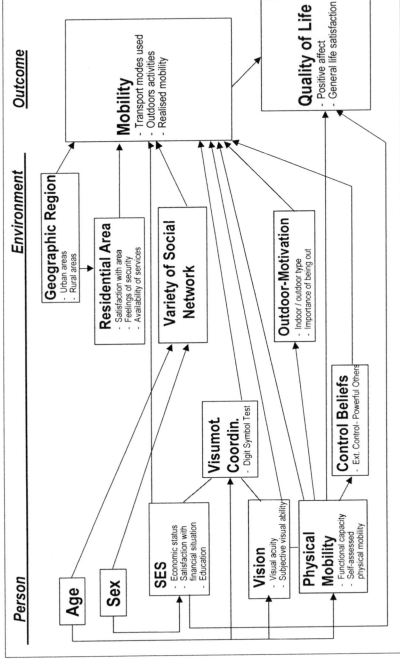

Note. MOBILATE Survey 2000

12.2.1   Results of structural equation modelling

12.2.1.1   Overall model fit evaluation

The postulated system of relationships was tested simultaneously as a structural equations model using the statistical analysis package AMOS 4.0 (Arbuckle 1999). Full information maximum likelihood (FIML) estimation was chosen to address the problem of missing values. An important issue for model testing are possible violations of the multivariate normal distribution required by the maximum likelihood estimation algorithm. Severe violations of the normal theory estimators (maximum likelihood, generalized least square) may lead to a too restrictive χ^2 goodness-of-fit test, underestimation of fit indexes such as the Normed Fit Index (NFI), Tucker-Lewis-Index (TLI) or the Comparative Fit Index (CFI) and biased parameter estimates, yielding too many significant results (West, Finch, & Curran, 1995). As AMOS does not offer an output routine to determine or test for multivariate non-normality when full information maximum likelihood estimation, examined the univariate sample moments for all variables included in the model. Although univariate tests identified significant deviations from a normal distribution for all variables at hand, this may well be due to the large sample size and should lead to a careful consideration of additional distribution moments (kurtosis, skewness) to assess the degree of non-normality in our data. Following the recommendations of West, Finch and Curran, we propose that a distribution substantially departs from normality if skewness equals or exceeds a value of 2 and kurtosis reaches values as high as 7 or over. Maximum values for skewness were found for satisfaction with area (-1.51) and satisfaction with life (-1.11), indicating substantial asymmetry of these distributions in favour of positive evaluations. Maximum scores for kurtosis were identified with respect to the model variables income per person (2.75) and satisfaction with area (2.71). As none of the variables in the model exceeds the indicator values for univariate non-normality presented above, we presume our model to meet the distributional preconditions necessary for adequate model estimation. It should be noted, though, that tentative multivariate normality remains an assumption rather than a demonstrated fact.

The comparison between the hypothesized and empirical covariance structures resulted in a highly significant chi-square ($\chi^2 = 6960$; df=280; p<.001), suggesting a misfit between the theoretical model and the empirical data. However, judgements based on the chi-square statistic may be considered overly conservative and could therefore easily lead to the rejection of theoretical models which represent the empirical data fairly well. As this is especially true with large samples, non-significant global model tests are assumed to be rather rare events and should not be regarded as the only criteria for model evaluation (Byrne, 2001, p. 81). For this reason, additional indicators of a valuable model fit have been proposed.

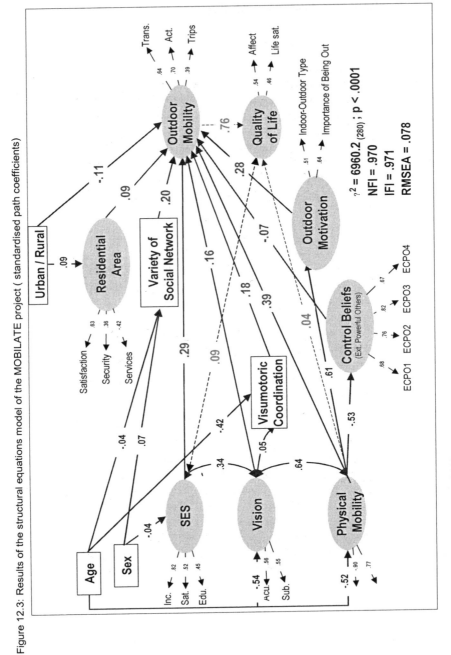

Figure 12.3: Results of the structural equations model of the MOBILATE project (standardised path coefficients)

Note. MOBILATE Survey 2000

All of the most commonly-used fit indices fell within an acceptable range. The 'Normed Fit Index' (NFI), the 'Incremental Fit Index' (IFI) as well as the 'Tucker-Lewis-Index' (TLI) and 'Comparative Fit Index' (CFI) showed values of 0.964 or above.

Evaluation of the 'root mean square error of approximation' (RMSEA) has remained somewhat controversial in the respective literature. According to Browne and Cudeck (1993), an RMSEA of 0.078 as found in the present model test would point to considerable misspecification of the hypothesized model. In contrast, MacCallum and colleagues (1996) consider scores below 0.080 as indicators of still a good model fit. Given that our model is based on pronounced cultural heterogeneity of the included countries, we suggest that our model represents the empirical data reasonably well.

12.2.1.2 In-depth consideration of measurement models

All observed variables showed highly significant relations (p<.001) with the respective latent constructs they were hypothesized to be related to. Nevertheless, most of the indicators were determined only moderately by the latent factors and may have been insufficiently reliable measurements of the proposed latent dimension.

- The construct 'socio-economic status' appeared to be most closely related to a person's financial situation, both in terms of available income (.82) and with respect to individual satisfaction with the financial situation (.52). Moderate relationships were revealed between the latent dimension socio-economic status and the level of education (.45).

- The objective measurement of visual acuity and self-assessed visual ability were nearly equally predictive of the latent construct 'vision' (.56 and .55). Due to the only moderate correlation between objective and subjective measures for visual ability (r=.33), the interpretation of the underlying dimension obviously should not be reduced to functional optometrics only.

- Both the ADL-score (-.90) as well as the self-assessed physical mobility (.77) proved themselves to be very good predictors of our proposed construct of physical mobility (Correlation between ADL and physical mobility=-.70).

- Key features of the residential area a person lives in comprised the availability of services in the near vicinity, residential satisfaction and the feeling of security at night. These features should result in a positive overall evaluation of the residential area. Empirically, only satisfaction appears to be a reasonably valuable predictor for the hypothesized common factor 'good area to live in' (.63), whereas only 18% of variance in the structural equipment variable (availability of services) and even less (13% of variance) in the security variable could be accounted for by the proposed underlying dimension.

- The Locus-of-Control construct 'external control-powerful others' was measured by four scale items, with a minimum factor score of .67. The latent dimension 'ec-po' was best indicated by the notion that 'other people generally make sure that nothing goes wrong in my life' (.82).

- A basic motivation for outdoor mobility should be present in both the importance of being out as well as in the description of oneself as an outdoor- or indoor type. These two indicators correlated modestly (r=.32), pointing to the fact that being out may still be an important and pleasant activity even if one considers him- or herself to be a homebody. Moreover, impairments to physical mobility may limit actual outdoor activity, although such activities may have a higher value and attractiveness due to reactance mechanisms. In our present model, the importance of being outdoor (path coefficient of .64) appears to be the slightly more dominant predictor of the latent construct outdoor motivation (.51 for indoor-outdoor-type, respectively).

- Of the three different variables used as indicators for the latent factor 'mobility', only realised outdoor mobility stood out in a negative manner. About half of the variance of the other components could be explained by the assumed mobility factor. The variety of outdoor activities (path coefficient of .70) and the options of transport modes (.64) could be regarded as the dominant aspects of the multi-facetted construct 'mobility'.

- The construct 'quality of life' was indicated by the amount of positive affect experienced and the self-rated life satisfaction. Both variables showed only moderate systematic covariation (r=.28), and seemed to be equally, albeit only to a relatively small absolute degree, determined by their shared latent construct 'quality of life'.

12.2.1.3   In-depth evaluation of the structural model

Our model expects gender and age to have only mediated (instead of direct) influences on mobility. One of the mediating variables for both gender and age is the variety of the social network. Being female should support the variety of social contacts, whereas increasing age is hypothesised to have an opposite effect on the social network. The path coefficients for our data confirmed these assumptions, although the effects were very small (age: -.04; gender: .07, but still significant), and the overall determination of the variety of the social network was not substantial ($R^2=0.01$). A second mediator of gender effects on mobility and quality of life was thought to be the factor 'socio-economic status'. With a path coefficient of -.04, this assumption was not confirmed by the data. According to the theoretical model, the constructs linked to body and cognitive functioning appear to be strongly effected by age. 29% of variance of 'Vision' and 'Physical mobility' (27%) could be accounted for by the age variable. The influence of aging on fluid intelligence/visumotoric functioning was estimated by a path coefficient of -.42 and can therefore also be considered substantial.

The remaining model variables were supposed to either directly effect mobility and quality of life, or to do so indirectly as well as by moderating other determinants of mobility or quality of life. In the following, the non-mediated structural influences on mobility are described.

As can be seen in Figure 12.3 all major model components (i.e., the latent factors, geographic region and visumotoric coordination) are theoretically linked to mobility directly. These direct influences are indicated by red regression weights in Figure 15.3. Of these determinants, physical mobility showed the strongest impact (.39), followed by socio-economic status (.29) and outdoor motivation (.28). Moderate relations could be found between mobility and network variety (.20), visumotoric coordination (.18) and 'vision' (.16). Minor influences on mobility were found for geographic region (-.11; indicating a higher level of mobility in urban areas) and aspects of the residential area (.09). 'External control beliefs' did not predict mobility very well (-.07). Together, the model accounted for a large proportion of the variability (86%) in the latent factor 'outdoor mobility'.

'Quality of life', as indicated by 'positive affect' and 'general life satisfaction' was hypothesized to be influenced directly by socio-economic status, physical mobility and the comprehensive mobility construct (indicated by green path coefficients). Surprisingly, socio-economic status failed to show substantial impact on quality of life (.05). Whereas only a moderate direct effect could be found for physical health (.22), the relationship between mobility and 'quality of life' was striking (.76).

Finally, for some components of the model, direct as well as indirect influences on mobility were assumed. Living in a rural area, for example, was shown to have a negative influence on mobility. Geographic aspects were also hypothesised to influence features of the residential area (e.g., feelings of security during the night). In this regard, living in a rural area shows a small but positive effect on the factor 'residential area' (.09), which positively affects mobility. Impairments to physical mobility were hypothesised to increase feelings of external control by powerful others, a relationship that is confirmed by the data (-.53). Moreover, reduced physical mobility was thought to alter the motivation for being outdoors: the data show a positive link between physical mobility and outdoor motivation (.61).

For reasons of completeness, it should be noted that all model variables showed either a direct, indirect or both influences on 'quality of life'. This section did not discuss all indirect and total effects at length. Nevertheless, as the value of an indirect path is indicated by the product of its direct sub-paths; it should be easy for the reader to estimate all indirect or total effects contained in the model from the path coefficients displayed.

Covariances were estimated for the error term of vision and the error terms of socio-economic status, physical mobility and visumotoric coordination. The disturbance term for vision failed to correlate significantly with the error term for visumotoric coordination, whereas statistically substantial relations could be found for the two remaining constructs (ses:.34; health:.64).

12.3   Summary and Conclusions

Out-of-home mobility is a complex phenomenon and simple answers are not possible when it comes to its explanation. Driven by the MOBILATE conceptual model of mobility, our own findings are able to add to the challenges related to the explanation of mobility on different levels. In addition, the issue of relations between mobility and quality of life has found new empirical substance through the MOBILATE project. In particular, the following points deserve emphasis:

- Out of socio-economic aspects, age and gender have inconsistent (and mediated) impacts on mobility and quality of life: Age and gender do not impact the variety of the social network and the socio-economic status, but age has a strong impact on visumotoric coordination and physical mobility: Increasing age negatively influences both health-related aspects. Admittedly, despite a relation between gender and socio-economic status, the latter is strongly related to outdoor mobility: A higher socio-economic status helps to maintain outdoor mobility. Related to socio-economic aspects, a broader variety of social network is moderately related to a higher level of outdoor mobility.

- Out of relations between mobility and health-related predictors, physical mobility showed the strongest impact on mobility when compared to all other predictors; in addition vision moderately influence mobility: Higher physical functionality and visual capability lead to a higher outdoor mobility.

- Living in an urban or rural area and further aspects of the residential area such as the availability of services, feelings of security and general satisfaction do not affect mobility in a substantial way.

- Out of psychological determinants, a high outdoor motivation has strong impact on a higher outdoor mobility, while visumotoric coordination only moderately influences mobility. On the other hand, control beliefs are not related to outdoor mobility in the expected manner.

- Quality of life as the ultimate outcome of the MOBILATE conceptual model is strongly related to outdoor mobility. Our results underline that outdoor mobility mediates various influences on the quality of life. On the most general level, our data support the assumption that higher outdoor mobility is positively related to the quality of life of ageing individuals.

Of course, a note of caution is in place when interpreting causal relations inherent in our findings due to the fact that the analyses were based on cross-sectional data. New data sets to come should thus be based on longitudinal observations. Going further, a challenge of forth-coming research will be to further improve the fit between theory (the conceptual model of mobility) and empirical observations. That is, besides the need to generate new empirical data over time, ongoing refinement of the MOBILATE conceptual framework will also be needed in the future.

References

Arbuckle, J.L. (1999). *Amos 4.0 [Computer Software]*. Chicago: Smallwaters.

Brown, M.W., & Cudeck, R. (1993). Alternative ways of assessing model fit. In K.A. Bollen & J.S. Long (Eds.), *Testing structural equation models* (pp.445-455). Newbury Park, CA: Sage.

Byrne, B.M. (2001). *Structural equation modeling with AMOS. Basic concepts, applications, and programming*. Mahwah, London: Lawrence Erlbaum Associates.

MacCallum, R.C., Browne, M.W., & Sugawara, H.M. (1996). Power analysis and determination of sample size for covariance structure modelling. *Psychological Methods, 1*, 130-149.

West, S.G., Finch, J.F., & Curran, P.J. (1995). Structural equation models with non normal variables. Problems and remedies. In R.H. Hoyle (Ed.), *Structural equation modelling: Concepts, issues, and applications* (pp. 56-75). Thousand Oaks, CA: Sage.

Enhancing Mobility in Later Life
H. Mollenkopf et al. (Eds.)
IOS Press, 2005

Chapter 13
The Mobility Rich and Mobility Poor

Heidrun Mollenkopf, Roman Kaspar, and Hans-Werner Wahl

13.1   Introduction

Mobility (the ability to move about) and traffic (the transportation of people, goods, and news) have become an ever more important precondition of ensuring the ability to lead one's everyday life, keep up social relations, take part in every kind of activity outside one's home, and seek out places that are either subjectively significant or objectively central to providing for daily material needs and health care. At the same time, mobility is increasingly jeopardised as a person ages. The findings presented in the preceding chapters confirm the importance of mobility for an independent lifestyle, on the one hand, and the various personal and environmental conditions it depends on, on the other. An individual's physical, economic, social, and technical resources, as well as the structural resources of the region he or she lives in, proved to be decisive components of out-of-home mobility. They constitute, however, only the basic preconditions for moving about. Therefore, in a last step, we attempted to examine characteristic connections between older adults' mobility and socio-structural, psychological, and structural variables, to distinguish subgroups of older individuals who differ in mobility and respective satisfaction. This enables us to identify groups that are particularly at risk of losing their possibilities to move about.

13.2   Identifying the 'Mobility rich' and 'Mobility poor'[1]

Besides the basic personal and environmental conditions of older people's out-of-home mobility, further variables such as an individual's motives for making trips, the importance assigned to going out[2], and psychological variables such as control beliefs and visumotoric coordination, for example, also play a decisive role. Control beliefs may influence outdoor mobility in a variety of ways. For example, the experience of being in control over one's life circumstances may strongly motivate an ageing individual to invest much time and effort in

---

[1] A revised and condensed version of this chapter has been included in Mollenkopf et al., 2004.

[2] To assess cognitive and affective environmental bonding, participants were instructed to indicate how important being out is to them on an 11-point Likert-type scale from 0 = 'absolutely not important' to 10 = 'very important'. Motivational environment-related attitude towards the indoor versus the outdoor home environment was assessed with a global self-rating of being an indoor/outdoor-type of person (staying at home versus being on the go as much as possible) (Mollenkopf, Oswald, & Wahl, 1999; see also Chapter 7).

maintaining a maximum level of out-of-home mobility.[3] Similarly, both high internal control beliefs and a high motivation for being on the go may overwrite adverse environmental aspects even when confronted with health decrements. Perceptual motor processing or visumotoric coordination (Oswald & Fleischmann 1995; Wechsler, 1958) has repeatedly been found to be a major indicator of basic cognitive functioning, frequently described in the literature as fluid intelligence or the mechanics of intelligence (e.g., Baltes, 1993). This cognitive ability is also an important ability underlying outdoor mobility related cognitive functioning.[4]

Therefore, in a further step of analysis, we examine characteristic connections between mobility, on the one hand, and socio-demographic, psychological,[5] and structural variables, on the other, to identify distinguishable subgroups of individuals who differ in their out-of-home mobility. For this purpose, we carried out a cluster analysis based on our model of mobility (see Chapters 11 and 12), including all three major indicators of out-of-home mobility as determining variables:

1. day-to-day mobility, measured in terms of trips as reported in the diaries,

2. variety of transport options used,

3. diversity of motives for undertaking outdoor activities (in terms of performed options).

As a further variable we included

4. satisfaction with one's mobility (range 0-10),

because a high extent of mobility does not necessarily result in high satisfaction. Instead, people with limited mobility in terms of few trips, low use of transport modes, and only few or no outdoor activities might be equally satisfied - at least according to theories suggesting disengagement (Cumming & Henry, 1961) or selective optimization with compensation (Baltes & Baltes, 1990) in old age. Low satisfaction, however, is assumed to indicate that people suffer from personal or environmental mobility restrictions and need support for improving their possibilities of moving about.

Analyses were performed using the SAS 8e software's FASTCLUS and CLUSTER procedures, using Ward's clustering algorithm. Using z-standardized scores of both the three mobility indicators and global mobility satisfaction as input variables, four clusters of outdoor mobility, similarly substantial with regard to group size, emerged.

In a second step, clusters were further described with respect to socio-demographic, health-related, psychological and regional variables. What we found were four clearly distinct subgroups of outdoor mobility (Figure 13.1).

---

[3] The instrument administered to the MOBILATE sample was the control beliefs questionnaire used in the Berlin Aging Study (Baltes, Freund, & Horgas 1999; Smith, Marsiske, & Maier 1996), in which the dimensions of 'Internal Control' (6 items), 'External Control: Powerful Others' (4 items), and 'External Control: Chance' (4 items) were assessed.

[4] Basic cognitive abilities in terms of perceptual motor processing or visumotoric coordination and working memory were assessed with the subtest provided in the Nuremberg Age Inventory (NAI) (Oswald & Fleischmann, 1995).

[5] Selected were those psychological variables which proved to be reliable across all countries as well as revealed substantial relation with the outdoor mobility indicators (see Chapter 7 on psychological aspects of outdoor mobility).

Figure 13.1: Four subgroups of outdoor mobility in old age (z-scores).

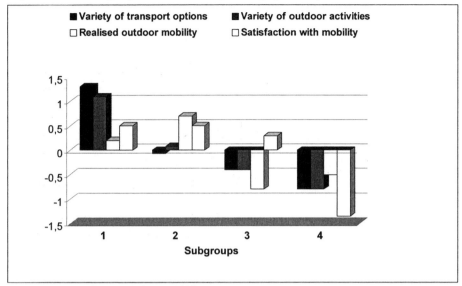

Note. MOBILATE Survey 2000

All scores z-standardized (M=0; SD=1) in order to facilitate comparison.

The first cluster (n = 887) had the highest mobility scores in terms of transport modes used, range of outdoor activities, and satisfaction with mobility. The frequency of trips in this group was also clearly above average, but not as high as that of Cluster 2. The broad use of available means of transportation perhaps led to a wide range of outdoor mobility in this group. Thus, Cluster 1 might be labelled as the 'High Mobility / High Mobility Satisfaction' group.

Cluster 2 (n = 1,320), which showed the highest level of day-to-day mobility, was as satisfied with their mobility as Cluster 1, although their use of transport modes as well as the variety of their outdoor leisure activities were clearly lower. As this subgroup still operated nearly completely in the positive range of scores, it might be labelled as the 'Medium Mobility / High Mobility Satisfaction' group.

The picture changes when it comes to the third and fourth subgroups. Satisfaction with mobility was still in the positive score range of Cluster 3 (n = 792) as well. However, all components of mobility were clearly lower than in the first and second Cluster. So this subgroup might be called the 'Low Mobility / Still Satisfied with Mobility' group.

Finally, Cluster 4 (n = 951) might be labelled as the 'Low Mobility / Unsatisfied with Mobility' group. All scores of this subgroup lie in the negative range of values with a particularly pronounced negative score regarding satisfaction with mobility. Interestingly, the narrow range of outdoor mobility of this subgroup (i.e., number of trips made) tends to be higher compared to Cluster 3, but the use of transport means and the outdoor leisure activities were clearly lowest of all groups.

When we now compare the four subgroups with respect to regional, socio-demographic, health-related, and psychological characteristics, we find sharp differences between the clusters, and practically all findings are in the expected direction (Table 13.1).

Table 13.1: Subgroups of outdoor mobility in old age (means; percentages).

	Subgroup 1 High Outdoor Mobility / High Mobility Satisfaction (n = 887)	Subgroup 2 Medium Outdoor Mobility / High Mobility Satisfaction (n = 1,320)	Subgroup 3 Low Outdoor Mobility / still satisfied with Mobility (n = 792)	Subgroup 4 Low Outdoor Mobility / unsatisfied with Mobility (n = 951)
Socio-Demographic variables				
Age (M)	65.2	66.5	70.2	73.5
Gender (%)				
Male	48.2	48.5	38.7	31.4
Female	51.8	51.5	61.3	68.6
Household size (%)				
Lives alone	23.4	24.0	27.0	44.0
Lives with others	76.6	76.0	73.0	56.0
Satisfaction with finances[1] (M)	7.5	6.9	6.7	5.7
Years of education[2] (M)	11.8	10.0	8.8	8.0
Car use (%)				
No car in household	20.3	33.9	46.7	68.5
As passengers	12.4	17.0	25.7	20.4
As driver	67.3	49.1	27.6	11.0
Health-related Variables (M)				
Physical mobility[3]	3.9	3.6	3.3	2.6
Satisfaction with health[4]	7.4	6.9	6.4	4.8
Psychological Variables (M)				
Working memory[5]	36.7	30.6	26.7	20.7
Control beliefs – powerful others[6]	2.1	2.2	2.5	2.9
Indoor-Outdoor-Type[7]	5.2	4.9	4.3	3.5
Importance of being out[8]	8.4	7.9	7.5	6.0
Geographic Variables (%)				
Region				
Urban	65.7	49.3	41.2	39.9
Rural	34.3	50.7	58.8	60.1
Country (%; rank order)				
1	Netherlands	Eastern Germany	Eastern Germany	Hungary
2	Finland	Italy	Western Germany	Italy
3	Western Germany	Western Germany	Netherlands	Western Germany
4	Eastern Germany	Hungary	Hungary	Eastern Germany
5	Italy	Finland	Italy	Netherlands
6	Hungary	Netherlands	Finland	Finland

Note. MOBILATE Survey 2000, means or percentages given; N=3934 respondents.

[1] Assessed on an 11-point scale (0=completely unsatisfied; 10=completely satisfied).
[2] Total amount of years of education.
[3] Assessed on a 5-point scale (1=very bad; 5=very good).
[4] Assessed on an 11-point scale (0=completely unsatisfied; 10=completely satisfied).
[5] Testscore (range 0-67).
[6] Subscale items assessed on a 5-point scale (1=not agree at all; 5=fully agree).
[7] Assessed on an 11-point scale (0=like being indoor best; 10=like being outdoor best).
[8] Assessed on an 11-point scale (0=not important at all; 10=very important).

With respect to age and gender, there was a descending order of mean age as well as a tendency of an increased proportion of women and of single living persons from Subgroup 1 to Subgroup 4. Satisfaction with one's financial situation and the level of education (total number of years) were highest in Subgroup 1 and lowest in Subgroup 4.

Not surprisingly, active drivers were most frequently found in Subgroup 1 (67.3%) while in Subgroup 4 only about every tenth person drives a car. The proportion of persons without a car in the household was highest in this group. Likewise, the proportion of persons who use a car only as a passenger decreased from Subgroup 4 to Subgroup 1. As well, there was a tendency for decreasing health from Subgroups 1 to 4. And finally, psychological variables also played a role as a characterising tool for these subgroups. Visumotoric coordination clearly and consistently decreased from Subgroups 1 to 4, while control beliefs / powerful others increased. In addition, indoor orientation increased from Subgroups 1 to 4, whereas the importance of going out decreased.

Taking these findings into account, Subgroup 4 appears to be at particular risk; the members of this group have already lost much of their outdoor mobility, and seem to be in need of immediate intervention and rehabilitation because they are most dissatisfied with this situation.

With regard to regional differences, older adults in rural areas were more frequently found in the low mobility groups 3 and 4. In terms of countries, the risk groups described above seem to be represented more strongly by older adults from Hungary and Italy, while the Dutch and Finnish elders were found predominantly in the 'mobility rich' group. Separate analyses for each country are needed to better understand the positive and negative conditions influencing out-of-home mobility of each country's older citizens.

In sum, the analyses point to the need to differentiate within the scope of older adults when outdoor mobility in later life is the target of study. Furthermore, our findings underscore the existence of specific groups deserving special attention with regard to stimulation, prevention, intervention, and rehabilitation. Singly living older persons, women, persons with impaired health and low economic resources, and rural older adults tend to be particularly at risk of losing their abilities to move about. An accumulation of such unfavourable conditions, as is the case in the 'Low mobility / unsatisfied with mobility' group, requires immediate intervention and social as well as technical support measures. Group 3 seems to exhibit beginning frailty, pointing to the need of pronounced preventive efforts to avoid further loss in out-of-home mobility. Persons belonging to Subgroup 2, showing moderate outdoor mobility and satisfaction in spite of a limited range of transport modes and outdoor activities, deserve attention and stimulation to enhance or maintain their out-of-home mobility, whereas the younger, healthier persons and active car drivers of group 1 seem able to cope very well with their needs in terms of outdoor mobility and activity.

Thus, improvements must focus as much on social and transport policy measures as on appropriate urban development planning. For older men and women, whose life space contracts with advancing age because of the growing risk of frailty, it is becoming increasingly urgent to create flexible, user-centred options for mobility that offer a genuine alternative to both the private automobile and traditional local public transport services. Neighbourhoods should have readily accessible stores, medical and care services, appropriate public transport, and other facilities that will allow older individuals to continue leading independent lives, maintain social contacts, and take advantage of recreational activities - in short: to continue dealing with daily demands and remaining full members of society.

References

Arbuckle, J.L. (1999). *Amos 4.0 [Computer Software].* Chicago: Smallwaters.

Baltes, P. B. (1993). The aging mind: Potential and limits. *The Gerontologist, 33,* 580-594.

Baltes, P. B., & Baltes, M. M. (1990). Optimierung durch Selektion und Kompensation: Ein psychologisches Modell erfolgreichen Alterns [Optimization by selection and compensation: a psychological model of successful ageing]. *Zeitschrift für Pädagogik, 35,* 85-105.

Baltes, M. M., Freund, A. M., & Horgas, A. L. (1999). Men and Women in the Berlin Aging Study. In P. B. Baltes & K. U. Mayer (Eds.), *The Berlin Aging Study,* (pp. 259-281). Cambridge: Cambridge University Press.

Cumming, E., & Henry, W. E. (1961). *Growing old, the process of disengagement.* New York: Basic Book Inc.

Mollenkopf, H., Marcellini, F., Ruoppila, I., Széman, Z., Tacken, M., & Wahl, H.-W. (2004). Social and behavioural science perspectives on out-of-home mobility in later life: findings from the European project MOBILATE. *European Journal of Ageing, 1,* 45-53. DOI: 10.1007/s10433-004-0004-3.

Mollenkopf, H., Oswald, F., & Wahl, H.-W. (1999). *Outdoor mobility in old age in two rural regions in Germany.* Unpublished Datareport.

Oswald, W. D., & Fleischmann, U. M. (1995). *Nürnberger-Alters-Inventar (NAI).* [The Nuremberg Age Inventory, NAI]. Göttingen: Hogrefe.

Smith, J., Marsiske, M., & Maier, H. (1996). *Differences in control beliefs from age 70 to 105.* Unpublished manuscript; Max Planck Institute for Human Development, Berlin.

Wechsler, D. (1958). *The measurement and appraisal of adult intelligence.* Baltimore: Williams & Wilkins.

Chapter 14
Summary and Conclusions

Heidrun Mollenkopf, Fiorella Marcellini, Isto Ruoppila,
Zsuzsa Széman, and Mart Tacken

At the end of this book we look back on the original research aims and the main questions and we reflect on the experiences made during three years of international comparative research. Thus, this final chapter serves to point to the main challenges, to summarize the main findings, and to draw the main conclusions of this research. We start by recapitulating the most important general results of the research project (section 14.1). Next, we discuss the methodological and practical challenges that a cross-cultural study such as the MOBILATE project has to face (section 14.2). And finally we discuss the findings with respect to conclusions and implications for prevention and intervention measures, for social and transport policies, urban planning, and future developments in transport technology (section 14.3).

14.1 Overview on the main MOBILATE findings

14.1.1 The basic goals and background of the MOBILATE project

In the research proposal the MOBILATE consortium has formulated the main aims of the project:

- The study's first objective was to provide a comprehensive and detailed *description and explanation of the actual out-of-home mobility of older people* by means of a broad interdisciplinary data set, including mobility-related personal as well as environmental aspects.

- A second objective of the research endeavour was to *describe and explain individual change and constancy* in mobility patterns in old age as a function of chronological age. In this regard, a 5-year follow-up data collection of persons first investigated in 1995 allowed us to describe change and constancy as well as inter-individual variability in these patterns (Mollenkopf et al., 2003).

- In addition, we addressed the question of *whether new cohorts of older people reveal different mobility patterns* as users of transport technology compared to older cohorts with differing technological experiences and resources (Ruoppila et al., 2003).

- The final goal of the research was to identify how subjective well-being, a key indicator of life-quality in old age, depends on outdoor mobility as well as on mobility-related personal and environmental factors.

- Through this research and the conclusions drawn from the results gained we aim to *contribute to the enhancement of the mobility of older people.*

With our general theoretical model we assumed that out-of-home mobility is based on the interaction between individuals, the transport modes they use, and their immediate surroundings, significant others, and family. The consideration of living environments, neighbourhood environments, spatial environments (including transport facilities), as well as technological environments are thus crucial factors for a comprehensive understanding of out-of-home mobility.

Comparison of five countries from different parts of Europe with different climatic and geographic conditions, institutional arrangements, population density, and cultural traditions is difficult. However, the aim of this research was not to compare the regions studied. Instead, the findings reflect older adults' out-of-home mobility possibilities and constraints conditional on diverging personal and social background, health status, and social networks in different regional conditions. When interpreting the findings, it should be kept in mind that elderly people are not an undifferentiated group and therefore their mobility patterns and needs may vary. The MOBILATE sample reflects this heterogeneity.

An essential focus of this study was on how environmental resources impact on the outdoor mobility of elders. Therefore, particular emphasis was placed on the contrast between rural and urban regions: it was presumed that environmental resources (and hence, out-of-home mobility) differ greatly between rural and urban regions in each country.

In order to take into consideration the specific national peculiarities, middle-sized cities were chosen in proportion to each country's characteristics: In *Finland, Jyväskylä,* the bustling centre of business and culture with about 77,900 inhabitants (in 2000) in the middle of the country was chosen. In *Germany*, where history has brought about rather different social and environmental conditions that can affect mobility, cities in the western and eastern parts of the country were chosen. Both *Mannheim* and *Chemnitz* are industrial cities with diversified settlement structures, comparable cultural infrastructures, universities, sports facilities, and diversified public transportation systems. In *Hungary* the city of *Pècs* was chosen. With its 180,000 inhabitants Pécs is the biggest town in South-west Hungary, seat of Baranya County. The *Italian* research was carried out in *Ancona,* a middle sized town in Central Italy (Marche Region) located on the Adriatic See (south of Venice). In *the Netherlands,* the investigation took place in *Maastricht,* a middle-sized city in the Southern part of this country near to the border with Belgium and Germany.

For the same reason, inside rural regions of each country, villages or areas were chosen which are characteristic for the respective country. They should not be very unusual for the participating countries. Instead, they should e.g. have a typical number of inhabitants per km, or a typical share of people over the age of 65 years. The rural areas chosen were: *Karstula, Kivijärvi and Nilsiä in Finland, the District of Jerichow (Saxony-Anhalt) and the District of Vogelsberg (Hesse) in Germany* (only villages having less than 5,000 inhabitants), the village *Jászladány in Hungary*, the municipalities of *Mondavio, Montefelcino and Orciano in Italy*, and the municipality of *Margraten in the Netherlands.*

The national samples were randomly drawn from the respective population registers. In the German rural areas, respondents were chosen by random route procedure. All samples consisted of men and women aged 55 years or older (born 1940 or before), disproportionately stratified by gender and age (persons aged 55 to 74 years and 75 years or older, with approximately equal numbers of men and women in each group). Thus, the samples allow conclusions to be drawn regarding the situation of older adults as well as of very old men and women in different urban and rural areas which would not have been possible with a proportional sampling. To correct for oversampling towards older persons and males, all descriptive and comparative analyses were done with weighted data.. The total sample included in the MOBILATE survey (MS 2000) consisted of 3,590 persons.

The stratification has brought comparable sub-groups, as regards the age means of the different strata. Only younger female respondents in the Dutch urban area were significantly older than all respondents of the respective sub-groups due to the different sampling procedure in the Netherlands (about one third of the respondents to be interviewed in the urban area of Maastricht were chosen from the users of the transport on demand system in Maastricht (VoM); see Chapter Methodology).

The MOBILATE respondents were similar to the general population of elderly:

Most of the younger respondents aged 55 to 74 years were still married, whereas the situation changed with increasing age: while the majority of older male respondents was still married, female respondents were more often widowed. Only in the western German urban area, less than half of the older men were still married; about every second was already widowed. Regarding differences between the European regions, highest proportion of divorced persons were found in the Finnish sample, while in the Italian sample hardly any respondent was divorced. The most diversified pattern was found in the Dutch sample where a lot of respondents had never been married or lived separated from their partners.

Urban elders were better educated than those living in the rural areas, with the exception of the Dutch areas. Moreover, men and younger respondents reported a better education than women and those who belong to the older age group. Respondents in eastern Germany reported the most extended education. Italian respondents (except younger urban Italian men) were those being most deprived as regards their education: especially women in the Italian rural area reported the lowest amount of full-time education of all respondents.

Most of the participating elders were already retired. Occupations and therefore socio-economic status differed between the European regions and between men and women. Except for eastern Germany, women reported occupations which require a lower level of qualification compared to men. In addition, especially many Italian women had no profession, but reported to be housewives. The majority of Finnish rural elders reported to be farmers. In the Finnish city men worked (or still work) in upper white collar professions or as skilled workers, whereas Finnish women reported professions with a lower level of qualification or being a housewife. The same structure was found among western Germans, whereas eastern German women reported also professions which need a higher qualification, like skilled workers or craftsmen. In the western German rural area, a considerable proportion of men reported to be farmers, while in the eastern German sample only few men were farmers (due to the former socialist structure of economy). In addition, in both parts of Germany a comparatively high amount of men reported occupations which require a high qualification, such as academic professionals, or freelancers. On the other hand, the comparatively low level of education in Italy and Hungary is reflected by less qualified occupations of the Hungarian and Italian respondents. In the Netherlands the situation is different. Despite small differences between men and women as regards education, male respondents worked or still work in blue collar jobs, while the majority of Dutch female respondents were housewives. In the past, the labour market participation of Dutch women was generally low.

Independent from profession, almost every respondent who had reached the respective retirement age in the different European regions was retired, except for some Hungarian people, who still worked due to the very low pensions in Hungary. Of those who had not reached the retirement age, especially men were still working, mainly in full-time jobs (up to 60% of the respective respondents). The highest employment rates for men was found in both Finnish areas, while the lowest employment rates were reported in the rural Italian and Hungarian samples. The highest unemployment rates were found among eastern German men. Female respondents worked less often, except for the Dutch and especially the Finnish areas. In addition to being retired or still working in a full-time or part-time job some respondents pursued additional work. Especially a lot of Italian respondents reported to take care for a relative or to be engaged in voluntary work. Voluntary work was most common in the Netherlands.

The socio-economic background becomes apparent in the older people's personal income: The lowest income was reported by Hungarian participants, while respondents living in both parts of Germany and the Netherlands reported the highest income. For this reason it is not amazing that Hungarian elders were most unsatisfied with their financial situation. Also Italian respondents had a comparatively low income. In the Dutch sample no systematic differences were found between urban and rural areas, men and women, or younger and older respondents, whereas in some European regions under investigation (Finland, Italy) such differences became apparent. Almost every older and therefore retired respondent got the main income from a pension, while some younger respondents still got income from a full-time job.

Because of the vast heterogeneity of the elderly people and the socio-geographical diversity of the regions studied, the most important aspects of mobility - transport behaviour, leisure activities, use of services, etc. - have been analysed in relation to variables such as gender, age, income, health status (personal aspects) and the country and residential area they live in (environmental aspects). In fact, transportation opportunities vary greatly, not only between the northern and southern or eastern and western European countries, but also within the same country.

14.1.2   The mobility patterns of older men and women in urban and rural areas

Mobility in terms of trips and journeys

One of the starting points of the MOBILATE project was that outdoor mobility is realised - and thus can be measured - by the trips and journeys people perform, either by foot or by any other means of transportation. The extent of this concrete travel behaviour or *realised mobility* was assessed by *mobility diaries* in which the respondents documented their trips per day and per person over the course of two days (the day before and after the interviews).

Three out of four persons made at least one journey over the two interview days. Most involved single journeys, i.e., from home to a destination and back home (consisting of one or several trips). About a quarter of the sample made no trip at all during the interview period. This proportion was especially high in the Dutch research areas. The average number of trips for the whole sample was 2.1 trips a day.

The extent of mobility did not differ between the urban and rural regions in most countries, except for Hungary and the Netherlands. In these countries, people living in the cities reported a significantly higher level of out-of-home mobility compared to those living in the countryside.

In Finland, eastern Germany and in particular Italy, men reported a significantly higher number of trips per day than women, while in western Germany, Hungary and the Netherlands, no such differences were found. Younger respondents in general reported a higher level of actual outdoor mobility when compared to older persons.

There were no differences between people living alone and those living with others regarding trip-making behaviour, even controlling for age. With increasing age the mean number of trips made decreased, but across all age groups, the number was quite similar. Children could support elder mobility by driving the car or by acting as companion, but having children made no difference in the mean numbers of trips undertaken. This shows clearly that living with other people or having children is not decisive for the number of trips made. Nonetheless, the social context obviously influences trip-making behaviour. People without important persons living outside the household made fewer trips (trip mean 1.8 a day) than people with a social network outside the own household (trip mean of 2.2).

The spatial range of mobility was also rather small: 44% of the trips were within a distance of one kilometre and an additional 24% were within 3 kilometres.

A time analysis of trip-making behaviour over the course of the day showed two peaks: the first in the middle of the morning and a second one in the middle of the afternoon. In Italy, the morning peak was a little earlier and the afternoon peak a little later than in the other countries. All countries had a clear dip during lunchtime except Finland where such a dip did not take place. Shopping was the most common motive for trip making, followed by visiting friends or relatives and going out for a stroll.

The private modes of transportation, including cars, bicycles or going by foot, were the most common forms of travelling. Simply going by foot was most common, followed by using a car as a driver or a passenger. Public transport seems to play a role when no other alternatives are available or when the system is very well organised, with a high frequency of traffic and a dense network of stops.

Measuring mobility using a trip diary is a feasible idea and common practice in transport research. However, there was relatively low variability in the number of trips in our sample. This may have contributed to the result that our model for explaining different aspects of outdoor mobility, which postulated that socio-demographic aspects, health aspects, characteristics of the environment and the social network are important, could explain only 15% of the variance in the actual number of trips (taken over a two-day observation period). Nevertheless, among the different types of predictors examined, socio-economic factors had the biggest impact on actual mobility behaviour: younger and male respondents with a higher income reported a higher number of trips, which can be due to the fact that younger males were more likely to still be employed. Conversely, aspects of the environment and the health (except visual acuity) were not decisive for one's outdoor mobility - an unexpected result. Everyday mobility seems to be independent of environmental features of the near vicinity (availability of services, neighbourhood safety) or personal variables (health), which run contrary to our assumptions.

Mobility in terms of transport options and outdoor activities

In the beginning of this report we argued that in modern societies where mobility is associated with freedom, autonomy, flexibility, and variability, outdoor moblity is much more than just getting from one place to another. The assessment of outdoor mobility of men and women living in modern industrialized countries should cover as many of these mobility-related aspects as possible. Therefore, we suggested a comprehensive model of outdoor mobility that included - in addition to the extent of *realised mobility* per day and per person based on the concrete travel behaviour reported in the mobility diaries - two further integral kinds of mobility: *Options of transport modes* (the amount of transport modes used shows the variety of options a person has at hand), and *Options of outdoor activities* (the range of outdoor activities performed shows the variety with respect to this aspect of a person's mobility). The use or performance of more or less options does not necessarily mean that a person is more or less mobile in a quantitative sense, but that he or she can use a certain variety of modes or can pursue a certain variety of activities and thus is more or less mobile (flexible) in a qualitative sense.

Transport options

The greatest variety of transport modes was reported by older Finnish people, both in the urban and rural areas, when compared to all respective regions. Moreover, both urban and rural Dutch respondents reported a comparatively broad range of transport modes available. The smallest range of transport modes was reported by Hungarian and Italian elders, especially those living in the rural Italian area, which is possibly due to differences in the infrastructure and to mobility habits in different cultures. For example, public transport is less available in the Italian countryside, and older Hungarians reported the lowest availability of private cars compared to all other respondents.

In all participating countries, older people in urban areas had significantly more transport modes available than those living in rural areas, which is an expected result due to the higher availability of public transport in cities. In all countries, men reported more transport options than women. This is probably due to the fact that more men drive - which will change in the near future. As expected, younger respondents used significantly more transport modes than older respondents in all countries under investigation. Regardless of age, Hungarian elders were deprived in terms of available transport modes.

Out of the different types of predictors employed in the analyses, the region a person lives in had the greatest impact on the variety of transport options used in all countries. This result confirms our assumption that public transport is less available in rural areas in general. Besides region, higher income and education, better health and better visu-motoric coordination were important prerequisites for using a large variety of transport options as well. However, health did not have a consistent impact on the number of transport modes used in different countries. The assumption that the social network could offer a reason for taking trips and could facilitate out-of-home mobility, only found partial support: although those with a larger social network and those living together with other persons reported a larger variety of transport options, the social network's contribution to this variety was not important. Aspects of the environment such as the availability of services and facilities or feelings of security when outside during the night did not play a decisive role either. Finally, outdoor motivation was not a significant predictor of the variety of different transport modes used (with the exception of Italy, where those respondents who evaluated themselves as being an outdoor-type reported using significantly more transport modes).

Leisure activities

When studying leisure time activities, one must be aware that especially with regard to older people there is no commonly accepted definition of leisure. In the MOBILATE project we selected a nomothetic approach to assess leisure activities. The subjects were asked to select from a rather long list of different groups of activities those they participated in. This selection of options can not cover all the possible leisure activities elderly people may pursue in different countries and environments, but included the most common alternatives, as well as a few activities which are frequent in only one or the other of the participating countries. It has to be pointed out that our leisure activity data do not describe the frequency or intensity of the pursue of the different leisure activities the elderly people engage in, but whether they pursue the activities and whether this is important to them.

Elderly people appear to be rather satisfied with their leisure activity possibilities. In the urban locations they were more satisfied in this regard than those in the rural environments, where the oldest age group in particular was less satisfied with their leisure possibilities.

At-home activities head the list of leisure activities. Among the outdoor activities, meeting friends elsewhere and going out for a walk were ranked first. Women performed more indoor activities whereas men were more active outdoors. Participation in indoor and outdoor activities was strongly related to health. Moreover, the more means of transport people were able to use, the more they went out. In a more comprehensive analysis, level of physical activity explained most of the variance, followed by the available modes of private transport (car and bicycle), and income. Subjects with better health showed higher satisfaction with the possibility of participating in different leisure activities, as expected. The better their health, the more likely people were to take part in both indoor and outdoor leisure activities.

Older people in the Dutch areas pursued the most *outdoor activities*, and western German and Finnish elders also pursued a large variety of outdoor activities. Older Hungarians and Italians had the lowest level of outdoor activity. When distinguishing the urban and rural areas under investigation, no clear pattern was visible: in the Finnish, Hungarian and Italian areas, more outdoor activities were reported in the cities, whereas virtually no rural-urban differences were found in Germany. In the Dutch rural area, more activities were reported compared to the urban area. As already stated, the rural Dutch area was very suburban, which might have led to the fact that Dutch rural elders reported significantly more outdoor activities compared to their urban counterparts.

Differences between men and women in number of outdoor activities were not readily apparent, with the exception of Italy: Italian men reported many more outdoor activities than Italian women. Italian women reported the lowest level of outdoor activities of all respondents. Though, a similar level of outdoor activities in all other countries does not automatically mean a similar structure of activities - they might differ due to cultural traditions.

Clear differences were found when analysing the number of activities by age: unsurprisingly, the younger elders (aged 55 to 74 years) reported a significantly higher level of activity when compared to older persons (aged 75 years of age and older) in all regions studied. Every fifth person would like to be more active. Meeting friends, making small trips, gardening and visiting a theatre or concert were mentioned most frequently, but were often prevented by the persons' state of health.

Among the socio-economic variables, only income per person had an impact on the variety of outdoor activities, while environment-related predictors were less important (at least compared with transport modes). Only high quality neighbourhoods supported a variety of activities. The respondents' health and visu-motoric coordination were much more important for pursuing outdoor activities compared to other predictors, which accords well with the assumption that being able to move is an important prerequisite for being active outdoors.

Although social network had no impact on the variety of transport modes used, it did influence outdoor activities: older people with larger social networks and those living together with other persons reported significantly more outdoor activities. As expected, outdoor motivation and satisfaction with leisure activities were additional predictors of outdoor activities. Though, this pattern of predictors differed between the individual countries under investigation.

14.1.3   The prerequisites and problems of older men's and women's out-of-home mobility

The general theoretical model of the MOBILATE research project has described out-of-home mobility to be based on interaction between an individual and his or her living environment. The first finding is perhaps a trifle obvious: having good health, accessible public transport, and being able to use a car are most important for out-of-home mobility. These factors are strongly interrelated and play decisive roles for out-of-home mobility and for older people's satisfaction with their mobility possibilities. In rural areas, a car becomes particularly important, because many important facilities and services are otherwise not accessible.

Personal prerequisites of mobility: health

Among *personal resources*, health can be seen as the most important one and its lack or weaknesses as the main risk factors causing difficulties and obstacles for mobility outdoors. Better health was related to a greater number of journeys made per day, especially in Finland and Italy. Health is also perhaps the most universal factor effecting on outdoor mobility generally, independent of country, region and gender. With increasing age and decreasing health the use of all transport modes was reduced and outdoor mobility decreased.

Different analyses showed health to be also an important factor affecting participation in leisure activities. This could be expected because health is a crucial condition particularly for participation in any kind of outdoor activity.

Long journeys (lasting at least one week) were as well more often undertaken by healthier persons. The effect of health on the number of long journeys was stronger in urban than in rural areas, except in Finland. Also, considerable differences between countries were found: German urbanites travelled most, Hungarian and Italian rural elders least. Urban elders in good health made about the same number of long journeys than healthy elders in the rural areas, but persons with poor health status in the cities made fewer trips than their rural counterparts.

Personal prerequisites of mobility: psychological resources

Psychological resources have typically been neglected in outdoor mobility analysis or have been considered only in a marginal sense in earlier research. In the MOBILATE study, psychological resources were explicitly addressed, assuming them to have a three-fold effect on outdoor mobility. First, basic functioning at the cognitive level (operationalised as visumotoric coordination/processing speed) was expected to directly influence the performance of outdoor-related behaviours. Second, a range of personality- and person-environment-related constructs (i.e., control beliefs, coping styles, place attachment) was expected to serve as a mediating force regarding out-of-home mobility. Third, it was assumed that out-of-home mobility may also serve as an antecedent variable for major psychological outcomes such as emotional adjustment (e.g., positive affect).

All of these hypothesis could be basically supported. Processing speed or control-beliefs were related quite consistently with mobility outcomes at all research sites. Mobility outcomes were stronger related to the importance of being out than to indoor place attachment, and positive affect revealed itself to be more consistently related to mobility than negative affect. The findings were quite consistent and make a substantially new contribution to intercultural research on the out-of-home mobility of older adults.

Environmental prerequisites of mobility: regional and neighbourhood resources

Country-based differences regarding different outdoor mobility aspects can be at least partly explained by differing environmental conditions such as the population density or the density of the road and other traffic routes. These affect the distances and times to get services, to participate in outdoor activities, and to meet relatives and friends. Finland and the Netherlands represent the both extremes among the countries that participated in the study. The supply of different transport modes and outdoor leisure activities have the greatest distances in Finland and the shortest in the Netherlands. Nonetheless, our study showed that the elderly people mainly lived less than 100 meters from their nearest neighbour. This means that elders could usually rely on others for help or a simple interaction. In fact, nearly all the elderly respondents stated that they can reach their neighbours within five minutes at most.

Most of the elderly people in all the countries had also good access to fundamental services (which can be reached in 15 minutes) such as food store, doctor, pharmacy, bank, post office, bus or tram stop, etc., except for Finland. The services which were rated the most important by elderly people were food store, pharmacy, doctor, and except for Hungary and Italy, bank. This shows that above all older people look after their primary needs: food, health and savings. The presence of a bus or tram stop, which was the most widespread service of all together with the food store, both in the rural and urban areas, was also one of the least important ones. This indicates that the availability of a bus or tram stop alone is not equivalent to a service meeting the needs of older people.

The Hungarians were the most satisfied with their services, both in the urban and rural areas, even though in the latter case they were not always frequently available, except for the food store. Generally, elderly Hungarians, especially those living in the rural area, obviously do not attach great importance to services or have resigned or adapted their expectations to the situation.

The most unsatisfied were elderly people living in the rural area of eastern Germany; this finding seems due to the lack or infrequent presence of services rated by them as fundamental. The Italian elders did not seem greatly satisfied either, even though the important services were usually well diffused. The reason could lie in the poor quality of Italian services. Finally, despite the poor availability of services compared to other countries, the Finns showed a good degree of satisfaction.

The mode of transport most often used in all countries to reach services was walking. The car was fundamental in Italy. The bicycle was used most in Hungary, followed by eastern

Germany, Finland and the Netherlands. Public transport such as bus or tram was not used much, either in the urban or rural areas. The worst situation observed with regard to means of transportation was in Hungary. This was confirmed by the infrequent ownership of a car, and by the greater use of bicycles and buses. Hungarian elders also had the greatest difficulty reaching services.

Even if most older people did not have difficulties in reaching services, it is interesting to note that the reasons which prevent accessing services were mainly linked to health conditions both in the urban and rural areas. Also great distances were considered a barrier in both urban and rural locations. Security was not a problem for most elderly people. Older men and women in Finland felt most secure. The highest percentages of insecurity were found in the Hungarian rural area, both by day and night. Also the Italians generally felt less secure than the Dutch and Finns.

The Finnish and the Dutch older persons were least tied to a particular place, and the Italian respondents were most strongly tied. Dutch elders showed the weakest tie to their home both in the urban and rural areas, although generally speaking, indoor place attachment was quite high in all countries. The tie was weaker between the elderly people and their outdoor environment, except in the case of the Netherlands. Dutch elders attributed more or less the same importance to being out as they did to their home. This is perhaps due to the less 'housebound' mentality of an open country such as the Netherlands, contrary to what happens elsewhere, as in Hungary, where the difference between the tie with the home and the importance of going out was the highest among all the countries studied. Finland had the highest values for both localities regarding the attachment to the home and the importance of the outdoor environment. These results were confirmed by satisfaction with the living area, which in Finland was the highest among all the countries for the urban area and the second highest for the rural area.

In spite of the mobility-related problems of today's elders uncovered by the study, it seems that the elderly people were all quite satisfied with their living area. It can be assumed that this is also due, at least in part, to the strong emotional bond created by elders with their environment over the years.

Environmental prerequisites of mobility: social resources

The social context can be both a stimulus and a form of support for mobility. Having a partner with a car makes it easier to go out, particularly for people who don't have a driving license. Among the participating countries, the average size of households was largest in Italy, and the lowest proportion of persons living alone was also found here - less than half that of people living alone in the other countries. They were most likely to live in multi-generation households, which also may have many practical and emotional advantages. For all countries, the proportion of living alone in old age was much higher for older women than for older men, due principally to their higher life expectancy.

In breakdown by settlement (rural vs. urban areas), only Hungary had a proportion of persons living alone that was lower in the rural than in the urban environment; in the other countries, the opposite pattern occurred, although to varying degrees. The rural environment also favoured multi-generation households.

The average number of children was much higher in the Netherlands and Finland than in the other countries. Older Hungarians reported the highest number of important relationships outside the household, reflecting the heterogeneity of the relationships. This statistic was the lowest in the two parts of Germany. Older people in Italy and the Netherlands had an average number of important relationships and the Finns an above average number.

The elders' social networks outside the house consist mainly of close relatives, namely their children. The two most important persons outside the respondents' households were children, regardless of where the respondents lived. If the older people were already living with children, then they reported other persons as being important. In the rural areas under investigation, important confidants lived closer to the older persons than was the case in the cities. In the Italian regions, the most important persons lived very close to the respondents, while in the Finnish, western German and Hungarian regions, the most important persons lived further away.

Those important persons who lived within the elders' immediate reach (less than 15 minutes away), were mainly reached by foot everywhere. If the confidants lived further away than 15 minutes, they were mainly reached by car, except for the Hungarian elders. Because only few of them had a car available, they mainly used their bicycles or public transportation.

The distance between the older persons and their social networks had the strongest impact on personal contact frequency; the closer they lived to important persons, the more frequently they met each other.

In general, hindrances could not be found in the social context. Living together or having children were not very decisive for out-of-home mobility. Instead, poor health was a more relevant obstacle than social factors. On the other hand, the presence of an out-of-home social network was in fact a stimulus to go out. With regard to problems meeting people outside the home, the most difficulties were reported by Italian respondents, the least difficulties by Dutch elders. Impairments in health status and lack of a car (except among older people in Hungary) were most often behind the problems in maintaining social contacts. Again, the distance to these important persons seemed to cause problems, especially in rural Finland where the distances between persons were very great.

14.2   Methodological challenges of a cross-cultural project

During the three-year multi-disciplinary cross-cultural research project MOBILATE: Enhancing Outdoor Mobility in Later Life, a number of theoretical, methodological, communication, and practical challenges had to be met.

The first, fundamental challenge was a *theoretical* one concerning the phenomenon 'out-of-home mobility.' Our basic starting point was that out-of-home mobility involves the person, the transport modes, and the environment which all interact with each other: how individuals cope with outdoor mobility, what motives they have, what transport modes are available, and which physical and social resources or obstacles in the living environment help or hinder the achievement of out-of-home mobility goals.

On the basis of the literature and on our earlier findings (Mollenkopf, Marcellini, & Ruoppila, 1998; Mollenkopf, Marcellini, Ruoppila, & Tacken, 2004), we identified as many factors as possible that might explain outdoor mobility: individual factors pertaining to the person, such as age, gender, economic resources, health, cognition and personality were expected to explain a large share of mobility among older people. In addition, variables describing the social context and social network were included, as well as variables describing the physical environment, such as the distances and access to services, the mode of transportation used to achieve outdoor mobility goals, and the outdoor activities elders are interested in and participate in. The interdisciplinary project was thus based on findings from the social sciences, psychology, the health sciences, environmental gerontology, and environmental or urban planning. Every one of these disciplines has its own theoretical system and own concepts which cannot be easily translated into concepts from other branches of sciences. Because the project partners came from different fields of science, it both stimulated but at the same time made intense communication between researchers necessary .

Interdisciplinarity, and the different disciplinary traditions that it entails, also results in a number of problems that have to be solved concerning *theoretical concepts and methodological approaches*. It is well known, for example, that similar concepts may have different meanings in the various disciplines. Discussions concerning quality of life, satisfaction with different spheres of life, outdoor mobility, health, leisure, social network, all very crucial concepts in the MOBILATE project – have been necessary, frequent, interesting and many-sided - and at the same time rather time-consuming. Many of the core concepts, although often used, could not be easily defined in a multicultural context, like concepts of family, socio-economic background and educational background.

The different scientific background of the cooperating partners led to different analytic approaches as well. In psychology, emphasis is placed on employing reliable scales, whereas the use of single questions is a more common practice in the social sciences. In the MOBILATE project, the partners achieved consensus regarding the planning of the project, including questions regarding assessment, such as the inclusion of single questions and psychological tests into the questionnaire and selection of topics for the diary. Because different disciplines employ various statistical methods, the analysis and the results reported varied by location. This kind of reporting illustrates the many different ways the MOBILATE dataset has been analysed, but at the same time requires from the reader more than if the analyses in different chapters of this book had been made statistically similarly.

Over the course of the study, theoretical discussions often arose due to differences between scientific cultures, and the theoretical traditions of social scientists working in *different cultural contexts*. These differences may make the theories, concepts and measures selected, although made in agreement, unsuitable for some participants. This happens unintentionally and usually goes unnoticed, especially if all of the partners have been working together from the very beginning of the project; such was the case in the MOBILATE study. Whether or not these biases have affected the findings can only be decided when the results have been calculated, the findings published, and critics review the work.

An important and *methodologically* demanding new approach to studying older people's out-of-home mobility included a series of psychological measures in the research. They were aimed to describe the individuals' own resources (or lack of them) for outdoor mobility. The individual's goals and ways of coping with environmental obstacles to out-of-home mobility were central to this point of inquiry. The selected psychological tests had not been previously translated into the language of all participating countries. Thus, it was necessary to analyse their internal consistency and validity to rule out cross-cultural differences. The internal consistencies of all tests in the participating countries were high or at least satisfactory for group comparisons.

Cultural comparisons based on psychological test results are admittedly very difficult. However, in the MOBILATE study, the test results were not intended for comparison between countries; rather, the approach was to identify those psychological factors most predictive of out-of-home mobility among elderly people. If the significance and explanator value of different psychological predictors vary between countries (and if methodological confounds can be excluded), this reveals possible cultural similarities and differences regarding the relationship between psychological resources and outdoor mobility. In this respect, it must be emphasized that similar theoretical and methodological problems like those of the MOBILATE study discussed above are met and solved with various degrees of success in every cultural comparative research project. Our general conclusions regarding theoretical and methodological issues are that the MOBILATE project has added quite a lot to the available knowledge of ageing and particularly to out-of-home mobility in old age, not only in the participating countries but hopefully in the whole of Europe.

There were different types of *communication problems* during the MOBILATE project caused at least in part by language barriers. English was used as a working language, but it was not any participant's mother tongue. Communication thus became a continuous effort in order to ensure common understanding between research partners.

One important language question is the *translation* of questionnaires as well as other tests and measures used. Translations and back-translations do not ensure that the meaning of an item or question is preserved. If, e.g., the questions presented in an interview do not have the same meaning in each of the languages - Finnish, German, Hungarian, Italian, Dutch - used in this project, comparable measurements cannot be obtained and valid inferences cannot be drawn. Hence, some of the problems that arise in this kind of research can be avoided by careful discussion of the meanings of particular concepts in the different languages. To avoid inconsistency and misinterpretations caused by translations, they were double-checked using German as a second language because it could easily be understood by most of the participating researchers, as well as by an expert translator in each institute. Thus, in the beginning of the MOBILATE project, considerable amounts of time were devoted to performing translations and checking them. Pre-pretests and pretests were employed to identify possible misunderstandings in the questions presented as well as items or questions that might be interpreted in more than one way. At this early stage of a research project, it is essential to pay attention to cultural and linguistic differences. Cultural sensitivity and patience are required, which is not at all an easy task in a project with a very strict timetable.

For interdisciplinary projects like MOBILATE, researchers must meet, especially in the preparatory phase and again in the analysis and writing phases of the project. However well one plans the research, new questions, new methodological solutions and new interpretations always arise; this is the nature of research. It is a living process. Frequent meetings between researchers are a necessary part of gleaning findings of scientific or practical importance from the rich data available.

Happily, the communication between research sites and the responsible offices and officials in each different participating city or municipality was very unproblematic. In every country and in every locality, these people helpfully complied with all requests and supported the MOBILATE project in many other ways as well. This phase, which included for example the sampling of subjects, was concluded rapidly, effectively, and without error.

Data collection was organised differently in each participating institute. The Finnish partner selected and trained the interviewers, senior female psychology students, and monitored quality of interviewers' work during the assessment process. The other participants used outsider organizations with high expertise in interview-based research. These interviewers were also trained carefully by the experts of the MOBILATE project and monitored on a random basis in every country. There was some discussion regarding whether interviewers (who were not psychologists) were qualified to administer psychological tests. In the end, it was decided to allow interviewers to administer them. They received additional instructions written by psychologists about the meaning and goals of the psychological tests in the MOBILATE context as well as guidelines regarding how to react in difficult cases. In every setting, the interviewers had either thorough theoretical and practical knowledge of interviewing techniques or experience as an interviewer in research institutes conducting these kinds of surveys. The majority of interviewers in the outside research institutes were about the same age as our younger respondents, whereas the psychology students were young. It is possible that this different approach may have affected the findings, especially regarding the psychological test results. We cannot be sure if the instructions and coding of the tests were based on exactly similar criteria in different participating institutes either.

The MOBILATE project has faced a number of *practical problems*, such as a lack of financing, a shortage of time, incompatibilities between computer programmes, poorly functioning software programmes for coding the interviews, as well as human errors in building up the database. Some of these problems could have been foreseen but not all. The MOBILATE project was accomplished on the basis of the original plan although only half of the funding applied for was actually granted. In hindsight, the researchers were too optimistic regarding what could be accomplished on limited funds, resulting in financial and time-budget pressures. Moreover, different traditional holiday periods in different participant countries and unforeseen acute illnesses and maternity leaves of absence can hamper executing a small project like MOBILATE, which had only one principal researcher in every country.

To sum up, interdisciplinary cultural comparison studies like MOBILATE need to be monitored carefully and require a great deal of coordination. The exchange of information and opinions from all participants is a must. This is one of the most important prerequisites for good scientific reporting; however, all of this is easier said than done. Comparative data reporting requires enough time for discussions, thinking and rewriting.

Although interdisciplinary comparative survey-research in five countries has been difficult and demanding, *this kind of project is also rewarding.* One of the main lessons is that when many countries are compared, it is absolutely necessary not to gloss over or conceal different theoretical, methodological and practical problems, but to discuss them openly. Open discussions may result in fresh insights into one's own familiar society and culture, not to mention insights into the foundations of an academic discipline whose theories and concepts as well as analytical tools are too often taken for granted. The comparative research design makes it possible to observe similarities and differences in the responses of senior citizens living in different societal and environmental contexts. Whenever analysis reveals that old people behave differently or have different opinions or have different difficulties regarding their out-of-home mobility, such as in their ability to access daily necessities, friends, services and leisure activities, these differences can be interpreted in terms of the cultural, political, economic, and social differences within their societies. Similarities may lead the researchers to question the theories and methods that have been used. The similarities may also lead to deeper analyses and to notions of far-reaching similarities in social systems that are superficially different. Hence, comparative analyses may reveal essential similarities in human behaviour – here, in the MOBILATE project, regarding relations between ageing and out-of-home mobility – regardless of context.

The lively interaction between researchers (although mostly by email) has greatly broadened the researcher network of each young and senior scientist who participated in the project. In particular, it has increased the knowledge and skills of those doing interdisciplinary cross-cultural research, abilities which can be used in new projects covering different EU-member states. For young researchers, participating in this (albeit very demanding and difficult) enterprise teaches skills that are urgently needed in future research. Handbooks on cross-cultural interdisciplinary research alone are not sufficient; knowledge on this topic can only be gleaned from participating in projects from the very beginning to the very end of the research process.

The results and experiences of the comparative interdisciplinary MOBILATE project suggest that new theories and concepts as well as new methodological approaches can be developed if the work undertaken by multi-national teams is based on openness and fosters the creativity of the individual members in the group. Comparison of the familiar with the unknown makes the familiar unknown and thus leads to new questions, and ultimately to new answers. Errors have to be analysed and reported so that in the future, at least some of the same errors can be avoided, and possible difficulties can be foreseen.

Taken together, despite the theoretical and methodological challenges, all the questions and issues raised by the project were solved successfully. Everyone involved in this project contributed with his or her special knowledge and skills. We have added a lot to the available knowledge base of ageing and especially to outdoor mobility prerequisites and obstacles in old age. One very important and positive contribution of this type of research is that young researchers have had the opportunity to begin broadening their network of colleagues and learn to 'think European'.

14.3   Conclusions and Outlook

Mobility (the ability to move about) and traffic (the transportation of people, goods, and news) have become an ever more important precondition of ensuring the ability to lead one's everyday life, keep up social relations, take part in every kind of activity outside one's home, and seek out places that are either subjectively significant or objectively central to providing for daily material needs and health care. At the same time, mobility is increasingly jeopardised as a person ages by age-related decrements of health.

The findings of the MOBILATE project have confirmed the importance of mobility for an independent lifestyle, on the one hand, and the various personal and environmental conditions it depends on, on the other. A person's physical, economic, social, and technical resources, as well as the structural resources of the region he or she lives in, proved to be decisive preconditions of out-of-home mobility. Further variables like a person's motives for making trips, the importance assigned to going out, and psychological variables such as control beliefs and cognitive abilities, also play a substantial role for moving about.

Unfortunately, the preconditions for mobility do not hold fully for all ageing European citizens. It is true that satisfaction with mobility-related aspects such as leisure activities, accessibility of services and facilities, public transport, travelling, or overall mobility, was generally high among the older adults who participated in the MOBILATE study. However, there were clear differences between subgroups and between urban and rural localities. Low satisfaction scores seem to indicate that people suffer from personal or environmental mobility restrictions and need support for improving their ability to get around.

In all countries, satisfaction was lower in rural areas, except in the Netherlands and western Germany. In Italy and western Germany, public transport in the country was evaluated particularly negatively. In Hungary, people living in the rural areas did not feel they had adequate opportunities for pursuing leisure activities, and in eastern Germany, both urban and rural respondents bemoaned the lack of services and facilities. These evaluations clearly indicate a discrepancy between what people want or need and what is available to them.

The situation was better in the cities studied. Essential services such as a grocery store, pharmacy, medical doctor and public transportation were accessible within 15 minutes for more than 85% of older adults living in urban areas. This means, however, that at least one out of seven persons aged 55 years or older could not reach basic facilities. Moreover, 15 minutes can constitute a serious problem for persons who are mobility impaired and cannot rely on a car.

Based on our findings, the following conclusion can be derived:

- For elders, whose life space contracts with advancing age because of progressive frailty or the inability to overcome environmental obstacles, it is crucial that the areas near their homes have readily accessible stores, medical and care services, appropriate public transport, and other facilities that will allow them to realise their mobility and activity needs, to maintain social contacts, participate in community life and, in general, continue leading independent lives.

Beside the structural differences between urban and rural areas, differences within the scope of older adults need to be considered when outdoor mobility in later life is the target of study. We found characteristic connections between mobility and socio-structural, psychological, and structural variables, and identified clearly distinguishable subgroups of persons who differ in their mobility, each with quite substantial sizes.

The first, highly mobile and highly satisfied group consisted mainly of the 'young' old, of men, healthy and better educated persons, and active car drivers. They had the highest mobility scores in terms of transport modes used, range of outdoor activities, and satisfaction with mobility. The performance of trips in this group was clearly above average as well.

The second group showed the highest level of actual day-to-day mobility, was as satisfied with their mobility as the first group, although use of transport modes as well as variety of outdoor leisure activities was clearly lower. Satisfaction with one's financial situation and the level of education (total number of years) were lower as well, but still on par with the average, or even slightly higher.

Satisfaction with mobility was in the positive score range of the third group. All components of mobility were, however, clearly lower compared to the two first groups. Members of this group seem to exhibit beginning frailty, pointing to the need for pronounced preventive efforts to avoid further loss in out-of-home mobility.

Finally, the fourth group was the counterpart to the first one: it consisted mainly of the old-old, of women, single living persons, and those with the least education, greatest health impairments, and most restricted financial situation. All of the scores in this group lie in the negative range of values with a particularly pronounced negative score regarding satisfaction with mobility. Interestingly, the narrow range of actual out-of-home mobility of this subgroup (i.e., number of trips made) tended to be higher compared to the third group, but the use of transport means and outdoor leisure activities were clearly lowest of all groups. The proportion of persons who used a car only as a passenger and/or persons without a car in the household was highest in this group. Not surprisingly, only about every tenth person of this group drove a car.

Psychological variables also played a role for characterising the groups. Visu-motoric coordination clearly and consistently decreased from the first to the fourth group, while external control beliefs increased. In addition, indoor orientation increased from the highly mobile and satisfied to the almost immobile and dissatisfied group, whereas the importance of going out substantially decreased.

Taking these findings into account, the members of the fourth group appear to be at particular risk; they have already lost much of their outdoor mobility, and seem to be in need of immediate intervention and rehabilitation because they are most dissatisfied with this situation.

With regard to regional differences, older rural adults were more frequently found in the low mobility groups. In terms of countries, it seems that the risk groups described above tend to be represented more strongly by older adults from Hungary and Italy, while the Dutch and Finnish elders were found predominantly in the 'mobility rich' group.

From these findings, a second conclusion can be derived:

- Single living older persons, women, persons with impaired health and low economic resources, and rural older adults tend to be particularly at risk of losing their abilities to move about. An accumulation of such conditions, as is the case in a considerable share of the older European population, requires immediate intervention and social as well as technical support measures. Persons exhibiting beginning frailty or decreasing sensory abilities need pronounced preventive efforts to avoid further loss in outdoor mobility. Persons showing moderate outdoor mobility and satisfaction in spite of a limited range of transport modes and outdoor activities require stimulation to enhance or maintain their mobility. Thus, specific focus group programmes for the prevention, intervention, and rehabilitation of mobility impairment must be developed and applied to persons at risk. Further support and stimulation must focus as much on transport policy measures as on appropriate social policy measures. For older men and women who have no social, economic, or technical resources at their disposal for overcoming personal or environmental limitations, it is crucial to create flexible, user-centred options for mobility that offer a genuine alternative to both the private automobile and traditional local public transport services. Separate analyses for each country are needed to better understand the positive and negative conditions influencing the outdoor mobility of each country's older citizens.

Our identification of groups deserving special attention with regard to stimulation, prevention, intervention, and rehabilitation hold true for all countries that participated in the MOBILATE project. Though differentiation between countries is often sensible, the most frequent and most important problem jeopardizing older people's mobility - and, thus, autonomy and well-being - is universal: among the personal, technical, and environmental conditions enabling mobility, an individual's health can be seen as the most essential and general one. With decreasing health, all kinds of movement - physical or by any means of transportation - become increasingly demanding, and environmental obstacles require continual efforts. When asked about the main reasons for not being able to meet relatives, friends or other important persons, for not reaching shops and services, not pursuing important leisure activities, and not being able to use public transportation, the older study participants usually first mentioned their bad health and second the distance. Both can be seen as interrelated, because longer distances need more effort to cover. People with good physical mobility and few problems performing activities of daily living made more journeys per day and covered larger distances than persons with poor mobility or functional difficulties. At the same time, they were clearly more satisfied with their possibilities of going out than the less mobile persons.

The obstacles and difficulties caused by poor health can be compensated for at an individual and technical level.

- At the individual level, many technical aids can be used beginning with glasses, artificial joints and limbs and ending with motorized wheel-chairs with different specialized aids. Sports and gymnastics programmes, tailor-made to the individual's ability yet attractive for all kinds of elderly interest groups can strengthen physical mobility, support healthy ageing, and at the same time initiate and enhance social integration.

- New technological information and communication systems (ICT) can be used to eliminate or circumvent some of the mobility problems experienced by elderly traffic users. ICT can make driving easier by improving in-vehicle technology (cruise-control, anti-collision equipment, way-finding, etc...), intelligent infrastructure (dynamic route information, warning for icy or slippery roads) and better information on the available alternatives in public transport (location of nearest stops, travel information, planning a trip).

- One of the possibilities ICT offers is its application in demand responsive transport. This type of transport relies on ICT for the organisation and functioning of the system, as well as for the communication between users and vehicle operators. The Dutch case shows that it works: it can be a useful alternative for the specific mobility problems of older people, but its introduction should be very well-prepared, user-friendly, and provide up-to-date information on the system.

- ICT can also reduce the need for transportation because of the increasing role of tele-activities. This is a two-edged sword, however, because older people should be encouraged to maintain their mobility, especially their physical mobility, as a matter of principle. The relation between health and mobility is reciprocal: health not only affects mobility, but mobility also affects health.

- Public transport could be an alternative to other modes of transport, but our findings suggest that this mode is chosen only when there are no other options, when access is easy, buses run frequently, and service is excellent. In this respect we found particularly great differences between countries and regions. Thus, a main European policy goal should be to create equal opportunities for meeting older persons' outdoor mobility needs.

In addition to distances that are difficult or impossible to overcome, several other spatial, technical, and social aspects constituted hindrances to getting around.

Spatial elements include certain, well-known conditions that are critical to mobility, such as bad roads, narrow or lack of sidewalks, lack of pedestrian crossings and cycle lanes, quickly changing traffic lights, busy roads, parking problems, and unsafe routes or places. The design of the public transportation system was also frequently mentioned among the technical problems older people experienced in the context of travelling. Virtually all of these difficulties dealt with riding a bus. For example, people reported that buses ran too infrequently. They also encountered problems reading timetables and route maps, and felt there were not enough seats or shelter at bus stops.

Several social features of the traffic system and the larger social context, however, were even more important than typical kinds of traffic conditions. Feelings of insecurity, lack of courtesy demonstrated by fellow travellers, heavy traffic, dangerous traffic situations, and financial costs were felt to be the most stressful of all.

Many of these aspects interfering with older persons' outdoor mobility have been known for many years. Therefore, we can only reiterate what measures must be undertaken:

- Improvements should include 'universal' or 'barrier-free' design features which are not only decisive for disabled or handicapped traffic participants, but also offer better conditions for ageing men and women and other mobility-impaired groups like children or people travelling with children. Well-tended and clearly designated pedestrian routes, pedestrian crossings, rest areas, traffic calmed areas, sufficient parking places near important destinations, and easy access to public buildings constitute basic preconditions for a safe and relaxed participation in traffic. Technical solutions include pedestrian crossings, traffic lights, easily accessible public transport (e.g., low-floor buses), demand-responsive transport, etc...

- Elderly people did not give highest priority to technical improvements, though. Rather, the context of travelling was most important. Therefore, improvements must focus on the organisational and social aspects of the traffic system. In order to provide elders with a high degree of spatial and social participation, we need mutual consideration, courtesy and help from younger passer-by's, public safety, and reasonable travel costs.

- If physical and sensory decline reduce the use of fast modes of transportation, walking becomes perhaps the last available option for moving about, especially for the oldest old. This means that the residential environment of older people should offer the most important services within walking distance and build a secure street network for pedestrians. Moreover, one must note that most of the oldest people, in particular old women, live alone. For them, escort services and companions can be a solution for feelings of insecurity or for a lack of self-confidence.

Outlook

Based on our findings, we envision two diverging tendencies: on the one hand, there will be a growing proportion of the older population who will be healthier, better-off, better educated, and physically more active than previous generations. The vast majority of them will own and drive a car, will be able to use all kinds of other transport modes, and profit from the latest technological developments to improve their mobility, travelling, and interpersonal contacts.

On the other hand, the demographic ageing of the population will result in a growing quantity of very old people who may suffer from physical disability, cognitive impairment, or sensory disorders (such as vision or hearing impairment). For these people's quality of life, outdoor mobility will be very important as well. As our findings showed, age-related loss of mobility does not necessarily indicate less desire to be mobile nor is mobility loss due to irremediable health problems; rather, it is often due to obstacles and hindrances in the environment and in the transport system.

Older people are not an undifferentiated group and therefore their needs vary. Thus, a new balance is necessary between the demand of specific user-groups and adequate supply, through a reorganization of transport policies and services in relation to current changes and to the needs expressed by elders. The car will still be widely used by the older population, so the industry will have to design cars that meet older people's real needs and their gradually declining performance. Closely connected with the greater presence of older car drivers is the problem of traffic safety, which can be increased with new technological aids, both in the car itself and in the infrastructures. Often older drivers compensate for their slower reactions, avoiding long journeys or motorways. New technologies such as ICT can offer much support in this direction.

Improvements in public transport could counterbalance the use of the car, since public transport better meets the needs of elders with reduced mobility. It can be assumed that the current 'ageing of ageing' will increase the number of people with reduced psychophysical performance, who today are often excluded from the present transportation system, even though they have the potential to use it. Greater accessibility and diffusion of accessible transport (e.g., low-floor buses) must be considered. Flexibility in transport is very important and can be carried out by adapting the existing system or implementing door-to-door solutions which respond to the needs of older people with reduced capacity or who live in isolated areas.

Infrastructures must also be modified, improving the connectivity and integration between means of transport and traffic safety, especially for pedestrians.

And finally, it is becoming increasingly urgent to combine social policy, traffic and urban planning, and technical development. Not only should neighbourhoods have readily accessible stores, medical and care services, and other facilities, not only should public and private transport become more appropriate for ageing users' needs, nor is it sufficient to solely improve vehicle technologies or to implement intervention strategies in order to improve older persons' mobility. Rather, the whole interrelated socio-technical system has to be shaped in a way that will allow the elderly to continue leading independent lives, maintain social contacts, and take advantage of recreational activities - in short, to deal with daily demands and remain full members of society.

References

Mollenkopf, H., Marcellini, F., & Ruoppila, I. (1998). The Outdoor Mobility of Elderly People – A Comparative Study in Three European Countries. In Graafmans, J., Taipale, V. & Charness, N. (Eds.), *Gerontechnology. A Sustainable Investment in the Future* (pp. 204 – 211). Amsterdam: IOS Press.

Mollenkopf, H., Marcellini, F., Ruoppila, I., & Tacken, M. (Eds.)(2004). *Ageing and Outdoor Mobility. A European Study.* Amsterdam: IOS Press.

Mollenkopf, H., Marcellini, F., Ruoppila, I., Baas, S., Ciarrocchi, S., Hirsiaho, N., Kohan, D. & Principi, A. (2003). The MOBILATE Follow-up Study 1995-2000. Enhancing Outdoor Mobility in Later Life: Personal Coping, Environmental Resources, and Technical Support. *DZFA Research Report No. 14.* Heidelberg: German Centre for Research on Ageing (DZFA).

Ruoppila, I., Marcellini, F., Mollenkopf, H., Hirsiaho, N., Baas, S., Principi, A., Ciarrocchi, S., & Wetzel, D. (2003). The MOBILATE Cohort Study 1995 – 2000: Enhancing Outdoor Mobility in Later Life. The differences between persons aged 55-59 years and 75-79 years in 1995 and 2000. *DZFA Research Report No. 17*. Heidelberg: German Centre for Research on Ageing (DZFA).

ANNEX

Enhancing Mobility in Later Life
H. Mollenkopf et al. (Eds.)
IOS Press, 2005
© *2005 The authors. All rights reserved.*

The MOBILATE Consortium

The German Centre for Research on Ageing at the University of Heidelberg
(DZFA) Department for Social and Environmental Gerontology
Dr. Heidrun Mollenkopf (Coordinator), *Prof. Dr. Hans-Werner Wahl,*
Dr. Frank Oswald, Dipl. Soz. Stephan Baas, M.A. Dinah Kohan
Heidelberg, Germany

INRCA, Istituto Nazionale Riposo e Cura Anziani, Dipartimento Ricerche
Gerontologiche
Dott.ssa Fiorella Marcellini, Dott.ssa Sabina Ciarrocchi, Dott.ssa Cristina
Gagliardi & Dott. Andrea Principi
Ancona, Italy

University of Jyväskylä, Department of Psychology
Professor Isto Ruoppila & M.S. Nina Hirsiaho
Jyväskylä, Finland

Delft University of Technology, Faculty of Architecture
Dr. Mart Tacken, drs. Ellemieke van Lamoen & ir. Remon Rooij
Delft, The Netherlands

Hungarian Academy of Sciences, Institute of Sociology
Dr. Zsuzsa Széman & Csaba Kucsera
Budapest, Hungary

The European countries involved in the study

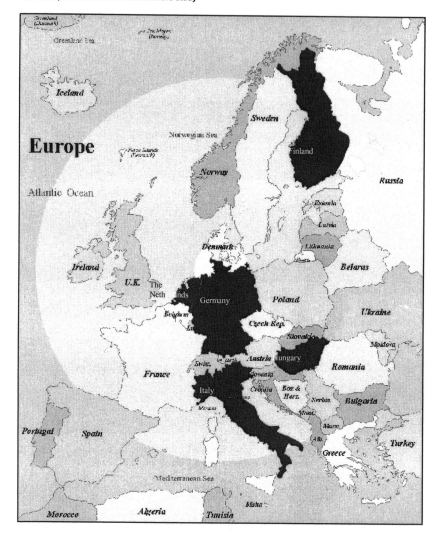

The MOBILATE Diary[©]

The **MOBILATE** Project:
Enhancing Outdoor Mobility in Later Life

1st day:_____

2nd day:_____

ID-number:_____

[©] **The MOBILATE Consortium**

Please complete this form for every journey that you took yesterday and will take tomorrow!

Please do not forget to include the journey home!

1 journey =   leaving one's apartment

and returning to one's apartment

(or other sleeping accommodation)

Thank you very much for your time and effort!!!

Day nr. __   Date __ / __ / 2000 (dd/mm/00)   made no trip ☐   ID resp. _____

Departure at home   __:__ hh/mm

Describe your journey from the trip leaving home till your trip back home. You can do this by mentioning the purpose (motive, activity in list A) of your trip, the means of transport and some more detailed characteristics. Start with the first activity →, tell then how you made this trip. After this you describe the next trip for a new activity.... → 2 : *each activity a new line*

	Motive or activity	how did you go? by... (more answers possible)							where	travel alone y/n
	LIST A	foot	bicycle	car driver	car pas-senger	bus	tram	special transport (fill in: elderly bus, or call bus, etc.)	LIST B	
1 first										
2 then										
3 then										
4 then										
5 then										

Arrival back home __:__ hh/mm

if arrival is on a different day, date ____/____(dd/mm)

How was your journey?

☐ comfortable   why? _____(LIST C)

☐ not comfortable   why? _____(LIST D)

NEXT JOURNEY

LIST A: Activities

1 working

2 meeting friends, relatives, acquaintances

3 helping someone (in household, baby sitting)

4 shopping (e.g. bakery, supermarket, hairdresser, travel agency)

5 attending (e.g. bank, post, authority)

6 health care (e.g. doctor, pedicure, massage)

7 drinking coffee, lunch (in restaurant, bar)

8 visiting cultural event (e.g. concert, theatre)

9 activities in association, voluntary work

10 gardening

11 sport activities (e.g. bowling, folk dance, ball plays, tennis)

12 religious services, cemetery

13 strolling, walking tour, cycle tour, hiking (home – home)

14 short trip, holiday

15 accompanying someone (e.g. bring away, fetching up)

16 fishing, picking berries, mushrooms

17 education (e.g. courses, vocational training, senior academy)

18 back home

LIST B: Destinations

1 near home, neighbourhood (less < 1 km

2 own urban area or village (between 1 and 3 km)

3 own city or municipality (3 km – 10 km)

4 neighbouring city or within region (10 – 30 km)

5 neighbouring city or within region (10 – 30 km

6 further away (more than 30 km

LIST C: Comfortable conditions of the trip

C1 broad and plain sidewalk
C2 traffic calmed area
C3 seats for rest
C4 traffic islands and zebra crossing
C5 good traffic light settings for pedestrians
C6 enough and good information on public transport
C7 friendly advice at ticket booth
C8 good connections, short waiting time
C9 help of other people with getting in and out bus or tram
C10 easy boarding and getting off bus or tram
C11 tactful driver of bus or tram
C12 immediately a seat in bus or tram
C13 public transport stop near destination
C14 nice talk with other travellers
C15 good parking place near home
C16 good parking place near destination
C17 favourable traffic light settings for car driver
C18 separate foot and cycle path
C19 cycle path available
C20 light traffic
C21 quit in shops and shopping streets
C22 nice other road users
C23 I had company
C24 Other reasons: ....

LIST D: Discomfortable conditions of the trip

D1 rough and narrow sidewalk, stairs
D2 sidewalk full of parking cars
D3 no seats for rest
D4 broad roads with heavy traffic
D5 too short go (green) on traffic lights
D6 bad handling of ticket machines
D7 not enough information in schedule or at ticket booth
D8 bad connections
D9 full loaded buses or trams
D10 problems with boarding and getting off bus or tram
D11 buses and trams drive too fast and brake too jerkily
D12 problems with my health
D13 far, strenuous trip, strenuous slope
D14 empty streets (anxious for hold-up, uneasiness for darkness)
D15 badly lighted streets and squares
D16 problems with parking
D17 problems with getting in and of the car
D18 no cycle path
D19 negative influence of the weather
D20 heavy traffic
D21 too many people on the way in shops and streets
D22 heartless and unfriendly road users
D23 company was missing
D24 Other difficulties: ....

Addresses

Dr. Heidrun Mollenkopf
Co-authors: Stephan Baas, Roman Kaspar, Frank Oswald, Hans-Werner Wahl
German Centre for Research on Ageing
at the University of Heidelberg (DZFA)
Bergheimer Strasse 20
D-69115 Heidelberg, Germany
Phone: +49 6221 548115 / Fax: +49 6221 548112
e-mail: mollenkopf@dzfa.uni-heidelberg.de

Dott.ssa Fiorella Marcellini
Co-authors: Sabina Ciarrocchi, Cristina Gagliardi, Andrea Principi, Liana Spazzafumo
INRCA, Istituto Nazionale Riposo e Cura Anziani
Dipartimento Ricerche Gerontologiche
Via S. Margherita 5
I-60100 Ancona, Italy
Phone: +39 071 8004 788 / Fax: +39 071 35941
e-mail: f.marcellini@inrca.it

Professor Isto Ruoppila
Co-authors: Tarjaliisa Raitanen, Nina Hirsiaho
Department of Psychology, University of Jyväskylä
P.O. Box 35
SF-40351 Jyväskylä, Finland
Phone: +358 14 2602 852 / Fax: +358 14 2602 841
e-mail: ruoppila@psyka.jyu.fi

Drs. Mart Tacken
*Co-author:*Ellemieke van Lamoen
Faculty of Architecture, Delft University of Technology
P.O. Box 5043
NL-2600 GA Delft
Phone: +31 15 278 1367 / Fax: +31 15 278 3694
e-mail: m.h.h.k.tacken@bk.tudelft.nl

Dr. Zsuzsa Széman
Co-author : Csaba Kucsera
Institute of Sociology
Hungarian Academy of Sciences HAS
Welfare Mix Team
Uri U. 49
H-1049 Budapest
Phone: +36 (1) 224 67 44 / Fax: +36 (1) 2246745
e-mail: szemanzs@hu.inter.net

Author Index

Baas, S.	43, 195, 257, 279
Ciarrocchi, S.	221
Gagliardi, C.	11
Hirsiaho, N.	11, 77, 141
Kaspar, R.	173, 289
Kucsera, C.	11, 195, 221
Marcellini, F.	11, 43, 221, 257, 279, 295
Mollenkopf, H.	1, 11, 43, 195, 221, 243, 257, 279, 289, 295
Oswald, F.	43, 173, 257, 279
Principi, A.	221
Ruoppila, I.	11, 43, 77, 141, 257, 279, 295
Spazzafumo, L.	221
Széman, Z.	11, 43, 195, 221, 257, 279, 295
Tacken, M.	11, 43, 105, 141, 243, 257, 279, 295
van Lamoen, E.	105
Wahl, H.-W.	43, 173, 257, 279, 289